Continued on back end papers

*Now available in a lower priced paperback edition in the Wiley Classics Library.

Planning Pharmaceutical
Clinical Trials

Planning Pharmaceutical Clinical Trials

Basic Statistical Principles

WILLIAM M. WOODING

A Wiley-Interscience Publication
JOHN WILEY & SONS, INC.
New York · Chichester · Brisbane · Toronto · Singapore

Library of Congress Cataloging in Publication Data:
Wooding, William M.
    Planning pharmaceutical clinical trials: basic statistical
principles / by William M. Wooding.
        p.   cm.—Wiley series in probability and mathematical
statistics. Applied probability and statistics.
    Running title: Clinical drug trials.
    "A Wiley-Interscience publication."
    Includes bibliographical references and index.
    ISBN 0-471-62244-3 (cloth: alk. paper)
    1. Drugs—Testing—Planning.   2. Drugs—Testing—Statistical
methods.   I. Title.   II. Title: Clinical drug trials.   III. Series.
    [DNLM: 1. Drug Evaluation—methods.   2. Clinical Trials—methods.
3. Research Design.   4. Statistics.   QV 771 W891p 1993]
RM301.27.W66 1993
615.5'8'0287—dc20
DNLM/DLC
for Library of Congress   93-3453

Printed in the United States of America

10 9 8 7 6 5 4 3 2 1

To Nina, Barb, and Beth

Contents

PART V.   DETAILS OF SAMPLE SIZE ESTIMATION   427

Chapter 15.   Sample Size Estimation   429

APPENDIX   472

BIBLIOGRAPHY: SELECTED BOOKS FOR REFERENCE   518

INDEX   531

Preface

NATURE OF THIS BOOK

This book is principally concerned with the planning of clinical trails that are designed, run, and analyzed in or for the *pharmaceutical industry*. Such trials may be planned to evaluate ethical (prescription) drugs or OTC (over the counter) and proprietary products. In some cases, studies are run that employ procedures not involving drugs.

A clinical trial or clinical study is an *experiment* designed to assess the safety and efficacy of one or more medical treatments, such as new drugs, using human beings as the patients or subjects. Such a trial is an exercise in applied science, and its design and execution, as well as the analysis of the resulting data, must therefore conform as closely as possible to the principles and procedures of good scientific experimentation.

In this country, most clinical studies designed to evaluate drugs that have not previously been accepted for human treatment must be preceded by extended animal toxicological studies and must not be undertaken without the knowledge and approval of the U.S. Food and Drug Administration (FDA). Most trials of treatments contemplated for sale by the pharmaceutical industry are conducted for three major purposes: (a) to ensure safety of the treatment, (b) to test its efficacy against a disease, symptom, or disability, and (c) to satisfy requirements of the FDA that are necessary before a drug can be marketed in interstate commerce.

The principal concern in this book is with the initial stages of a clinical study, the *experimental design* or structure of the experiment, and the general planning of the trial. However, some knowledge of analysis is necessary for adequate planning, including the selection of an appropriate experimental design. Consequently, two of the 15 chapters deal with elementary applied statistics, and there is one chapter devoted to the very important topic of sample size estimation (the number of patients required). We emphasize also that our concern lies almost exclusively with the *scientific* and *statistical* aspects of industrial clinical trials. Details of the management of a trial (other than the careful execution of the planned procedures), many regulatory matters, as well as other activities not concerned, directly or indirectly, with experimental design and statistics, are not covered at all, or, at most, are discussed only briefly.[1]

EXPECTED AUDIENCE

This book was written principally for persons in the pharmaceutical industry who plan, run, and analyze industrial clinical trials. Many will be physicians, nurses, and CRAs (clinical research associates); perhaps also there will be some biologists, pharmacologists, chemists, or physical chemists. It is assumed that you understand the fundamentals of undergraduate algebra and that many of you have done some kind of scientific research. You will require no prior knowledge of experimental design or the statistical analysis of data to study and understand the information presented here. There are no mathematical proofs, and although theory is sometimes necessary, it has been kept to the minimum needed to assure reasonable understanding. If you have had a course or two in statistics, it will be helpful, but it is not essential to your understanding of the material in this book.

There are many books dealing with applied statistical analysis, but relatively few about experimental design. I know of *no* other books on planning and design that are intended exclusively for this audience. And, in fact, there are only a handful of works on truly elementary statistical analysis for a medical audience. Yet the majority of clinical studies in this country—undoubtedly thousands every year—are sponsored by industry and run by medical and paramedical scientists. Although some of these trials are "farmed out" to statistical consulting firms, many, probably most, are designed, supervised, and analyzed in house.

If you are fully or partially responsible for clinical studies sponsored by your organization, your knowledge and experience have no doubt been recognized by your employer. This being so, there is *no one* better qualified than you—no statistician, no nonmedical scientist, *no one*—to plan the studies, supervise their execution, and report the results. But unless you are also a professional in experimental design and statistics, you are likely to require some additional assistance in those fields. The major purpose of this book is to attempt to supply that assistance.

THE CLINICAL STUDY TEAM

During the Renaissance, it was possible to be a generalist in science and what passed for engineering. Because so little was known in each field, one person could learn virtually all there was to know about a number of spheres

---

[1]We do include a short chapter on the role of the FDA, Chapter 3.

of knowledge. One could be a competent scientist and excel simultaneously in other disciplines as well. Leonardo da Vinci was an outstanding example of this phenomenon—a "man for all seasons," indeed. But, unfortunately, such versatility is almost impossible today.

Most modern professions are so complex that most of us can do no more than become reasonably proficient in one specialty. And at least in science, engineering, and medicine, even a moderate acquaintance with more than a small proportion of one's field is becoming increasingly difficult to acquire as our knowledge of the world and the rest of the cosmos increases. Thus, in your profession, the ideal is probably a breadth of training beyond that possible for one busy person to achieve.

Planning, executing, and analyzing a clinical study requires familiarity with a variety of scientific and medical fields. It is highly unlikely that any one person today can be familiar with all of the needed disciplines. The solution is teamwork. A moderate-sized or large study may require the cooperative work of medical and paramedical personnel, statisticians, chemists, biologists, pharmacologists, and perhaps others. But although your primary background may be medical and/or pharmacological, you yourself should possess some further skills. To plan and manage clinical studies, you should have or acquire enough background in experimental design and statistics to do a satisfactory job of designing your trials and seeing to the analyses of the resulting data. Therefore, unless you are already an experienced biostatistician, take two steps: Read this book, but also obtain the help of a biostatistician to work with you. Unfortunately, a great many monitors design and analyze studies in the pharmaceutical industry without statistical help, often to their eventual sorrow. Please don't emulate them. Find a biostatistician, either an employee or a consultant, and make use of his or her services from the first day of planning.

Following this advice and reading this book will not make you a statistician if you are not one already, but it will help you to obtain a working understanding of the statistical principles and procedures necessary for the conduct of successful clinical studies.

CONTENT AND SCOPE OF THE BOOK

As noted, this book emphasizes experimental design rather than statistical analysis. However, the design (i.e., the structure) of an experiment and the analysis of the resulting data are interdependent, so that it is not possible to prepare an adequate study plan without knowing something about the statistical tests that are required by the design. An elementary treatment of statistical analysis from the point of view of clinical work is therefore given in Chapters 13 and 14. Should you need or desire further information about the analysis of data or about applied statistics in general, you will find many books dealing with these topics. Some of these are listed in the Bibliography.

Elementary texts largely devoted to experimental design are much less common.

Part I comprises three introductory chapters. After a brief introductory chapter, Chapter 2 discusses the nature of scientific experimentation, along with some general information about clinical trials. Chapter 3 is devoted to the major requirements and facilities of the Food and Drug Administration (FDA) with respect to clinical trials.

Part II consists of four chapters describing the essential steps in the planning of a clinical study. The first three of these (Chapters 4, 5, and 6) consist of an introduction to study planning and describe briefly the principal phases of that process, with examples. The fourth, Chapter 7, consists of a brief description of the process of protocol writing and the preparation of clinical report forms, or CRFs.

Part III, consisting of Chapters 8 through 12, is a detailed catalog of the experimental designs most commonly used in clinical work. These are the core of the book, and describe the nature, use, and randomization procedures needed for a variety of experimental designs.

Part IV comprises two chapters, Chapters 13 and 14, on elementary applied statistical analysis. Chapter 13 presents some fundamental principles and a little necessary theoretical background, and Chapter 14 describes five basic statistical procedures in detail (the two common t tests, two rank tests, and a contingency table test (a chi-squared test).

Finally, Part V consists of a single chapter, Chapter 15, which presents details of the estimation of sample size (numbers of patients or subjects needed in a trial).

A class of very widely used statistical techniques, the analysis of variance (ANOVA), is not described in this book. However, the multifactor factorial designs, data from which are most easily analyzed by the use of that technique, are described in Part III, and the estimation of sample size for these designs is covered briefly in Part V. Further information on the use of ANOVA, factorial designs, and the corresponding sample size estimates are available in many of the professional books and textbooks listed in the Bibliography.

Most chapters end with a summary, and many include a list of periodical references. Citations to these are enclosed in parentheses. The Bibliography at the end of the book lists recommended books and other publications, some of which are also cited in the text, in brackets.

Readers often prefer examples in a professional book to be taken from "real life." In an industrial milieu, however, this is nearly impossible because of the proprietary nature of the information. Thus, in this volume, all of the examples but one are "made up." They are also substantially shorter than most actual trials would be, because their object is to illustrate the subject matter. In many cases, I "synthesized" the data representing the responses by the use of random, random normal, and random binomial numbers.

Whether or not you expect to do any of your own statistical calculations, you may find it helpful to work through some of the examples to be sure you understand them. And if you do plan to carry out some of your own computations during your regular work, using a computer, you should first practice the procedures by hand (i.e., with a pocket calculator). *No one* should use a computer for statistical techniques without first being very familiar with them.

Although this is a professional book and does not include student problems, like many good textbooks, it does contain a substantial amount of intentional repetition. Sometimes a topic is introduced in an early chapter and then expanded later. Sometimes important points are simply repeated for emphasis in succeeding chapters or sections of chapters. There are two reasons for this. First, I believe repetition to be pedagogically effective. Second, it is possible that you may use the book as a reference manual, perhaps never reading it entirely, or doing so once, and then referring to various sections from time to time.

APPENDIX TABLES

The tables in the Appendix were prepared or adapted particularly for the sample size and statistics examples given in the book (Chapters 5, 14, and 15). As a result, several tables are abbreviated, and there may be times when you will not find them extensive enough to be useful for your own trials. In most cases, however, you or your statistician will find the full tables you may need in Beyer [47], Fisher and Yates [48], Pearson and Hartley [51, 52], and Rohlf and Sokal [53].

Some professional books devote some space near their Appendix tables describing their use. In this book, such information is given in the text when the need arises, but because of your possible use of the book as a reference manual, a short explanation of the use of each table is also given in the Appendix.

IDEAS AND SUGGESTIONS

Do not modify the procedures described here for your own work unless you are statistically knowledgeable. As one example of a common error, after you have established the sample size to use (which must be done before a trial begins), do not alter it during the trial.

After reading this book, you may feel that there are topics that should have been included, clearer explanations of some points, additional examples, and the like. If so, I would be delighted to hear from you. If there should be a second edition, I will try to incorporate as many of your suggestions and ideas as possible. So, if you wish, write to me in care of the publisher.

BOOKS FOR REFERENCE

References to the Bibliography are given in square brackets, [ ], in the text. Some that are especially recommended are marked with asterisks with their listings. You will have a fine reference library if it is possible to obtain all of those so marked. As a minimum, I strongly suggest that you obtain the following five, and keep them readily available. The bracketed numbers refer to their Bibliography listings:

Subject	Authors and Reference Number
Experimental design	Cochran and Cox [11]
Statistical analysis plus	
some design	Snedecor and Cochran [38]
	Colton [20]
Reference	Beyer [47]
	Moses and Oakford [49]

Acknowledgments

Many people helped me in the preparation of this book. Professor J. Stuart Hunter, a very old friend and one of Wiley's Advisory Editors, was first. Stu introduced me to Wiley's Senior Editor, Bea Shube. In turn, Bea graciously gave me an initial push. But she retired, and I was without an editor for some months. At last, Kate Roach, the present Senior Editor, came upon the scene, and she has been my guide for most of the last 4 years (I am not a speedy writer). Kate has been of more real help than I could have reasonably expected. In addition, at Wiley, Beth Pappas solved numbers of problems for me. Finally, Bob Hilbert, Associate Managing Editor, and an anonymous copy editor, were most helpful and obviously very hard workers. I am very grateful to all of these competent and gracious people.

In the beginning, I recruited nine volunteers who devoted significant portions of their time to reading the manuscript and offering suggestions. Joseph P. Soyka, M.D., Vice President and clinical trial Monitor at Wallace Laboratories (where I was employed for many years), helped with many invaluable suggestions and several times corrected my errors. Joe is not only a fine physician who is broadly experienced in clinical trial work, but he also possesses an excellent grasp of the statistical and experimental design aspects of his work. Jack M. Becktel, a very old friend and a biostatistician with many years of experience in clinical trials at the Veterans' Administration, was an indispensable statistical and experimental design devil's advocate. My brother Bob Wooding and his wife, Alma, and my daughter Beth and her husband, Rick Kontur, each spent many hours helping to ensure that my grammar, syntax, sentence structure, and general understandability were acceptable. Professor Joseph Suchar, Chairman of the Science Department at Green Mountain College in Vermont and a math and computer science professor, made a number of helpful suggestions. I must not forget to mention Dr. Lloyd S. Nelson, who supplied me with a great deal of information about Michael's test. And last but by no means least was my wife, Nina, who faithfully read and reread every chapter and table, most in several revisions. Without the help of all of these generous people, it is likely that the book would still be in progress.

I am grateful to the Biometrika Trustees of London for permission to reprint Tables A.1 and A.2, adapted from E. S. Pearson and H. O. Hartley, *Biometrika Tables for Statisticians, Volume I*, 3d ed. (1966). Thanks are also due to the Longman Group, UK, Ltd., for permission to adapt Tables A.3 and A.4 from Owen L. Davies, *The Design and Analysis of Industrial Experiments*, 2d ed. (1956). The American Society for Quality Control kindly permitted my use of the material in Tables A.6, which was taken from T. L. Bratcher, M. A. Moran, and W. J. Zimmer, "Tables of Sample Size in the Analysis of Variance," published in the *Journal of Quality Technology*, 2, No. 3, July 1970. Dr. Lloyd Nelson, for that Society, granted permission for the use of Program AP.1, which was published in the same journal. And, finally, I owe thanks to John Wiley & Sons, Inc., for its permission to use Tables A.8, derived from Joseph L. Fleiss, *Statistical Methods for Rates and Proportions* (1981).

Last but not least, four anonymous readers recruited by Wiley deserve very sincere thanks. All of them clearly spent many hours reviewing the material. Although their opinions were not always unanimous, their comments were most encouraging and truly helpful. This book reflects many of their ideas and critiques. One of them, in particular, was unusually committed, clearly taking a great interest in the project. The many helpful comments and rigorous detection of my errors were responsible for a much-improved book.

Of course, as always, any errors or discrepancies remaining in the book are my responsibility.

PART I

Preliminary Considerations

CHAPTER 1

Introduction

1.1 TYPES OF STUDIES COVERED

The clinical studies discussed and exemplified in this book are limited to industrial trials, and these are usually evaluations of drug treatments, although other kinds of treatments can be handled in the same way. Such trials are most often run to obtain information about the safety and efficacy of candidate treatments for ethical, OTC (over-the-counter), or proprietary uses. The purposes of a trial are usually to evaluate marketability of a drug or other treatment and to satisfy FDA regulations. At least in the United States, some trials are relatively small or medium-sized affairs, although others are larger and may last for a number of years. A typical new drug may be in the clinical trial stages for as few as 2 or 3 years, but usually for no more than 10. As to numbers of patients, some studies, those in so-called Phase III, utilize several hundred or a few thousand patients, but most use fewer than that. This is in contrast, for example, to some studies sponsored or run by NIH (National Institutes of Health) or the Veteran's Administration, which may often involve thousands of patients. In addition, trials run by pharmaceutical companies rarely involve long-term data collection, such as the measurement of mortality rates needed in cancer studies.

Relatively small trials, lasting for a few years at most and sponsored by pharmaceutical firms, probably comprise the major proportion of *all* clinical trials run in the United States. The remainder are principally tests of materials or treatments sponsored by one of the National Institutes of Health, the Veteran's Administration, or by persons or organizations engaged in academic research. There are some specialized studies run both by industry or other agencies, such as evaluations of genetically engineered organisms. There is also some research done by academic institutions under grants from the pharmaceutical industry.

In this book, we will be concerned chiefly with the fundamental technical and scientific aspects of trial planning, and with a very few but necessary topics in statistical analysis. We will not be concerned with the logistics or other ancillary activities in which you will necessarily be involved. The principal theme of this volume is **the design of experiments,** or **experimental designs.**

1.2 EXPERIMENTAL DESIGNS

Most introductory courses in statistics, especially those offered in medical, nursing, and scientific curricula, focus almost exclusively upon statistical analysis, covering experimental design only lightly and incidentally, if at all. But today, in most industrial organizations, the analyses of data from clinical trials is nearly always done by professional statisticians. The medical and paramedical personnel responsible for the overall planning, execution, and reporting of clinical studies have neither the time nor the training for this activity. On the other hand, we believe that only those responsible for the overall planning of a study can adequately plan it. The word *planning* in this book includes the important activity called **experimental design.** Experimental design is closely related to statistical data analysis, but, at least in its applied form, it is easily and intuitively understandable and usable without a professional background in statistics. Unfortunately, there are only a handful of professional books that treat this topic in depth for personnel in the pharmaceutical industry (see the Bibliography).

In spite of this, it is true that the effective choice of a design, the estimation of sample size for common kinds of trials, and the interaction with the statistician, does require some knowledge of statistical analysis; therefore, this book treats that subject briefly. As to the estimation of sample size, it is important, as one of those responsible for a study, that you be able to set the specifications that are necessary before estimates can be made, because the sample size will have a major effect upon the precision and reliability of the results of your study. To summarize, we believe that you must have a good knowledge of experimental design, sample size estimation, and related processes, such as randomization, in order to confidently handle the overall planning and execution of a clinical study. Although you should work closely with the statistician, you should make the principal decisions in these areas, and he or she should be principally responsible for the data analysis and to act as your advisor.

Clinical trial design is a branch of experimental design, and experimental design is based upon the principles of statistics. Even if you have had no courses in statistics, however, I believe that you will find the material on design in this book easy to understand. On the other hand, for those of you who have had the good fortune to have been exposed to one or more well-taught courses in statistics, it is my hope that this book will broaden your comprehension of the applications of that material to clinical trial design.

There are good reasons for you to have some understanding of statistical analysis as well as of experimental design, although it is very likely that a biostatistician will perform all or most of the final statistical analyses of your data. The most important reason, as we will continue to emphasize, is that the kind of design chosen and the analyses that must be used are strongly dependent upon each other. And, because the design must come first, choosing a design and the kinds of response (measurements) that will be used essentially dictate the kinds of data analyses that must be done, often between rather narrow limits.

The basic selection of a design and the kind of measurement(s) to be made are directly connected with the objectives of a study. These decisions must be made by one of those responsible for and knowledgeable about the nature of the study from a medical and scientific point of view. Therefore, you, not the statistician, must make these choices. Of course, a good statistician will also possess a working acquaintance with a wide variety of experimental designs, the kinds of randomization required, and the nature of the sample size estimation to be made (number of patients required); therefore, you should make your choices only after careful consultation with such a person. Of course, all of this implies that you yourself must have a good knowledge of design, along with some knowledge of sample size estimation and of the basic principles of statistical data analysis.

Even today, several decades after statistics and experimental design were introduced into the processes of clinical trials, large numbers of the trials are run using inefficient or totally incorrect designs, having either too few or too many patients, using incorrect randomization procedures, and planning for too many and perhaps statistically inappropriate methods for the response measurements. The principal purpose of this book, even beyond the emphasis upon design, is to try to convey enough knowledge of the correct procedures to ensure that medical, paramedical, and other professional but nonstatistical personnel can run successful, properly planned trials.

1.3 THE BIOSTATISTICIAN

In spite of the inclusion of a small amount of material on analysis, however, teaching you to "be your own statistician" is emphatically not one of the purposes of this volume. If your experience and training in statistical analysis is not extensive, I can think of no better way to risk your falling into one of the many traps that abound in statistics. And the use of a computer for statistical analyses without knowledge of the statistical processes involved merely makes it possible to fall into many more such traps in a given time. All of this aside, you undoubtedly have enough to do in keeping up with your own profession without being asked to acquire a detailed background in another. Therefore, it is essential that a professional biostatistician, either staff or consultant, be available for the statistical work.

The purpose of the inclusion of the statistical chapters, instead, is to supply you with enough information and understanding to allow you to choose your designs with open eyes, to understand the sample size estimation processes you will need to use for most trials (Chapter 15), and to work and communicate effectively with the biostatistician or consultant. Of course, if you do have a thorough background in statistics, or plan to acquire one, that is all to the good. But in that case, the material in this book is only introductory.

If you are not well-experienced in applied statistics, it would be useful and would increase your understanding if you can find time to do some of the analyses illustrated in Chapters 12 through 14 when they are needed for your data. But show your work to the statistician for comment. Remember, that is one reason why he or she is there.

In fact, you should become well-acquainted with the biostatistician and confer with him or her early and often. By "early," I mean that you should be sure that he or she is involved in the planning of any trial from the very beginning. *This is of major importance,but, unhappily, the statistician may frequently be introduced to the study only after it has been completed and a data analysis is needed*. In addition to other benefits of involving the statistician in your project at the very beginning of your planning, doing so will help to ensure that your design will be one that is compatible with an appropriate and efficient data analysis. You should also involve the statistician in the preparation of your randomization scheme, the selection of response measurements, and the estimation of sample size (numbers of patients or subjects needed), all of which are interconnected.

1.4   READING MATERIALS

As suggested earlier, although there are a number of professional books and textbooks devoted to various aspects of clinical trials, most of them are not concerned with industrial trials, despite the fact that there are many more such trials run than in any noncommercial category. Whether a book is concerned with industrial or other kinds of clinical studies may not be obvious from the titles or advertising. In addition to the sparse coverage of industrial trials, some of the available volumes concentrate upon organizational matters, and are short on technical and scientific activities, publishers' blurbs to the contrary. Additionally, by far the greater proportion of texts and professional books on applied experimental design are written from the points of view of chemistry, engineering, or the behavioral sciences. Industrial clinical studies are different than experimental work in these fields in their requirements for the types of design, the kinds of analyses used, and the nature of the difficulties that occur. And, finally, industrial clinical studies are different in many ways from noncommercial clinical trials, and because most of the available texts are written from the point of view of the latter, there is a further narrowing of the choice of appropriate books. This book attempts to fill part of that gap. Of course, you are encouraged to do as much additional reading in statistics and experimental design as you have time for.

That is the primary reason for the Bibliography and its recommendations found at the back of this book.

To furnish a basis for a small library related to your work that you may wish to acquire, the Bibliography includes selected available texts and useful professional books related in one way or another to clinical studies. Its arrangement and use in this book are described in the Preface. References to the periodical literature appear at the end of each chapter, and their arrangement and use are also described there.

Four books listed in the Bibliography, Pocock [4], Bolton [7], Hill [22], and Mainland [25] percent some material similar to that given here. Although I recommend these highly, they do not specialize in experimental design. Hill and Mainland, probably among the first authors in this field and very famous, are not new (I believe their last editions are those listed—1963 and 1966). Pocock is recent, and his very helpful book does approach the goals of this volume, although it is not a substitute, as it is broader and less specialized. Bolton's book is a fine elementary statistics text and is written from the point of view of pharmaceutical studies. However, it contains only two chapters on design. I recommend that you examine and purchase all four, if possible, but if you prefer to choose one, Pocock is recommended.

You will probably wish to read some of the available journals regularly. I especially recommend *Controlled Clinical Trials*, the official journal of the Society for Clinical Trials. There is no journal exclusively devoted to clinical trial design, or even to experimental design in general, although there are several professional statistical organizations, all of which publish journals. You may wish to look into membership in the Society For Clinical trials or in one of the others devoted to clinical studies and related activities. And you may also wish to consider membership in one or more of the statistical organizations, such as the Biometric Society or the American Statistical Association.

Because you must undoubtedly spend some of your time writing and editing reports and other technical documents, there is a section in the Bibliography that includes a few books related to that subject. I find all of those listed extremely helpful in my preparation of reports for clients. I feel that no writer outgrows the necessity for good guides to writing. The section on Graphical Data Display is included for the same reason. Finally, I must mention the Computer Software section. Each of the few items listed there is either the best (in my opinion) or the sole representative of its kind.

1.5 KINDS OF CLINICAL TRIAL DESIGNS

This section presents a brief introduction to some experimental designs commonly used in clinical trials. Much more detailed information and examples of these and others will be discussed later (Part III).

ONE-FACTOR PARALLEL
K-TREATMENT DESIGN
(FIVE PATIENTS PER TREATMENT)

Treatment 1	Treatment 2	Treatment 3	. . .	Treatment K
—	—	—		—
—	—	—		—
—	—	—		—
—	—	—		—
—	—	—		—

Figure 1.1   One-factor parallel *K*-treatment design.

There are a number of ways to classify the many different types of experimental designs. In clinical trial work, the most commonly used nomenclature groups all possible designs into one of two categories, parallel and "crossover" (changeover). A **parallel** design is one in which each patient receives only one of the treatments. A **changeover** design is one in which each patient receives two or more of the treatments. A variety of different usages have made the term "crossover" ambiguous, which is why I have placed it in quotation marks. In this book, that term is reserved for the two-period, two-treatment crossover design, whereas the term changeover is used as the general designation just defined.

1.5.1   Parallel Designs

Figure 1.1 is a schematic illustration of the structure of a *K*-treatment parallel design. Each treatment has been assigned at random to five patients or subjects.[1] The symbol *K*, which stands for the number of treatments used in the design, is used instead of a specific number to indicate that any number of treatments might be used, the last one being the *K*th. In the figure, a treatment is defined as one level of a variable (it could be one of *K* drugs being compared), which is imposed upon one group of patients by the experimenter. In a well-designed trial, there will be at least two treatments

---

[1]For brevity, we will hereafter use the term "patients" to mean either patients or subjects. A subject is a healthy volunteer, usually taking part in Phase I trials for safety testing. A patient is an ill person.

($K = 2$), because the usual purpose of a design is to *compare* two or more of them. Designs using a single treatment are not advisable unless they are absolutely necessary, because they can lead to incorrect conclusions. The reason is that, in such a case, the results for the treatment must be compared with something that has not been part of the same experiment. This kind of comparison (historical control) has been found to be notoriously unreliable.

Example 1.1: A Four-Treatment Parallel Design

In the following example and elsewhere in this book, a placebo is used as one of the "treatments," and this is commonly done in industrial trials. In many cases in clinical work, however, it may be impossible to use a placebo, because failing to provide a treatment believed to be efficacious is unethical, particularly if there is reason to believe that one or more of the active materials will be successful.[2] In such cases, an active drug of well-known efficacy (i.e., a **standard**) may be the only control possible.

Suppose an investigator is planning a four-treatment parallel design to evaluate a new antihypertensive drug. Assume the questions of interest are, "Does the test drug work? How does it compare with a currently available drug? As a check, is the experiment giving reasonable results—is it to be trusted?" These questions could be addressed if two standards consisting of known antihypertensives, a placebo, and the test drug are each randomly assigned to one of four separate groups of patients in the same experiment. With this arrangement, if the results for the standards show a reduction in blood pressure relative to the placebo, the last question would be answered affirmatively. Comparisons of the new drug with the placebo and with the standards would then give the investigator an idea of its relative efficacy, thus answering the first two questions. By running the three controls, the standards and the placebo, *concurrently* with the test drug, confidence in the results is greatly increased.

When treatments are assigned randomly to patients, as is assumed here, it becomes a matter of chance which patient receives a given treatment, under the minor restriction that (often, as in Figure 1.1) an equal number of patients is assigned to each. It is assumed that the average effect of a given drug will be the same regardless of which randomly selected group of patients happens to receive it. Of course, this assumption is unlikely to be strictly true, but in practice it works, on the average. It is also assumed that the treatment given to any patient in no way affects or is affected by the treatment given to any other. This may seem obvious but is not always so.

The dashes in Figure 1.1 represent one set of **responses,** or **measurements,** that will be obtained when the trial is run. However, it is common to use

---

[2]There are other situations in which the use of a placebo is acceptable. If the withholding of a treatment known or believed to be effective can result in no harm or discomfort to the patient, it may be judged ethical to use a placebo. Again, many clinical trials in industry use subjects (healthy volunteers) rather than patients (ill individuals), and often, in such cases, there is not ethical objection to the use of a placebo.

several different responses for each patient. These all may either measurements of the same kind, such as a series of readings done at intervals, or a variety of responses, such as blood pressures, white counts, urinary volume, and pain scores, perhaps with all of these repeated from time to time. In such cases, the data might eventually be tabulated separately, as represented in Figure 1.1, for each measurement or interval. Note, however, that when multiple responses or repeated responses are used in these ways, it may be necessary to compensate for them during planning by adjusting the sample size upward. For this reason, as well as the desirability of keeping the study as simple as possible, it is advisable to use as few different responses, or as few repeated measurements on each patient, as possible.

Although Figure 1.1 shows an equal number of patients assigned to each treatment in the design, this arrangement is not essential. There are occasions when unequal numbers might be desirable. When the trial is over, of course, even if the original group sizes were equal, there might well be unequal numbers of response data available for different treatments simply because of patient dropouts, or "noncompleters."

There are many different kinds of parallel designs; this example is just one of them. Others will be introduced as we continue.

1.5.2   Changeover Designs

Example 1.2: A Four-Treatment Changeover Design
A **changeover** design with K patients, each of whom receives four treatments, is diagrammed in Figure 1.2. The four treatments are given to each patient sequentially; a different treatment is used, for example, during each of four weeks. Figure 1.2 represents a **randomized blocks** design of a particular kind (in which the patients form the **blocks**—Chapter 11). In each block (patient), the order of the four treatments is randomized. Randomized blocks designs that are not changeovers can also exist (Chapter 10). As in the case of the parallel designs, there may be more than one kind of response, but one is again represented in Figure 1.2 for clarity. Also, as for the parallel designs, this illustration shows only one of the many different kinds of changeover designs.

Losses of data in changeover designs in which the patients are the blocks can be more serious than in parallel designs, because the loss of a patient early in the trial can mean that all or most of the data in that block may be lost. On the other hand, if a patient drops out after completing all but one or even two of the four treatments, or neglects to use one of the treatments for some other reason, the rest of the data in the block may be salvaged during the analysis. Of course, such losses of data being about a reduction in the precision with which the analysis can be done; for example, the ability to detect differences between two treatments will be reduced, so that the analysis will be as sensitive as it would otherwise have been. In such a case, the **statistical power** of the analysis will be reduced. In addition to reducing

TWO-FACTOR CHANGEOVER
DESIGN (RANDOMIZED BLOCKS)

K Patients, Each Receiving
Same Four Treatments

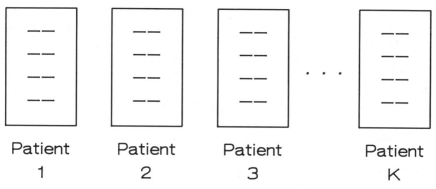

Patient 1   Patient 2   Patient 3   Patient K

Figure 1.2 Two-factor changeover design (randomized blocks).

power, under some circumstances, missing data can seriously bias an analysis (i.e., bring its validity into question).

Both the parallel and the changeover designs will be discussed at greater length in Part III.

1.5.3 Other Classification Methods

Within the categories of parallel and changeover designs, there are many different arrangements. In fact, this method of classification is not very useful because it is so broad; it was discussed principally because it is widely used by those engaged in clinical studies.

Experimental designs can be designated as **one-way, two-way, three-way,** and so forth. A one-way design has only one **factor.** The term "factor" is related to "treatment," but is broader, referring to any controlled experimental entity introduced by the experimenter that may affect the response measurement. One way to understand this is to think of an experimental design as embodying **experimental units** to which the treatments are applied; later, these produce measurement values. This concept will be discussed in more detail in a moment.

You may remember that, in mathematics, variables can be classified into **independent** and **dependent** kinds. Dependent variables are **functions** of independent variables; in an experiment, the values of the dependent variables may be thought of as being controlled by those of the independent ones. An experimental design illustrates this idea in less abstract terms. The factors (and other entities, such as experimental errors) are the independent variables, and their values affect the values of the responses or measurements, which are the dependent variables; we say that the responses are functions of the factors.

To put it even more concretely, Figure 1.1 illustrates one factor, meaning all four drugs taken together, which I called "treatments." Let us assume that these treatments consist of several different nonsteroidal antiinflammatory drugs that are being tested by assigning them at random to patients with rheumatoid arthritis. This group of drugs comprises an independent variable; in this design, it is the only one. It is a variable because it can take on several "values" or **levels;** you can think of each separate drug as a level of the single factor, antiinflammatory drugs. One dependent variable, a response or measurement, might be a grip-strength measurement. It is a dependent variable because its value may be affected by the drugs—affected differently or perhaps not at all, depending upon which drug is being used.

A changeover design, such as that in Figure 1.2, must have at least two factors. In the figure, the factors are **treatments** (perhaps four different drugs) and blocks (patients). You might ask, "Why don't the patients in the parallel design of Figure 1.1 constitute a factor?" The reason is that in that design, the patients are the experimental units, that is, the basic units to which each treatment is assigned, one treatment to each. But in a changeover design, such as the kind of randomized blocks design in Figure 1.2, the patients are no longer the experimental units. Each patient constitutes a **block,** and each block is divided into four **experimental units** (often called **plots** in the jargon of experimental design). Thus, in this way of looking at a design, an experiment or trial includes one or more **factors;** each factor is divided into two or more **levels** or **treatments;** and each treatment is applied to one or more (usually more) **experimental units.** But in this special case, the patients are now a factor, with as many "levels" as there are patients, completely analogous to the drugs factor. Each experimental unit "contains" one level of each of the factors, patients and drugs.

1.5.4 Crossed Parallel Designs

Example 1.3: A Crossed Parallel Design with Two Factors
A parallel design can also possess more than one factor. Figure 1.3 shows a **crossed** design in which there are two factors, drugs and doses. In this design, the experimental units are patients. The treatment each patient receives comprises one of the nine combinations of the three drugs and three doses. Note that the term **treatment** in this case represents a *combination* of a drug and a dose. Three patients receive each treatment combination, so that there are 9×3, or 27, patients in all.

TWO-FACTOR (TWO-WAY) CROSSED PARALLEL DESIGN

(Three Patients Assigned to Each Treatment Combination)

	Drug 1	Drug 2	Drug 3
Dose 1	---	---	---
	---	---	---
	---	---	---
Dose 2	---	---	---
	---	---	---
	---	---	---
Dose 3	---	---	---
	---	---	---
	---	---	---

Figure 1.3   Two-factor crossed parallel design.

Figure 1.3 shows the three drugs as comprising the columns of a two-way table, and the doses as the rows. There could be more than two factors, of course. For example, a third factor could be represented by a separate table for each level of that factor, and so on. In the usual factorial design used in clinical studies (see Chapter 9), the term **crossed design** refers to one in which each level of each factor is used with every level of each of the others, and the factor represented by rows and columns could be reversed without altering the meaning of the diagram. If there were a third crossed factor, each level of this factor would be used with each of those of the other two. In the complement of a crossed design, called a nested design, although more than one factor is used, the arrangement is different; it is hierarchical, like a military or industrial organization chart. That is, each factor and its levels directly accompany only that "above" it. In a nested design, you cannot reverse the roles of the rows and columns without changing the meaning or structure of the design. Nested designs are not used often in clinical trials, and are not treated in detail in this book.

1.5.5   Other Designs

More extended and detailed discussions of some of the wide variety of available designs are given in Part III. We show methods of randomizing for each and, in some cases, we mention the kind of analyses to be done, because, to emphasize a point, the kind of design determines both the kind of randomization and, although sometimes within broader limits, the appropriate analysis.

1.6 STATISTICS

1.6.1 Introduction

Two chapters in Part IV of this book are devoted to statistical analysis. Part V (Chapter 15) is concerned with the estimation of sample size (the numbers of patients needed in a trial). To understand and use the sample size procedures described there, knowledge of the statistical material in Part IV is necessary, and you must have some familiarity with the experimental designs described in Part III. In most cases, you will probably have arranged for the biostatistician to do most of the analyses needed for your trials, and he or she can also do the sample size estimations. However, this important topic requires much judgment on the part of the person(s) responsible for the trial, which you may feel should not be done by anyone else. It is therefore important that you fully grasp the ideas in Chapter 15, even if you become familiar with the contents of Part IV only to the extent needed to understand that of the sample size procedures. We are not urging you to carry out the sample size procedures unless that is your wish, but we feel that it is most important that you understand them thoroughly. Of course, there are other topics in the two chapters on analysis (Part IV) with which it is recommended that you become familiar. For one example, you should have sufficient grasp of the nature, purposes, and variety of the available procedures for data analysis to allow you to make well-informed choices among experimental designs, randomization methods, and response measurements during the planning stages of your studies.

1.6.2 Sample Size Estimation

To obtain an estimate of sample size, it is necessary, among other things, that you specify how small a difference you wish to detect between any two drug treatments. In addition, except for the smallest trials, unless you have data available from a very similar experiment, or there are special circumstances like the availability of *recent* data from a very similar trial, you should run a small **pilot study** before beginning your main trial. The purpose of this is to supply an estimate of the **standard deviation(s)** or "experimental error" value(s) for one or more of the responses (measurements),[3] such as blood

---

[3]In clinical trial work, responses or measurements are frequently called **parameters.** This use of the term is avoided in this book because it is also used in statistics, with a somewhat different connotation.

pressure, degree of pain, or the like. The standard deviation and related matters are discussed several times in succeeding chapters, and thoroughly, with examples, in Chapter 14. An estimate of the standard deviation is necessary in order to make sample size estimates. Unfortunately, the use of pilot trials to obtain such estimates of the standard deviation is not common in industrial clinical trial work. Yet they often turn out to be important time-savers, and sometimes prevent an entire trial from being discarded. Estimating the sample size a priori reduces the likelihood of using greater numbers of patients than necessary, with a consequent substantial loss of money and time, and at the same time, it avoids the repetition of a trial that is not large enough to demonstrate a possible difference of a desired magnitude between two treatments.

Chapter 15 should provide sufficient guidance to help you to make adequate sample size estimates for most of your trials. Discuss the matter with the statistician if you have any trouble understanding the procedures. Some of the more complex cases are not described in this book, but references to the literature and available computer software are given, and, with the help of your statistician, those should be all that is necessary to apply them. The point is that you, as well as the statistician, should become involved in this activity, even if you have nothing to do with the subsequent data analyses. Unfortunately, published volumes devoted to this subject are very few; I know of only two books currently in print. These are listed in the Bibliography: Cohen [27] and Kraemer and Thiemann [28]. There are several useful published papers, however (see citations in Chapter 15).

1.6.3 Statistical Data Analysis

The first of the two statistical chapters in Part IV, Chapter 13, is principally devoted to the basic ideas needed to understand and use the statistical analysis procedures described in Chapter 14. Chapter 14 describes five of the simplest and most common methods used in analyzing clinical trial data. Perhaps the most important item in these chapters is the explanation of the basis of **hypothesis testing** (sometimes called significance testing: the process of comparing treatments or treatment combinations). In addition to explaining these frequently misunderstood concepts, these chapters again emphasize the dependence of the kind of analysis necessary upon the design.

The methods used to analyze your data depend not only upon the design selected, but also upon other factors. As is sometimes supposed, it is not true that data resulting from the execution of *any* design can be analyzed—at least not correctly, effectively and efficiently. To assume that your statistician will be able to deliver a precise, powerful, and statistically unbiased analysis regardless of the nature of the design you have used is certainly a compliment to his or her ability, but, unfortunately, it is empty flattery. There are cases in which your data may not be analyzable at all, because you have used the wrong randomization procedure or otherwise biased the data beyond repair.

With these in mind, you should choose a design and response method(s) that are practicable for your use and that call for an analysis capable of the precision and validity you need. Next, you must use the correct randomization for that design. If, as is usual, the trial uses several different kinds of responses, it may be necessary to use several different kinds of analyses. Dichotomous responses (yes/no, improved/not improved, etc.) require quite different kinds of analysis (and usually much larger sample sizes) than measurements using scales with several integer values (such as mild, moderate, severe, or a five-point scale), or truly continuous measurements, like temperatures, pressures, weights, volumes, lengths, or the like.

Finally, as mentioned earlier, you should be certain that a statistician is involved in the planning of your trials at the very beginning.

Although the two chapters in Part IV were written to help you understand the principles and some of the procedures of the statistical analyses you are likely to encounter most frequently, reading them will be very far from sufficient to supply the statistical knowledge that you would need were you to plan to do your analyses without the assistance of a statistician. Therefore, if you do not already possess a professional background in applied statistics, you are certainly urged to become as familiar as possible with the material in those chapters, but, again, it is strongly recommended that your analyses be done for you by your biostatistician. You cannot afford to take the attitude that these are things for you alone to decide, and are not the statistician's business. Although you may be *responsible* for your trials, you need not and cannot do everything yourself. Therefore, you should have enough knowledge of what others are doing to ensure that it is done properly. At times, I still encounter medical monitors who appear to believe, and sometimes tell me, that I am unable to understand many medical concepts (certainly true!), while simultaneously assuming that the statistical aspects of their work are either self-evident, requiring no special training or experience, or are highly theoretical and impractical.

You should include descriptions of all important aspects of the design of your trial, as well as descriptions of the proposed analyses themselves, in the protocol. The latter are best written by the biostatistician. Of course, there is no disadvantage in writing them yourself from notes provided by the statistician, as long as you ask for a critique when you are done. The preparation of the protocol with regard to the items and activities with which we are concerned in this book will be discussed in Chapter 7.

1.7 PERSONNEL AND FACILITIES

This section contains a brief discussion of the personnel and the kinds of specialized equipment that are needed for a department devoted to the planning, execution, and analysis of clinical trials.

1.7.1 The Biostatistician

It is possible to arrange with a statistician or statistical group employed by your company, a consultant or a consulting firm, to handle all your statistical design and analysis work with almost no attention from you at all. Some monitors and others responsible for clinical trials do this. But it is inadvisable to place all your experimental design and statistical activities in the hands of a consultant and then give those matters no further attention. Unless you make it your business to become familiar with what such individuals or organizations are doing with your projects, and to be critical of their activities if necessary, the probability of success for your studies will be reduced. It is quite important that you and others in your department interest yourselves in experimental design and statistics to a reasonable extent, and to develop an understanding of the purposes behind the designs among which you will choose.

If it is economically feasible, hiring a company biostatistician or setting up a department of medical statistics on the premises is a most efficient arrangement. On the other hand, for smaller firms, for divisions of larger organizations without such facilities, or for those requiring only occasional statistical assistance, using an independent consultant can be a practical plan.

The following is relevant if you do not yet have a company biostatistician who is knowledgeable in medical statistics, and have not yet made arrangements to obtain the services of a well-qualified biostatistical consultant.

How do you obtain statistical help? If you and your associates know nothing about experimental design or statistics, you will be unable to evaluate the capabilities of your biostatistician. One of the purposes of this volume is to help you to make an informed choice. With this knowledge, even if the statistician or statistical department will not report directly to you or will not be a part of your own section or department (and, in fact, it is advisable that they be separate), you should try to take a hand in its organization and the hiring of its personnel. You will be much more familiar with what is required than others in your company who are less closely involved with the firm's clinical trial work.

Inevitably, as for all professional people, statisticians come in a variety of levels of competence. Academic qualifications are highly desirable but do not guarantee proficiency. Many statistical curricula, at least to date (with a few significant exceptions), have not included sufficient knowledge of applications to provide effective performance in industry, especially in the field of clinical trials. Until work experience supplies the lack, their graduates will be less than completely helpful. In fact, it is difficult for a university to provide such training, because, quite aside from the enormous amount of work required of the student, which leaves little time for internship, there are many different fields of application of statistics, differing from each other in many ways, including the appropriate designs and methods of analysis. Especially if yours is a small organization, one method that you might consider is to use consultants until you have had sufficient experience with statistics and experimental design to hire, or advise your company in hiring, a full-time professional. You might even consider employing a consultant for the purpose of recruiting an adequately qualified biostatistician as a permanent employee.

It is *not* a good idea for the statistician to report to you or to anyone in the medical department or the Monitors' group. There will be times when you or members of your department may not agree with the biostatistician on a statistical matter, or when there is some lack of understanding on his or her part regarding a medical or pharmacological point. The statistician should be an independent-minded person who is willing to persist in any such arguments, and you should encourage such behavior. It is not reasonable to purchase the services of an expert and then ignore the advice you have bought. Of course, because you will presumably be responsible for your project, you will need to overrule him or her at times. When you do, however, be careful. If you have done your job at the hiring stage, and the matter is statistical, you should expect the statistician to have better judgment. It is important that you recognize this. A rare but important skill of a good supervisor is the ability to recognize and hire people who are more capable than they at their particular jobs. If you know as much or more than anyone working for you about their specialties, why employ people with any special qualifications at all?

If you plan to do a bit of statistical work yourself, or if you were unable to avoid having the statistician on your own staff, you will need some computing facilities. If your company is currently setting up a statistical department, you can help. If the statistician is a consultant, and you do not plan or are unable to obtain such equipment and software, be sure the consultant has them, can do the data analyses, and can write an intelligible report for you.

1.7.2 Computers

Given sufficient time, every statistical procedure normally employed in the assembly and analysis of drug trial data can be done without a computer, using a pocket or desk calculator. However, most of the statistical procedures used today can be done so much more rapidly with a computer than without one that the latter would be unthinkable. As in many other fields of human activity, planning and scheduling of the work of a modern medical department is based upon the expectation that computers will be available.

Despite its advantages, however, there are some dangers connected with the use of a computer. First, a statistical program in the hands of someone who does not fully understand it can produce a greater degree of misapplication of statistical processes than is possible in any other way—and much more rapidly. Second, it is necessary to select suitable "packages" of statistical programs, and, unfortunately, despite advertising claims, not all of those available are suitable for clinical work. Some do not include procedures especially necessary for the analysis of clinical trial data, with their frequent "unbalance" due to patients who do not complete a course of treatment. Some, unbelievably, include inaccurate or incorrect methods. The best ones are intended for the use of professional statisticians and do not give advice as to the applicability of their methods. Furthermore, it is impossible, as suggested earlier, to use a statistical software package without a good knowledge of statistics. One of the best with which I am familiar emphasizes repeatedly that it is not its purpose to teach statistics. Beware of the program that claims that statistical training is not required to use it properly or effectively.

There are three common kinds of digital computers: **mainframes, minicomputers,** and **microcomputers.** Mainframes are the very large machines now principally employed, in industry, by medium and large company data-processing departments for handling the firm's financial, inventory, and similar business-oriented records, and by the military and government agencies. They can cost as much as several million dollars or more.

Minicomputers are smaller, requiring perhaps 100 to 400 square feet of floor space as compared to hundreds or thousands for the mainframes. They are also an order of magnitude less expensive, running perhaps between $25,000 and $100,000 when fully functional. Despite the space required and their cost, minis can be sophisticated and flexible. Until recently, they were the preferred machines for much scientific and technical work. But they are rapidly becoming much less common, because the power and speed of desktop machines have increased almost exponentially in the last few years.

Beginning in the mid-1980s, desktop microcomputers have become increasingly suitable for small and medium statistics departments, and today they can perform almost every function of the minis, often as rapidly. They are much less expensive and can satisfy all of the requirements of the average department running clinical trials. And for cases in which more commuting power is required today, the **networking** of groups of minicomputers "headed" by a "file-server" machine having very large disk storage capacity are becoming increasingly common.

Such networks also commonly use a single fast and sophisticated printer, available to all the computers in the group, saving the expense of having printers at each station in the network. Networks of small computers, called LANs, or local area networks, possess the additional advantage of allowing use of special software licensing, leading to lowered software costs. If your department or that of the statistician employs several people handling data storage for a study, and more than one or two statisticians are involved in the final data analysis, a network can replace, at less cost, the former use of a company mainframe or minicomputer connected to remote terminals. The mainframe was never the ideal facility for the statistician, because the statistical programming necessary was quite different than the kind normally handled by a company data-processing department. And the cost of getting and maintaining the necessary statistical software was not trivial for either the mainframe or the minicomputer.

A small computer, either an individual or part of a LAN, can fill needs other than those of a statistician. By using some of the vast variety of software available, it can be useful in report writing, preparing graphs and tables, and other office functions. Letter-sized optical character readers are not new, but they have been greatly improved and reduced in price during the last few years. With one of these, you can set up a system for reading properly designed clinical report forms, saving much manual transcription on the typewriter or word processor.

If you plan to purchase any computing equipment intended for statistical work you will need someone in the firm who combines a knowledge of the kinds of statistics needed for clinical trial work with a good background in the installation and use of microcomputer hardware, peripherals, operating systems, and statistical software, to advise you in your purchases and to help set up the equipment. The statistician or one of his or her staff may have this knowledge. An alternative is to obtain a consultant qualified in the kind of computing needed in clinical work (the biostatistician may be able to help you find such a person).

1.8   WRITING AND EDITING

The last of the important resources needed for your department, and certainly one of the most important, is facility in writing reports and other necessary documents. First, your biostatistician must be able to produce a report that is intelligible to statistical nonprofessionals (such as some of your top management, who may wish to sample some of your or the statistician's work). At the same time, he or she must also be able to make the same reports statistically sophisticated and informative for professional statistical readers, including those at the FDA. Finally, the reports must also be as medically sophisticated as necessary.

The ability to write lucidly and understandably should extend beyond your statistician. Not only you, but members of your staff who must help you produce interim and final reports of a trial, as well as help handle the everyday correspondence and other written material, should be good writers.

Technical, medical, and scientific personnel who are also skilled at technical writing are not always easy to find. The problem is not that intelligent technical, scientific, and engineering people do not have a competent grasp of grammar, syntax, and composition. Rather, the most common failure,—and it is really common,—is that many such people write material that is understandable only to members of their own professions. A typical example is some of the documentation that comes with your computer or your applications software, which can be appalling in its lack of clarity, and appears to have been written for someone who is already a member of the same profession as the writer and therefore already knows what is says.

1.9   SUMMARY OF THE CHAPTER

The chapter begins by reviewing the types of studies to be covered—that is, industrial safety/efficacy trials, usually done for the purpose of evaluating new drugs. It is pointed out that there are probably many more industrial studies carried out than any other kind.

In this book, we emphasize experimental design rather than analysis. You are urged to develop an early and close relationship with your statistician, and to work with him or her throughout the planning of a study. Although we believe that the readers of this book should be reasonably familiar with the principles and kinds of experimental designs, it is emphasized that this volume does not advocate that medical and paramedical personnel learn to "be their own statisticians," carrying out their own analyses in addition to performing their regular professional duties. In some cases, if there is time, there is, of course, no disadvantage in doing some of your data analyses with the guidance of a biostatistician. But although most of you will probably not have the time or opportunity to do this, it is important that certain common statistical procedures at least be familiar to you because of their connection with the experimental designs that you will select. In addition, a knowledge of these principles is important in sample size estimation, and it *is* important that you develop some knowledge of that.

There is a short discussion about the importance of having a biostatistician available, not only for the performance of the necessary data analyses after a study is completed, but also to help you in your understanding of some of the statistical aspects of your trials, and to assist or carry out the necessary sample size estimates during the planning of any trial. It is pointed out that the statistician should be a part of the team from the earliest planning session.

There is a discussion of the available literature, some of which is listed in the Bibliography.

A major section of the chapter is devoted to an outline of the more common types of experimental designs. These and others will be covered later in much greater detail. By using the common nomenclature of clinical trial work, the designs described are first classified as **parallel** and **changeover.** A parallel design is one in which each patient receives *one* **level** of *one* of the **factors** in the design. For example, if a factor consists of two or more different drug treatments, its levels would be one or the other drug. In a trial using a parallel design, each patient would receive one, and only one, of the drugs, possibly once or for a few doses, or perhaps repeatedly for a longer period of time. Changeover designs are those in which each patient receives more than one of the levels of the factor(s), each for a period of time, that is, perhaps several drugs, each given in a series of doses for a fixed period. There are many varieties of both parallel and changeover designs. Some common types of each are introduced.

Other methods of classifying designs that you may encounter are mentioned. These include **one-way** (one-factor), **two-way** (two-factor), and more. The idea of **experimental units** is defined to aid in understanding the arrangements comprising an experimental design. The ideas of **crossed** and **nested** designs are explained; the latter are of little use in clinical studies, but are mentioned to clarify the nature of the crossed designs.

The ideas behind some elementary statistical procedures, including sample size estimation, are introduced. Only two chapters are devoted to statistical analysis, and one to sample size, but it is important that this information be included, because of the intimate connections among the type of design chosen for a study, the kind of response(s) (measurements) planned, the nature of the analysis to be done, and the sample size to be used.

Brief discussions of the selection of a statistician (staff or consultant) and types of computing equipment follow. The chapter ends with a discussion of writing and editing, an important part of the activities of a clinical trial section in any pharmaceutical company.

CHAPTER 2

Nature and Purposes
of Clinical Testing

2.1 SCIENTIFIC EXPERIMENTATION IN MEDICINE

In *Webster's Ninth New Collegiate Dictionary* [71], the relevant definition of the term "experiment," in a context of scientific inquiry, is "an operation carried out under controlled conditions in order to discover an unknown effect or law, to test or establish a hypothesis, or to illustrate a known law." A properly done clinical drug trial is "an operation carried out under controlled conditions" and is run "to test or establish a hypothesis." Thus, it is a scientific experiment. A correctly used experiment is a marvelous tool of scientific research. In a properly done drug trial, an experiment can supply evidence of the efficacy and safety of a drug with a degree of reliability obtainable in no other way. Of course, "evidence" is not proof; there is no "proof" in science. Hence, most drugs that show promise require a *series* of trials in order to produce sufficient evidence of safety and effectiveness to justify their sale to the public. On the other hand, a single trial can be enough to establish a lack of either characteristic.

The appropriate use of experimentation in science can be summarized in these five steps:

1. Devise a hypothesis to describe what you believe to be an explanation of the phenomenon to be investigated.

2. Plan an experiment to test your hypothesis.

3. Perform the experiment.

4. Observe and record the results obtained. Determine whether they *completely* support the hypothesis (they must not contradict it in any way whatsoever). The experiment should be looked upon as an attempt to *disprove* the hypothesis, *not* to *support* it. Then, if the hypothesis still appears convincing, it becomes more believable.

- **CONSTRUCT A HYPOTHESIS**
  Based upon what is known or believed

- **DESIGN AN EXPERIMENT**
  Try to disprove the hypothesis

- **PERFORM THE EXPERIMENT**

- **OBSERVE AND RECORD RESULTS**

- **DO THE DATA SUPPORT THE HYPOTHESIS?**
  If so, the hypothesis is strengthened
  If not, revise the hypothesis and start again

Figure 2.1 The scientific method.

5. If the hypothesis is supported by the observations with no inconsistencies or contradictions, it then gains more strength. If, however, the outcome is different in any way than was predicted, it *must* be revised. The process then returns to step 2, using the revised hypothesis based upon the new observations, and repeating steps 2 through 5.

These general principles embody the **scientific method.** To emphasize its importance, it is summarized in Figure 2.1.

After you have obtained a set of results that appears to support a hypothesis, you will nevertheless almost always want to design and carry out similar but perhaps larger experiments to test it further. You will not be finished with this process until you are strongly persuaded, *based upon the evidence*, that your hypothesis is reasonable and accounts *without exception* for the observed values of all of your data. *Any data at all* that contradict it are sufficient to invalidate it unless you know that something went wrong with the experiment. On the other hand, although you may have accumulated sufficient data to be convinced of the validity of the hypothesis, you can never be absolutely certain that it is true. By "sufficient," I mean that such evidence must be convincing to any unbiased person who is professionally experienced in the disease or symptoms being studied, and in running clinical trials. Of course, you should recognize that the "truth" has not been discovered, but only that all the observed data are consistent with the hypothesis.

An essential part of the scientific method is to plan your experiment (step 2) as rigorously as possible, so that it will detect any flaws in the hypothesis if they exist. If, instead of trying to invalidate the hypothesis in this way, the experiment is arranged so that it tends to provide evidence to support it, you will not be testing it adequately; you will be deceiving yourself. The support comes when the final modification of the hypothesis at last survives the most demanding testing process you can devise. It then emerges as a reinforced method of prediction, which you may feel you can call a *theory* (a greatly strengthened hypothesis). This procedure is an idealization, of course, because it can be quite difficult to maintain the necessary objectivity. Nevertheless, it is important to approach this ideal as closely as possible. The crackpot drug treatments that surface from time to time, like laetrile as a cancer cure of DMSO as a panacea, when they are not simply cynical promotions, are usually the result of undisciplined investigations by sincere but misguided advocates who have either been unable to summon the necessary experimental objectivity and scientific skepticism, or truly have no understanding of the process of experimentation and the scientific method.

2.1.1   Use of Experimental Design and Statistics

We should point out that statistics and experimental design are not absolutely essential components of the scientific method. If they were, there would have been no important and validated results of clinical trials and other scientific experimentation in the past, before the use of these tools became widespread. However, after many years of crude experimentation, it became apparent to many workers during the past 30 years that experimental design and statistics furnished the best available methods of evaluating medical treatments. These techniques can make a final conclusion in a drug trial, for example, become available much sooner, with much less time and effort and fewer patients, than would be needed without them. They so greatly intensify and improve precision and accuracy in the clinical process that they have become the standard and essential approach. Today, it is unlikely that any drug firm could obtain regulatory approval if they have not been used, and, moreover, even if such approval were not necessary, competitive operation, good business, and profitable products would make their use necessary.

This book is about the use of experimental design and statistics in the planning, execution, and data analysis of clinical trials. Our emphasis is upon planning, which includes experimental design, rather than upon the execution of your trials, or upon their statistical analysis. Nevertheless, to an extent, we must include information about the analysis of your data and the estimation of sample size, both of which are statistical processes. This is so although there are many professional books and textbooks about statistics, and a few on experimental design (see the Bibliography for a sample of some relevant works). There are several reasons for this:

1. Any experimental design implicitly specifies the use of a particular class or a limited number of classes of statistical methods of data analysis, and you must be aware of this when planning your experiment. This point is not necessarily clear to the reader of the average statistical textbook or professional book.
2. Most books about statistical analysis are unnecessarily complex for users who need some statistical knowledge for clinical trial work but who need not become professional statisticians.
3. The use of methods of estimating sample size (numbers of patients) for a clinical study requires some basic knowledge of statistics, and this information is not readily available to nonstatistical professional people who need them only in a form that is easily understandable and applicable to clinical studies.

2.1.2   Development of New Medical Treatments

Traditional Methods

Thus, as noted, until very recently, the genesis and use of new treatments came about by means having little to do with the scientific method. For millennia, the majority of therapies appear to have evolved by one of three methods: accidental discovery of treatments with unmistakable efficacy; the use of hypotheses alone, without any experimentation; or the utilization of experimentation without **controls, randomization, blinding** (defined in next section), or adequate sample sizes. Treatments originating by one of the latter two routes frequently persisted for a very long time despite a lack of unbiased evidence of their efficacy. Bloodletting, purging, and the use of homeopathic dosages of drugs are examples. Failure of a treatment in any particular case was usually attributed by its practitioners to its misuse, to poor diagnosis, or to complicating factors. It is remarkable that medicine evolved at all in its earlier years, considering its notable lack of dependence upon disciplined, unbiased observation. Introduction of a new procedure seems to have not infrequently been accomplished through the force of personality of a sponsor (an "authority"). When a truly valid treatment did emerge through this process, it usually did so because it exhibited overwhelmingly obvious benefits.

From the eighteenth and nineteenth centuries and earlier, and even from the first half of the twentieth, with a few exceptions that are not generally widely accepted, there are few records of any serious attempts to conduct systematic and scientific experiments, such as our modern, randomized controlled clinical trials, to evaluate the efficacy or safety of medical treatments. And when a rare, serious, and well-conceived experiment did support a new treatment, the medical establishment and others were very often unbelievably slow in accepting the evidence. A famous example is the discovery by the East India Company in A.D. 1600, and again in 1747 by Lind on the basis of a controlled experiment, that citrus fruit juices would prevent scurvy among British seamen. Despite terrible outbreaks of the condition on long voyages in the British Navy, however, regular supplies of juice for the sailors were not made available until 1795 (see Meinert [3], p. 5). That is, the British Navy required almost 200 years to accept the evidence and put the idea into practice by supplying daily lime juice for the men. Part of this delay, at least, was a result of the stubbornness and unwarranted conservatism of the Naval medical practioners of the day.

Scientific Method
Only after World War II, for the most part, a century or more after rigorous experimentation in the physical and biological sciences had become widespread, did the value of controlled, randomized clinical trials finally begin to be recognized.[1] At long last, in the 1950s and 1960s, the benefits of such trials, incorporating the principles of good scientific experimentation, were tentatively acknowledged by some in the medical profession. But it was only in the mid-1970s that properly done clinical trials began to be widespread in the pharmaceutical industry. This accomplishment can be attributed, at least in great part, to the increased rigor of new food and drug law amendments and to vigorous establishment and enforcement of regulations by the Food and Drug Administration (FDA) requiring logical and scientific experimentation.

Example 2.1: The Scientific Method in a Drug Trial

Experimental Design and Response Measurement
Let's say that you have evidence, based upon preclinical work and observations made during *Phase I* safety trials (see Chapter 3) that a new drug developed by your firm may be useful in decreasing farsightedness without the use of glasses, presumably through some effect upon the muscles of the eye. The preclinical and Phase I trials have shown no evidence of serious toxicity. Now, using a series of small to moderate-sized *Phase II* trials, you wish to obtain further evidence of efficacy, as had appeared in the *Phase I* trials. Of course, you will also continue to observe and record any evidence of adverse effects, as you should always do throughout this and all other trials. In this example, however, we will be concerned with the measurements of efficacy. Your hypothesis (expressed as a purely scientific concept, not a statistical hypothesis) is simple: It states that the drug, given orally, improves the clarity of near vision when compared to a placebo. Of course, you will

---

[1]As an example, Isaac Newton was an accomplished experimenter as early as the latter third of the 1600s, and the Royal Society, of which he was president from 1703 until his death in 1727, encouraged experimentation beyond any other method as a tool of research.

derive your conclusions from this and any further trials with the help of statistical analyses (probably done by a statistician), using data from the trial.

Now you must design a trial to test your hypothesis. Your patients must be shown to be farsighted, the experiment will be double blind, and it will test the hypothesis using a randomized two-treatment parallel design, comparing the drug versus a placebo. As you will learn, this is an experimental design using one *factor* (drugs) at two *levels* (the test drug and the placebo, here classified as a "drug"). You are planning to do vision tests of all of your prospective patients before inviting any to participate in the trial, and then to select patients with simple farsightedness only (having no other abnormal visual condition). Each patient who agrees to take part will be randomly assigned to one of the two treatments, the drug or the placebo, will take that material orally for a month, and will then be reexamined. The assignments will be double blind. That is, neither the clinician administering the trial nor the patients will be told which treatment each patient receives, although all will be informed that it will be one of the two treatments, and will also be fully acquainted with the nature and purposes of the trial.[2] The *response* ("measurement") in this example will be a classification of the patients into successes and failures, that is, whether or not the examining physician finds improvement relative to each patient's original condition. There will be no further patient classifications, such as age group (beyond a limitation to adults), whether they use glasses, the degree of their farsightedness, etc., although all of these and similar characteristics will be recorded for reference during the initial interview.

You should note that several of the procedures in this example are not those most likely to be used in a well-designed clinical study. For example, it is not advisable to use a binomial response in a case where a numerical measurement or at least a score is feasible, especially as the principal or only response. Such measurements often yield much less information per patient (are less efficient) than other procedures, thus requiring more, typically many more, patients. Again, we use it here because it simplifies the explanation of this particular example, and the nature of the response is not the point in this example. In addition, it is poor practice to require an investigator to judge "improvement" or "success," thus requiring him or her to compare a presently observed condition with an original observation made in the past. Instead, it is much better to record a baseline response and the current response, and to use differences between these two measurements as the

---

[2]Many of these arrangements are described here to simplify the explanation of the example. Normally, if the patients are outpatients, it is usually better to arrange for each to visit the clinic at least once a week, even if you plan to use the final (fourth-week) measurement for the data analyses. This arrangement allows you to issue only a week's supply of the test materials at each visit and to collect unused doses more frequently (the FDA expects you to maintain a reliable count). You will then also be better enabled to track the patients' conditions for safety and other reasons, and reinforce them in their realization that you are seriously interested in their condition.

final response data for analysis. The difference can be calculated by the computer during the analysis of the data.

Sample Size
Your estimate of sample size, carried out as described later in the book, indicates that 49 patients be assigned to each of the two treatments. You therefore randomly select 49 to be assigned to each drug, following a procedure also described later.

The Trial and the Results
You then carry out the trial. The results are shown in Table 2.1. Thirteen of the 49 patients on placebo (about 27%) show improvement, and 30 of the 49 (about 61%) on the test drug improved (it is common for patients on placebo to improve during a trial). A statistical **hypothesis** ("significance") test was done to compare the results for the two treatments. Such a test assumes that the patients in the trial comprise a **sample** taken from a **population** of potential patients. It can produce the numerical **probability** of finding an observed difference between the two proportions of patients improved that is as large as that actually obtained if there really is no difference between them in the two populations, so that the observed difference is merely a matter of sampling variation.

The probability of the observed difference in proportions in Table 2.1 being as large as found, if there were really no population difference, was about 0.001 (i.e., very unlikely; about one in 1000 trials). During the planning of this trial, it was specified that any probability less than 0.01 (1 in 100) would be considered to support a conclusions that the two proportions were different. It was therefore reported that there was statistical evidence of efficacy for the test drug.

This may require a bit more explanation. The hypothesis testing process is important to everyone doing clinical studies, and is very widely misunderstood. When the patients are selected for the two groups comprising the trial, it is assumed that the measurements in each group comprise a sample from a large population, any of which could have been selected instead. Within that population, or **distribution,** there is considerable variation among the individual measurements, reflecting patient differences and so-called "random error." Each population has a **mean,** which is the average measurement for the

Table 2.1. Improvement of Vision in Farsighted Patients: Example 2.1

Drug Used	Successes	Failures	Totals
Placebo	13	36	49
Test Drug	30	19	49
Totals	43	55	98

entire population, and is, of course, unknown. This is called a **parameter.**[3] However, its value can be approximated by taking the average of a sample. It can be shown that the larger the sample, the more nearly the sample mean approaches the mean of the distribution.

After the patient sample is split into two groups, one for each treatment, if at least one of the two treatments affects the measurements, the theoretical population receiving that treatment will be different than the original population, inasmuch, at least, as it will have a different mean. The statistical hypothesis test consists in assuming initially that the two treatments are completely ineffective. This assumption is called the **null hypothesis.** The probability of a difference as large as that observed between the two sample means is then obtained by a simple calculation or obtained from a table. If that probability is unbelievably small, the investigator may conclude that the null hypothesis is very unlikely to be true, and that there really is a difference in the two populations, evidenced by the different means of the two samples. For this procedure to be scientifically and mathematically rigorous, the null hypothesis and its alternative, which *must* be accepted if the null hypothesis is rejected, must be established before the trial begins. Also, the magnitude of the "unbelieveably small" probability must be defined beforehand.

The meaning and use of hypothesis tests, even when presented in greater detail (as we will do later), are not very complex. However, it is critical that you understand them thoroughly. They underly the objectives and motivations of almost every clinical study. Not only are such tests necessary as means of presenting evidence of safety and efficacy for any submission made to the FDA for approval of a drug, but they are prerequisites for your understanding of what the statistician will be doing with your data, as well as for your own understanding of the methods of estimating sample size. This explanation will do for now, but it will be developed further in Chapter 13.

Example 2.2: Second Trial (Successes)

The experiment of Example 2.1 did not satisfy you. You thought about the fact that some patients on the test drug did not improve. Did such patients have anything in common? You wondered whether the use of glasses could have influenced the results and decided to investigate this point. You prepared a breakdown of the 43 successes in Table 2.1, ignoring the failures

---

[3]The statistical meaning of the term **parameter** is that it is a characteristic of a *theoretical* population, such as the mean, although it is commonly and incorrectly used to refer to the related quantity derived from the sample, such as the sample mean, or even, as is very common among clinical investigators, to a measurement itself. Statisticians refer to sample measurements and their means as **statistics,** which are *estimates* of a parameter. Some populations have only one parameter, while others have more. The so-called **normal** or **Gaussian** distribution, originally supposed to be the most common of all, can be plotted to form the familiar bell-shaped curve. It has two parameters, the mean and the standard deviation. The latter is a statement of the degree of variation among the measurements comprising the population.

Table 2.2. Improvement of Vision in Far-Sighted Patients: Example 2.2 (Successes from Table 2.1)

Drug Used	Glasses		Totals
	Yes	No	
Placebo	6	7	13
Test Drug	3	27	30
Totals	9	34	43

for the moment. Were there more successes associated with users of glasses, or vice versa? Your new tabulation is shown in Table 2.2.

Table 2.2 indicates that, in this trial, the test drug was successful with more patients if they did *not* use glasses (of course, none wore their glasses during the examinations). Ninety percent (27/30) of the test drug patients whose vision improved did not possess glasses, whereas only 10% (3/30) did. In contrast, there were 13 successes on placebo, and those with and without glasses were as evenly divided as possible—about 46% (6/13) and 54% (7/13), respectively. This table suggests, of course, that patients who were wearers of glasses were less likely to respond favorably to the new drug.

Example 2.3: Testing the Failures

Finally, Table 2.3, showing the failures, was constructed. The trial resulted in 55 failures (patients showing no improvement), 36 on placebo and 19 on the drug. Of the 19 on the test drug, 10, or about 53%, were users of glasses and nine (47%) were not. Of the 36 on placebo, 24 (67%) were not wearers of glasses, and 12 (33%) were. See Feinstein (1). This table, taken in conjunction with Table 2.2, again suggested that users of glasses were less likely to experience improvements in farsightedness with the test drug. Perhaps, you thought, such patients were more difficult to help, being on the average more advanced in their condition.

Table 2.3. Improvement of Vision in Far-Sighted Patients: Example 2.3 (Failures from Table 2.1)

Drug Used	Glasses		Totals
	Yes	No	
Placebo	12	24	36
Test Drug	10	9	19
Totals	22	33	55

Discussion of Examples 2.1, 2.2, and 2.3

Please note that significance tests of Tables 2.2 and 2.3 were not necessary, because a final conclusion would not be based upon this trial. Examples 2.2 and 2.3 are illustrations of "exploratory" work, done to suggest a direction for further trials. If these two tables were to be tested statistically, a special kind of hypothesis test for the entire set (Tables 2.1, 2.2, and 2.3) would have been necessary, because, in a sense, tests of the latter two were repetitions of part of the original tests in Example 2.1, and they were created as a result of observations made in that trial.

To summarize, it appeared that the test drug was likely, in general, to improve farsightedness, and particularly so if a patient was not yet a user of glasses. In spite of the fact that a substantial proportion of patients with glasses took part, presumably diluting the strength of the new drug's effect, you were encouraged by the fact that in the first (overall) experiment (Example 2.1), the test drug was shown to be superior in your hypothesis test. However, good science suggested that you run a new trial, taking the use of glasses into account in an overt manner, to try to reinforce your conclusions from Example 2.1 and confirm your observations in Examples 2.2 and 2.3, which you should at present regard as tentative.

In such a new trial, you should use two **factors** at two **levels** each: the two drugs as the first factor, and the use of patients who wear glasses vs. those who do not as the second.[4] You would use four patient groups. They would consist of patients without glasses assigned to placebo, patients with glasses also on placebo, and an analogous pair of groups assigned to the test drug.

There could have been several other questions that you might have wanted to ask, such as whether a patient's age would affect the performance of the drug, and whether the severity of the farsightedness would affect the performance of the drug, and perhaps others. However, this, again, is exploratory research, and should be done before beginning a final series of studies for the purpose of seeking approval of an NDA (New Drug Application). In any event, when all the preliminary exploratory studies have been done to your satisfaction, you will need one or more confirming trials, in which you do not expect to need to alter your final hypothesis. This trial or trials should be considerably larger than the preceeding ones, so that you can make your

---

[4]The new factor, the use of glasses, is not the same kind of variable as the drugs factor, but it is nevertheless amenable to a similar experimental design and analysis. In the first trial, you used the **drugs** factor alone and had the power of randomly assigning either drug or placebo to any given *patient* (this decision was made in each case by the use of a random assignment). This would be no longer true for the second factor, **use of glasses.** This factor is not a "treatment" in the same sense as **drugs,** because it is a characteristic of each patient and cannot be randomly assigned. Its use as a design factor, therefore, is similar to the arrangement used in a **survey,** as contrasted to an **experiment,** wherein the patients or subjects already have the characteristics being used as factors (remember the Surgeon-General's *Smoking and Health* report). Because of the lack of randomizations, results involving such a factor must be interpreted more carefully. This kind of factor is discussed later at length.

inferences from a broader base. You should not use any of the patients from the previous trials. Of course, because this final step will be more expensive than the earlier, smaller trials, you should be reasonably sure of the outcome beforehand.

We have assumed that you began your series of trials of this drug with some very small studies, immediately after the preclinical work indicated that they could be conducted safely. This *Phase I* stage requires an **IND** or **INDA** (Investigational New Drug Application) from the FDA, which will involve your supplying information from your animal work and seeking approval for your initial clinical studies. After obtaining approval to continue, you performed the early *Phase II* studies just described, in which you were concerned with efficacy as well as safety. Additional and larger Phase II studies would have then been likely to be necessary. The final trials just mentioned would then have been *Phase III*, and some of them would have been very likely to be multiclinic studies. You would hope at that point that these trials would be instrumental in persuading the FDA to approve an application to market the drug with specific approved claims. This would be embodied in your application for an NDA. The next chapter will describe the regulatory process in more detail.

2.2   ESSENTIALS OF A GOOD CLINICAL TRIAL DESIGN

There are many features of a good clinical trial design that are important, but there are three that should always be present except in very rare cases:

1. The use of concurrent controls
2. Blinding
3. Randomization

The need for these three characteristics is endorsed by almost all statisticians and experimenters experienced in clinical trials, as well as by FDA statisticians. Figure 2.2 may help to emphasize their fundamental importance. You should use them unless it is impossible to do so. If you are forced to omit one or more of them, the probability that the conclusions you draw from the data analysis will be valid will be substantially reduced. Furthermore, a trial lacking *any* of these features is fairly likely to be rejected by the FDA, and will be unconvincing to other informed critics, such as journal readers.

To summarize, a clinical trial is an experiment. Trials should virtually always use one or more concurrent controls, random assignment of treatments to patients, and double-blinding.

- ## CONCURRENT CONTROLS

  Placebo

  Standard

  Both

- ## BLINDING

  Patients
  Investigator(s)
  Both

- ## RANDOMIZATION

  Random Assignment

Figure 2.2   The essentials of a clinical trial.

2.2.1   Concurrent Controls

The phrase *concurrent controls* implies the inclusion in an experiment of a placebo (inactive material) and/or a drug, similar to the test drug, having a known effect. In the language of analytical chemistry, the placebo would be called a "blank" and the know drug a "standard." Both are forms of controls. The word "concurrent" means that your controls are included in the experiment and tested at the same time and in the same way as the other treatments; that is, they should be treated as additional drugs in the trial and data analysis, becoming additional levels of the treatments or drugs factor. It is usual when analyzing the data to compare each test material of interest with the controls, and probably with each other.

The use of "before and after" tests (omitting concurrent controls and comparing test products with baseline data only) is, unfortunately, common practice in industrial trials. There are rare occasions when such a technique must be used, but it is usually very poor science. It assumes that there has been no change from the time the baseline measurements were taken to the time when the final measurements are made after treatment. This is almost always a poorly supported assumption. However, this fact does not negate the value of using baseline responses consisting of the same kind of measurements as those used after treatment. It is common, and often enhances the sensitivity (statistical **power**) of a study, to use *differences from the baseline* as the data for analysis.[5] But the set of such differences should include differ-

---

[5]When this is done, there is a hidden assumption that should be recognized. It is the assumption that changes in the response at baseline occur at exactly the same rate as those occurring after treatment. In other words, the assumption is that the slope of a line formed by plotting the

ences from concurrent controls. It is the use of baseline data as a *substitute* for concurrent controls that is objectionable. An exception to this is the use of differences from baseline in certain types of *changeover* studies (mentioned in a moment). Note that the usual use of baseline data as a basis for generating differences for analysis in this way is not implied or specified by any statistical principles. It is merely good, logical scientific experimentation.

Another and even more extreme violation of good scientific practice is the use of so-called "historical controls"—results or data found in the literature or in another experiment done earlier—as a substitute for concurrent controls. This should never be done unless there is no other possible kind of control.

Exceptions to the use of a placebo include certain studies in which a "zero-dose" level may not be needed or may be impossible. Dose-ranging studies in which one factor (dose) comprises a series of quantitative levels (10 mg, 20 mg, 40 mg, etc.) are in this category. Such studies seek to estimate the rate of change in the effects of the drug under test as the dose increases, or to estimate the shape of the dose response, if it is not linear.[6] However, it is a good idea to use a zero level even in these studies when possible; it does no harm and furnishes an additional level of the factor. But there are also cases in which the use of a control is impossible. For example, this would be so if you were using the logarithm of the doses (there is no logarithm of zero), perhaps in the hope of obtaining a linear response when you believe that the original dosage units do not form a straight line when the effect of the drug is plotted against dose.

A typical single-factor parallel trial with three levels of the factor, designed to evaluate a test drug, might have the following as the three treatments: the test drug, a placebo, and a drug of known potency. Each of the three drugs would be assigned to a randomly selected group of patients. In some experiments, the use of a placebo will be ruled out because of ethical considerations, and there are times when a standard cannot be used, of course, but when both a placebo and a standard can be compared with the test substance, the conclusions drawn from the data analysis can be strengthened. Comparing the placebo with the standard will show whether the experiment was able to detect a known difference, and if so, confidence in the experimental procedure can be increased. If this occurs, the other two

---

baseline value for each patient against the response after treatment with the drug is 1.0. This may well be true or approximately so, but should not be assumed. In cases of doubt, the statistician should use a technique known as **analysis of covariance,** using the baseline data as the covariate, when analyzing the data. If certain additional assumptions underlying that technique are valid, it will then ensure that the correct allowance will be made for the baseline measurements. This technique is valid *whatever* the relationship between the baseline observations and those made after treatment.

[6]Such studies are important but are beyond the scope of this book. See Draper and Smith [34] or Snedecor and Cochran [38].

possible pairwise comparisons will carry more weight. Comparing the test drug to the standard will then provide an estimate of its efficacy relative to the known material, and comparing it to the placebo will allow an estimate of its absolute efficacy.

If you use baseline data, there is one important precaution of which you should be aware. It is common to use baseline data in a two-period crossover design (discussed in Chapter 12) in an attempt to eliminate so-called carry-over effects between periods. But Fleiss and others have recently pointed out that this must never be done, as it will introduce a severe nonconservative bias (2, 3).

To recapitulate, almost all good trials should use comparisons between one or more test treatments and at least one control (e.g., placebo and/or standard) whenever possible, to reach conclusions about both the safety and the efficacy of the test material. The use of both a control and a standard is recommended.

2.2.2 Blinding

The second critical characteristic of an effective clinical trial is *blinding*. The use of blinding means that the identity of the treatment assigned to a given patient is concealed from the patient, investigator(s), or both, although they may know the identity of the treatments being used in the trial. *Double blinding* means blinding both investigator and patient. *Single blinding* means blinding only one of them; in common usage, usually the patient or subject. Sometimes, blinding is extended to others who work with the data, including the statistician at the time of data analysis. Double blinding, at least, should be used in every trial in which it is physically possible. There are a few situations in which it cannot be used, but these are rare.

In the 1950s and 60s, when controlled, randomized trials were beginning to be used widely, there was considerable reluctance on the part of some investigations to use blinding. Its advocacy was sometimes taken as a reflection upon the reliability of medical opinion. But most of us are susceptible to bias in one way or another. It is a characteristic of human observation and thought, and no one can be sure it has been completely excluded from a measurement or evaluation process. I have heard it explained that, yes, obviously patients need to be blinded (exhuming many rational arguments), but experienced clinicians should not be required to take measures to prevent bias, because they are already unbiased. The best answer to this is that perhaps they are, but the remedy will do no harm, and in the remote event that they are wrong, it may save the day.

Blinding is not a statistical process, and cannot be said to be an essential part of *statistical* design, but it is most definitely needed for good *scientific* reasons, especially when, as in clinical testing, there are subjective or semi-objective responses. But it should also be used even in the case of most instrumental measurements. I do not think that many truly objective responses exist. Even the process of reading a sphygmomanometer or a meter needle can be biased for a physical reason, if for no other; for one thing, it is subject to parallax, especially when the observer is careless or fatigued. Such readings are also subject to a more subjective kind of bias involving parallax, because if the observer expects or hopes to get a high or low average, the reading will frequently tend to be higher or lower than otherwise. All that is required is a slight, perhaps unconscious, head movement. Some instruments must be read rapidly, which can make them subject to similar biases. An EKG can be recorded without influencing the results, but the process of reading it is seldom free of bias. Some kinds of X-ray readings are notoriously dependent upon the viewer. And in clinical trials, there are many, probably a majority, of measurements that are noninstrumental, such as scores and ranks, and that are very highly subjective. The measurement of pain on an n-point scoring scale, the joint-tenderness index sometimes used in the measurement of arthritic conditions, the counting of comedones in acne testing, the ranking (ordering) of relative degrees of edema or erythema —all are subject to observer (and patient) bias.

Therefore, because no one can guarantee freedom from bias when making measurements, you should plan to use double blinding in any clinical trial unless it is really impossible. Of course, as you probably already know, the FDA is quite strict about the matter, so perhaps my arguments are superfluous. But this was not always so.

2.2.3 Randomization

Randomizing Treatment Assignments
A third essential procedure in a clinical trial is the *random assignment* of treatments to subjects or patients. It will be discussed at more length in Chapter 6. Unlike the practice of blinding and concurrent controls, it use is a statistical requirement, as well as good science. But as was true for those procedures, especially the former, there was considerable resistance among investigators to its use in the early days of clinical trials. Articles appeared by advocates of nonrandomization, with many arguments presented against its use, similar to those given against blinding, including claims that it was unethical, because a patient could not control whether he or she received a placebo or an effective drug in a trial. Of course, that argument ignored the fact that there is no assurance at the start of many trials that the test drug itself is effective, and it also ignored the requirement of informed consent by patients. And all of the arguments against it ignored the fact that it was essential for a valid statistical analysis.

The insistence upon the use of these procedures on the part of statisticians and many medical officers in the FDA was a major factor in the eventual acceptance of the use of concurrent controls, blinding, and randomization.

Among the reasons for the use of randomization in the design of any experiment, a most important one is that only in that way can correct long-run probabilities be derived from the statistical hypothesis tests that will undoubtedly be performed on most of your data. Without an appropriate randomization procedure, your statistical tests will be of unknown and therefore questionable validity. Other reasons for randomization are the elimination of trends, a precaution against certain patient characteristics affecting the treatment comparisons, and others, but many of these are really other aspects of the first reason.

The random selection of patients to receive treatments means neither *haphazard* nor *systematic* assignment. The assignments must be made according to an explicit procedure. Before the use of randomization was generally accepted and enforced by the FDA (by the refusal to accept trial data based upon improperly randomized treatment assignments), it was common (as late as the 1970s) to make assignments according to systematic or predictable procedures like birth dates, odd and even numbers, and the like. These techniques are *not* random processes; in fact, they are *deterministic*. Moreover, many commonly used physical processes, such as drawing numbers out of a hat, throwing dice, the ping pong balls used for state lotteries, and the like, are also unlikely to be truly random. A really random sequence of numbers is one for which a priori it is a matter of pure chance which number may be drawn next. No known influence must govern the selection of a particular number in the series. This includes the provision that each drawing must not affect the probability of drawing any particular number during the next selection.

Even computers cannot generate truly random numbers. Because a digital computer operates on a deterministic basis, it is literally impossible for it to produce truly random numbers. Many computer programs use algorithms that can produce a very long series of *almost* unpredictably permuted members and then repeat the series. A program can be made to compose a different series each time one is called for. But the results are not quite random. Such computer-generated "random" numbers are often called "pseudo-random" for this reason. In spite of this, most statisticians doing practical work today do use this means of generation, relying upon programs that produce very long permutations before repeating. The reason for using the computer, despite its inability to produce a truly random series, is that although this method is not truly random, it is believed to be so nearly so that its convenience and objectivity outweigh that disadvantage. Some statisticians, moreover, doubt that the generation of truly random numbers is possible by any means. In addition to these problems, the pool of numbers from which one is chosen at each drawing is generally limited in practical work. This makes the "random" series somewhat less than truly random in any event, but we must do the best we can, and allow practical procedures, made as nearly random as possible, to guide the process.

There are many different kinds of randomization. The method used depends upon the nature of the design and the kind of statistical analysis that will be selected. Details of the appropriate randomization procedure will accordingly be discussed whenever an example of a particular design is given.

If a design consists of two drugs in a parallel study, in the simplest case (roughly equal numbers of patients to be assigned to each drug), randomization will provide a (long-run) guarantee that the probability of assigning a given drug to a particular patient is 0.50 (i.e., there will be a 50% "chance" of any patient receiving either treatment). If there are three drugs, again in the simplest case, each patient will have a probability of 0.33 of receiving any one of the drugs. In other words, in these situations, it will be equally likely that any patient will receive a given drug. Ideally, therefore, all patient groups (one for each drug) will be equal.

The use of equal group sizes produces an advantage when the statistical analyses are done. All hypothesis tests or confidence intervals (discussed later) involve calculation of the experimental error of the observations or responses. When the group sizes are equal, these errors are minimized, although, of course,they can never be eliminated. For slightly or moderately divergent group sizes, however, the increase in the error is not very great, and is usually of little consequence.

Nevertheless, there are some cases in which equal likelihood is not desired. The randomization procedure can then be altered so that something other than equal-sized patient groups will result. For example, in a study using two drugs and a placebo as treatments, you may sometimes wish to arrange for twice as many patients to receive placebo as either of the two drugs. If this were the case, you could use a randomization procedure that produces a probability of 0.50 of any patient receiving a placebo, and probabilities of 0.25 of receiving drug A or drug B.

Returning to the more common eventuality in which you want to produce at least approximately equal group sizes, let us assume that you are planning a trial in which there is a single factor, such as drugs, and that the study will use a parallel arrangement, in which each patient will receive just one of k different drugs. The use of equal group sizes implies that you want the probabilities of assignment of each of the k drugs to any patient to be as nearly equal as possible. There are two common ways to carry out this randomization. If it is essential for some reason that exactly equal numbers of patients be assigned to each drug, you must first be certain, of course, that the total number of patients selected is divisible by k, the number of levels of the factor (the total number of different drug treatments). You then repeatedly select patients randomly and assign him or her to a given drug until exactly $1/k$ patients have been assigned to it. You then no longer assign any patients to that drug, but continue with assignments to the remaining drugs until an equal number have been assigned to a second drug. You repeat this process until one less than k patient groups have been formed. The remaining patients will form a group equal in number to the preceding groups, and can then be assigned to the last of the k treatments.

In the simplest case of this procedure, in which $k = 2$ (two drugs), this reduces to a process in which you select either drug and randomly choose patients to be assigned to it until exactly half of them have been drawn. The remaining patients, a number equal to that of the first group, comprise the second group and are assigned to the other treatment.

This process does not produce a perfectly random set of assignments. The reason is the restriction introduced by the elimination of further assignments to one of the drugs when half of the patients have been assigned to it (or $1/k$ of the patients if there are more than two drugs). The other method involves no such restriction, but will usually result in somewhat unequal group sizes. To carry out this procedure, you simply randomly assign the k drugs, with equal probability, to your patients until the total preplanned number of patients has received assignments. The inequality in group sizes likely to occur here will tend to be proportionally less as the total number of patients planned becomes greater. Thus, this method might produce quite highly divergent group sizes and become impractical if you were assigning three treatments to a total of, say, 15 patients, but the divergence would be likely to be moderate or small, percentagewise, if the total was, say, 45.

Randomization does not guarantee perfection in the assignment of treatments to patients. For example, in the second method, in which the randomization is unrestricted, as indicated it is likely that you will obtain unequal treatment group sizes. Usually, this does not matter much unless the groups are quite small, as when some groups of two or three patients receive one treatment, whereas other treatments are assigned to two or three times as many. To minimize this difficulty, some designers restrict the randomization by constraining the process to ensure that all the treatments are used an equal number of times (usually once) each time the assigned number of patients reaches a sub-multiple of the number of treatments being used. This will reduce the possible inequality of group sizes to any desired degree. As an example, suppose you are designing a trial in which there are three treatments—perhaps a test drug, a placebo, and a standard. If you wish to "block" the assignments in this manner, you can identify the three treatments as A, B, and C, and create the six possible permutations of these three (you may wish to use the computer to do this if the number of treatments is greater than 3 or 4):

ABC	ACB
BAC	BCA
CAB	CBA

You now select one of these six permutations at random (this should be done by the computer or with the use of a table of random numbers). Suppose you obtain BCA. Your first "block" will then consist of treatments B, C, and A, in that order, to be assigned to the first three patients reporting to the clinic when the trial is run. You continue in this way until you have accounted for whatever number of patients you have planned to use altogether. *Note that each set of three treatments should be selected randomly; you must not attempt to arrange the selections so that all six permutations occur an equal number of times.* Of course, in the remote case that this happens by chance, you should not try to change the arrangement. Note also that you must use a sample size that is an integer multiple of the number of treatments in order to avoid getting incomplete blocks; in this case, 3, 6, 9, etc. Of course, you would be unlikely to use sample sizes as small as this in an experiment with three treatments. If patients are lost during the trial, the inequality of assignments will still be small.

Many trial designers stop here. They have ensured that there will be equal numbers of patients on each treatment after every third patient has been assigned. The statistician analyzes the data when the trial is complete, ignoring the blocking. But strictly speaking, this is incorrect, because the analysis does not then completely reflect the design, and the results can sometimes be distorted. Consequently, if you feel that you must block the randomization process in this way to avoid discrepancies in the treatment group sizes (although moderate inequalities are not serious), you should ask your statistician to take the blocking into account in his analysis of the "ANOVA model." This procedure creates a form of randomized blocks design, although, unlike the usual kind of blocks, these will not be known to be identified with any particular "nuisance variable." The analysis will suggest whether that is true or not.

The Population Sampled

The target population (the patients who you expect will eventually use the drug) must be defined explicitly in your protocol, as a guide to drawing conclusions at the end of the trial. The discussion so far has been concerned with the use of **random assignment** of treatments to patients or subjects. We have not mentioned **random selection** of the patients (or, for that matter, of the investigators or centers in a multicenter trial). The fact is that it is impossible to select patients or centers in a random manner, with the population defined in a practical way.

In some nonmedical surveys, political polls, for example, great pains are often taken to obtain representative samples of the populations of interest (usually random or stratified random samples of potential voters). But such populations never include future members, or present members as they will be in the future, so that any conclusions from the samples must be limited at least to members present, and their opinions, at the time of sampling. There are many other difficulties involved in obtaining a truly representative and random sample of a defined population for these purposes, and it may be that such samples are very rarely obtained. This may be tolerable in such activities as political polls, but it is almost never practical in industrial clinical trials. For one thing, the principal interest in clinical studies has reference to the treatment of *future* patients, after the drug has been approved and marketing has begun. Another is that the centers or investigators in medical trials are virtually always the best and most expert who can be found, who are willing to take part. They are never a random sample of the average practitioners who may prescribe the drug if and when it becomes available. Thus, the population of interest does not exist at the time of the trial. Finally, the patients selected will not represent all present and future patients who might receive the test drug, but rather only those available to and applying to each center used in a trial. Some examples that discuss this subject include Deming (4), Nelson (5), and Friedman, Furberg, and DeMets [2].

As a consequence, the random selection of subjects or patients in clinical trials is usually limited to the process of *assignment of treatments*. Only very rarely is random sampling of patients from any defined patient population ever possible or attempted.

The use of an appropriate randomization procedure makes possible the valid use of *statistical inference*, that is, induction. Statistical inference is the process of applying conclusions drawn from a statistical procedure, performed upon a sample, to the population that was sampled (the target population), that is, drawing conclusions about the general from the particular. The analogue of this in Sherlock Holmes' case (miscalled "deduction" by his creator) might have been the examination of a footprint conveniently located in some soft soil under a window, by means of which Holmes could almost invariably *induce* a variety of personal characteristics about the perpetrator, such as weight, economic status, and English social class.

Thus, with random sampling of the appropriate patient population impossible, no statistical inference can be legitimately made to the population, but only to the sample of patients (and the investigators) at hand.

Random *assignment* assures lack of bias in the distribution of the treatments to the sample, and makes valid statistical inference possible—but such inferences will be statistically valid for the patient *sample* only. It does nothing to ensure valid inference to the future population of patients and physicians who will use the treatments if the tests are successful.

Nevertheless, if it is your opinion that your sample of patients is typical of those with the condition you hope will be remedied by the treatment under test, and if you believe that your sample of investigators is representative of the population of physicians who will use your treatment, then you can reasonably extrapolate your results to these populations. But you must bear in mind that the *statistical* evidence will be valid only for the samples used in the experiment. What you will be doing is extrapolating these *statistical* results on a *logical* but not a *statistical* basis. Although you cannot use the outcomes of your statistical tests to make statistical inferences to the target populations of patients and investigators, you can nevertheless use these results as bases for drawing conclusions about those populations. Therefore, although you cannot sample randomly from your target population, you must not think that statistics is of little use in your work.

Thus, it becomes obvious that the inability to use **statistical** inference beyond the sample does not preclude the employment of **scientific** inference.

Generalization of the conclusions of your trial is still possible, and is facilitated by both processes.

2.3 THE NEED FOR CLINICAL TRIALS

Why is there a need for clinical trials? Why can't pharmaceutical firms release their new drug products as soon as they feel they are ready, as was done in the past?

In general, there are two answers to this question. The first one is that there was distribution of dangerous products in the preregulated past by some companies. This necessitated the original U.S. food and drug laws, which required only that products be safe before they could be sold. But it was later realized that the release of safe but ineffective products could also be dangerous to users, and therefore the original act was eventually modified to require both safety and efficacy.

The second answer to the question of why there is a need for clinical trials is that it is good business for your company to ensure that your product is as effective as you claim it is. It is similarly good business to do everything possible to be certain that your product is safe, or, failing that, that any hazards are fully disclosed. The most successful pharmaceutical organizations, in the long run, are those whose products are most reliable. Eventually, the results of clinical trials submitted to the FDA are publicly available, so it is possible for you or anyone else to compare your results with those of others who have tested similar products. You may also read, in the *Federal Register*, why if your competitor's application was rejected by the FDA, this action was taken; this, of course, may help you avoid a similar fate.

The next chapter is a summary of the regulations and procedures governing the interaction between the FDA and any person or organization planning to market a new drug. It is fairly general, and few details are given, because regulations can change rapidly; however, sources of up-to-date information are given.

2.4 SUMMARY OF THE CHAPTER

The chapter begins with a discussion of the nature of scientific experimentation, as it should be used in clinical studies. A brief review of methods used in the past to develop medical knowledge and practice follows, and is contrasted with the *scientific method*, which is widely used today. Examples of the use of this procedure during the early stages of drug development are given.

A discussion of good clinical trial design follows, emphasizing the use of concurrent controls, blinding, and randomization. Reasons for the need for clinical trials are then discussed.

2.5 LITERATURE REFERENCES

(1) Feinstein, Alvan R., *Science*, **242**, 1256–1263, 2 December 1988.

(2) Fleiss, Joseph L., *Controlled Clinical Trials*, **6**, 192–197, September 1985.

(3) Willan, Andrew, et al., *Controlled Clinical Trials*, **7**, 282–289, December 1986.

(4) Deming, W. Edwards, *The American Statistician*, **29**, 146–152, November 1975.

(5) Nelson, Lloyd S., *Journal of Quality Technology*, **22**, 328–330, October 1990.

CHAPTER 3

The Role of the FDA

3.1 BACKGROUND

In this chapter, we will be concerned with the drug regulatory activities of the Food and Drug Administration, and the ways in which they affect the development of new drugs (and, at times, the requalification of old drugs) by the pharmaceutical industry.

The definition of a drug in *Webster's Ninth New Collegiate Dictionary* [71] which is relevant in our context is "a substance intended for use in the diagnosis, cure, mitigation, treatment or prevention of disease . . . a substance other than food intended to affect the structure or function of the body."

With respect to the interaction of a pharmaceutical company with the FDA, a **new drug** is a substance that the sponsor wishes the FDA to sanction for marketing, accompanied by claims of efficacy for a specified purpose or purposes, as well as disclosures of any hazards of use. The material may or may not be new in the sense of having a new chemical structure or a new mixture of components. It may even have been marketed previously, or may be currently available, either for another purpose, or because it appeared before the present regulations regarding safety and efficacy were written. Any substance or mixture of substances will be regarded by the FDA as a new drug if it has not previously been approved as safe and effective under current regulations for the condition for which the sponsor wishes to make claims. If the "drug" is a mixture of materials, all of them deemed by the FDA to be "active" and not simply "vehicles" or carriers, the mixture must be safe for the proposed use and *each component must contribute to the effectiveness of the mixture*.

With some important exceptions, most of the vast current pharmacopeia created since the food and drug laws became effective is a result of efforts by the FDA and the pharmaceutical industry, rather than of foundation, academic, or government research. There are many cases in point. Not long ago, for example, there was no generally effective treatment for hypertension, and it was a major killer. With the development and trials by industry and approval by the FDA of the first beta blocker, hypertension, in general, became a minor annoyance (to the extent that patients can be persuaded to be diagnosed and to continue their medication). As another example, although penicillin was discovered by Sir Alexander Fleming in England (Fleming was an academic researcher), the drug did not become generally available to the public until after World War II, when several different forms of it were tested and manufactured industrially. Since then, of course, a very wide variety of other antibiotics has been developed, evaluated, and marketed by pharmaceutical firms. There are many more examples, including many OTC and proprietary drugs, such as analgesics, skin treatments, and others.

In all of these activities, the FDA, via the section formerly called the *Bureau of Drugs*, then the *Center for Drugs and Biologics*, and currently the *Center for Drug Evaluation and Research*, strongly emphasizes safety and the use of good statistical design and correct statistical analysis in clinical drug trials run by industry. In the process, pharmaceutical manufacturers have developed better and safer drugs, with the result that everyone benefits —the sponsors (manufacturers or marketers), who enjoy increased sales as a result of greater public and professional confidence in their products; the medical profession, which can prescribe with increased confidence; and the public, who are the recipients of a greater variety of more useful medications. Of course, there are occasional failures, mistakes, and accidents, but there has never before been so large, so safe, and so effective an assortment of medicinal products available to practicing physicians and the public.

3.1.1 Statistics and the Food and Drug Laws

In order for a manufacturer to comply with food and drug laws, the use of modern experimental design and statistics is essential. In the form of applied sciences, and with the exception of quite primitive work in probability and distribution theory, these techniques are products of the twentieth century. The *t* test was discovered and developed by "Student," the pseudonym of William Sealy Gosset[1] (1, 2), an Oxford-trained chemist and mathematician employed by the Guinness Brewery in Dublin. This was the first practical small-sample statistical procedure, and was published in 1908. Beginning at about that time and continuing until his death in 1962, the great genius Sir Ronald A. Fisher was responsible for using the factorial design in methods of analyzing factorially designed experiments, as well as a large number of other fundamental statistical tools that we still use today. His work inspired many others to use applied statistics and to develop additional methods and techniques. Without the work of Fisher and Student, most of the experimental designs and statistical analyses now used in drug development and required by FDA regulations could not have been developed. And without

---

[1]This is the correct spelling, although some of the literature spells Gosset's name with two *t*'s. See Kotz and Johnson (2).

the statistical design and analysis of experiments, drug development would be vastly retarded, and we would have much less assurance of both safety and efficacy for most pharmaceutical products developed during and since the 1960s.

The first important drug legislation in this country was contained in the U.S. Food, Drug and Cosmetic Act of 1938. This had little effect in encouraging the use of statistically valid clinical trials for drug products, however, and it was not until the 1962 Kefauver and Harris amendments to the Act, and, more recently, extensive new regulations promulgated by the FDA in 1969 and 1970, that effectiveness as well as safety was emphasized as a requirement for the approval of pharmaceutical materials. The Kefauver-Harris amendments were the first to specifically mention the use of "adequate and well-controlled investigations, including clinical investigations" as being among the criteria for the approval of a new drug product.

3.2 SUMMARY: REQUIREMENTS FOR APPROVAL OF A DRUG

3.2.1 Introduction

The material in this section is not intended as an official guide for dealing with the FDA. Rather, it is provided to help clarify the experimental design and statistical activities in which you must engage, partly as a result of the FDA requirements for the continued sale of an old drug or the initial sale of a new one. FDA regulations or rules change from time to time, and some of the information given here may change by the time it sees publication. For accurate information about the drug regulations, any proposed submissions, or other dealings with the FDA, you should consult your company's regulatory affairs department or the person designated as responsible for such activities, or contact the FDA yourself (with company approval).

The information in this section, as well as generally in this book, refers to trials both of ethical (prescription) and of nonprescription items (proprietary and other OTC drugs). Although the topics and examples given in this book are totally or almost totally concerned with drug treatments, some of the regulatory material and many of the techniques of clinical study planning and data analysis apply equally to medical treatments not involving drugs.

The processes of running clinical trials to qualify a drug (usually a so-called new drug) for sale to the public has been classified by the FDA into three stages. These are referred to as Phases I, II, and III. Postapproval trials fall into a category known as Phase IV, but this has not been official FDA terminology.

3.2.2 Phase I, II, and III Trials

Phase I represents the initial period in the testing of a new drug, begun after very extensive preclinical safety testing has indicated that the toxicity of the material is low enough to justify careful, small-scale clinical testing.[2] Before a sponsor (usually a pharmaceutical manufacturer) can begin Phase I trials, an Investigational New Drug Application (INDA, as defined earlier) must be submitted to the FDA. If there is no objection by the latter within 30 days, the work described in the INDA may begin (if the trials to be run are to be different than those described, information about the revision must be submitted before initiating them). Initial Phase I trials are usually very small, often involving as few as perhaps 4 to 10 subjects. The emphasis is upon safety of increasing doses, metabolism, and pharmacologic action of the drug. The sample will therefore commonly consist of healthy volunteers, *subjects*, rather than *patients*, although either might be used. In the most common kind of trial at the point, each subject is given one of the drugs, observations are made, and then, sometimes with a "washout" period, the next drug is given to the same subject in the same manner. If there are more than two drugs, this process continues until each subject has been given all of them and all necessary observations have been made. Random assignment is used if at all possible, often consisting only in the establishment of the order of giving the drugs to each subject.

During Phase I, these cautious small-sample tests may employ gradually increasing sample sizes, although they will never become very large. The total number of subjects or patients in phase I is generally no more than 20 to 80. If, in this series, no serious safety effects are found, the sponsor may then continue to Phase II trials. Just as for Phase I, a complete outline of all of the experimental work planned must be or have been submitted (any subsequent changes in the plans must be resubmitted). If, within 30 days, the FDA makes no objection that would delay or cancel the proposed work, the sponsor may begin Phase II.

Phase II trials emphasize both safety and efficacy, and are well-controlled, usually double blind, closely monitored, and randomized. They are likely to be substantially larger than those of Phase I. Of course, sample size (i.e., the number of patients) will depend upon circumstances, but will commonly range from as few as 20 to as many as 150 to 200 or more. As will be shown in Chapters 5 and 15, the sample size in any single well-planned trial will depend largely upon a statistical estimation process, based typically upon pairwise treatment differences in efficacy required by the sponsor as its principal criterion. Usually, sample size calculations are not done in terms of safety data, because there are literally never enough patients in a trial to ensure safety with a truly satisfactory probability. More often, there will be a series of small Phase II trials, with the sample sizes gradually increasing, but with the total number of patients in a single trial usually no more than a few hundred, so that the total sample for estimating safety will be quite large. If

---

[2] In certain cases, when there is very strong existing evidence of safety, toxicity testing before starting clinical trials may be reduced or eliminated, and, consequently, the trials started with Phase II or, very rarely, Phase III.

no serious toxicity effects have then surfaced, and there continues to be enough evidence of efficacy to justify continuing, the final and largest round of trials, those of Phase III, will begin.

Phase III trials constitute the final stage in the premarketing process for qualifying a drug for sale with particular claims. It usually includes two or more fairly large multicenter trials, although, as for Phases I and II, Phase III may begin with smaller trials, not necessarily multicenter. Both the sponsor and FDA, at this point, are likely to have been in agreement, based upon a conference at the end of Phase II, that there is substantial evidence of efficacy as well as safety, and that Phase III trials may begin. The large multicenter trials may involve relatively small numbers of patients per center, but can, in some cases, require as many as 20 or more centers, each with tens or even hundreds of patients. With such large samples, safety problems, if there are any, are more likely to emerge. The FDA normally requires at least two adequate and well-controlled Phase III trials prior to the approval of a new drug (NDA approval).

The Phase III series may continue for several years, include several thousand patients, and cost several million dollars. This, of course, is part of the reason why new drug products are often expensive. When the Phase III trials have been completed, the sponsor submits a New Drug Application (NDA), which must include description of all intermediate development work done during the IND process. If the FDA does not disapprove, marketing may begin.

3.3 POSTAPPROVAL ACTIVITIES

3.3.1 Phase IV Trials

Phase IV "trials" are open-label monitoring programs (not blind or double blind), and may often not be randomized. They can be controlled or uncontrolled, and are carried out after marketing has begun. They may be imposed by the FDA for postmarketing surveillance, or run by your company for marketing or promotional purposes. Their purpose may be to monitor both safety and efficacy, but especially the former, taking advantage of the very large "sample" sizes that will be available at that point. Phase IV is most often invoked for ethical drugs as part of the NDA process, or as an informal understanding between FDA and the sponsor. The subjects in these programs are patients for whom the new drug has been prescribed by practicing physicians.

There is another kind of Phase IV trial series, usually designated as DESI (Drug Efficacy and Safety Implementation) trials. These are true randomized, controlled trials. They are usually moderate to large single or multicenter studies, run at the behest of the FDA to provide evidence of efficacy for "old" drugs that may have been initially marketed before current laws and regulations were put into effect. There is ordinarily no question of safety in such cases, because of the long periods during which the materials have already been marketed. As may be imagined, there are many such drugs, and there are DESI studies still in progress at this writing.

3.4 WORKING WITH THE FDA

The interaction of the FDA with the pharmaceutical industry does not stop with the beginning of marketing. FDA may suspend sales of particular materials if there is evidence, in its opinion, of a safety or efficacy problem. Such bans may be abrupt, or, in the absence of an imminent health hazard, more protracted, sometimes allowing time for manufacturers to exhaust current stocks.

Certain investigators may be disqualified from taking part in any drug trials for limited intervals or undefined periods. In such cases, data from trials in which such investigators have been involved must be reevaluated. In other cases, additional trials and/or analyses may be required if the FDA believes that previous work has been poorly done or because it is not convinced of the safety or efficacy of a drug for other reasons. It is an unfortunate fact that, even today, substantial numbers of industrial drug trials (as well as many noncommercial trials) are designed, run, and analyzed using incorrect or inadequate designs, poor or careless execution, or unsuitable or incorrect statistical analyses. Other actions may be taken by the FDA on the basis of the drug regulations. Of course, any such action may be appealed.

There are aspects of your present or future dealings with the FDA with which you should be aware, and that bear especially upon the subjects of this book. Among these, you should know that the Center for Drug Evaluation and Research is very well-staffed with medical and scientific personnel, all of whom can advise the pharmaceutical manufacturer about the design and execution of the necessary clinical trials. For example, the center makes available a series of *Guidelines* that provides suggestions and advice for particular kinds of trials. To illustrate, it is usually necessary to run comparative bioavailability trials (often misnamed bioequivalence tests) when the dosage form of a drug is to be changed (e.g., from a capsule to a tablet), or the drug is reformulated, or a new manufacturer, such as one producing generic drugs, will produce it. For such trials, there is a group of guidelines outlining the experimental designs and other procedures and requirements, such as minimum sample sizes. Everyone involved and responsible for drug trials should have an up-to-date collection of these documents.

The FDA staff includes a large and experienced group of Medical Officers as well as Consumer Safety Officers (CSOs), one or more of whom will be assigned to your project from the beginning. It is to your advantage to know and consult with the Medical Officer whenever you need advice or help with a project. However, your principal contact with the Center, even when you wish to confer with others, will be the CSO, who is the traffic controller within FDA. In addition, depending upon policy, your company will generally require that you first clear such contacts with a designated company officer, usually in your company's regulatory of government affairs department.

In addition to these FDA Medical Officers, the staff at the Center for Drug Evaluation and Research includes a large, well-qualified, and experienced assortment of scientists: pharmacologists, chemists, biochemists, pathologists, statisticians, and others. You may wish to take advantage of the help you can obtain from FDA statisticians. One way to do this is to request a meeting with them to review the design and general planning of your trial, well before you begin. This is not required, and some companies do not meet with the FDA unless requested to do so, but such a meeting can be of substantial help to you, because you will either come away with suggestions that will increase your chances of final acceptance or with a general agreement regarding your experimental design as it stands.[3]

3.5 REGULATORY INFORMATION

3.5.1 Good Clinical Practices

There are large amounts of information available from the FDA for anyone desiring or needing it. It can be obtained by contacting the Center for Drug Evaluation and Research (CDER). Food and Drug Administration, 5600 Fishers Lane, Rockville, Maryland 20857. One current "packet" that should be obtained by anyone active or contemplating activity in the planning, execution, data analysis, or submission of results to the FDA is entitled *Good Clinical Practices*. This was assembled under the supervision of Alan B. Lisook, M.D., of the FDA, and includes the items listed in what follows as of mid-1992. They are presented here in the order in which they appear in the packet. Of course, the latest information may vary from the current material as new publications become available. Here is the list:

(a) *Information Concerning FDA Regulations*

(b) *Center for Drug Evaluation and Research Publications*

(c) *Clinical Investigations* (excerpt from the *Federal Register*, 9-27-77)

(d) *Protection of Human Subjects*; *Informed Consent* (excerpt from the *Federal Register*, 1-27-81)

(e) *New Drug, Antibiotic, and Biologic Drug Product Regulations*; *Final Rule* (excerpt from the *Federal Register*, 3-19-87)

---

[3]Of course, such a session will in no way guarantee final approval of your application.

(f) *Investigational New Drug, Antibiotic, and Biological Drug Product Regulations*; *Treatment Use and Sale*; *Final Rule* (excerpt from the *Federal Register*, 5-22-87)

(g) *Guideline for the Monitoring of Clinical Investigations* (1-88)

(h) *Investigational New Drug, Antibiotic, and Biological Drug Product Regulations*; *Procedures Intended To Treat Life-Threatening and Severely Debilitating Illnesses*; *Interim Rule* (excerpt from the *Federal Register*, 10-21-88)

(i) *FDA IRB* (Institutional Review Board) *Information Sheets*

(j) *FDA Clinical Investigator Sheets*

(k) Reprint of Alan B. Lisook, M.D., "FDA Audits of Clinical Studies: Policy and Procedure," *Journal of Clinical Pharmacology*, **30**(4), 296–302, April 1990.

(l) *Federal Policy for the Protection of Human Subjects*; *Notices and Rules* (excerpt from the *Federal Register*, 6-18-91)

(m) *FDA Compliance Program Guidance Manual—Clinical Investigators* (9-1-91)

(n) *FDA Compliance Program Guidance Manual—Sponsors, Contract Research Organizations and Monitors* (12-3-91)

3.5.2   Guidelines

In addition to the kind of material in the *Good Clinical Practices* packet, there is a considerable number of FDA *Guidelines* addressed to evaluations of specific categories of drugs and procedures. Any of these is available from the Legislative, Professional and Consumer Affairs section of the FDA Center for Drug Evaluation and Research (CDER), and other FDA and U.S. Government agencies. As examples, there are *Guidelines for the Clinical Evaluation of Anti-Anginal Drugs, Guidelines for the Clinical Evaluation of Bronchodilator Drugs*, and many others. Some of these documents are obtainable at no charge and others can be obtained at moderate cost. Listings are available from the FDA Legislative, Professional and Consumer Affairs at CDER. Before embarking upon a trial of any kind, it is advisable to obtain any relevant Guidelines.

3.5.3   Summary of Good Clinical Practices Documentation

The following are brief summaries of the documents included in the *Good Clinical Practices* packet:

(a) *Information Concerning FDA Regulations:* You are advised in this document to purchase *Title 21, Code of Federal Regulations*, and to subscribe to the *Federal Register*. A list, summaries, and costs of the several parts of

Title 21 are given. I might add that anyone concerned with any aspect of the planning, execution, or analysis of clinical trials, or with any regulatory affairs connected with them should have the *Federal Register* available.

(b) The list in the *Center for Drug Evaluation and Research Publications* is a general summary of titles, costs, and where to obtain a number of CDER publications, most of which are relevant to clinical trials and their regulation.

(c) *Clinical Investigations* is a description of the *Proposed Establishment of Regulations on Obligations of Sponsors and Monitors* from the *Federal Register*. It includes extended descriptions of the proposed rules and requests comments. Many of these rules were later adopted as final.

(d) *Protection of Human Subjects*; *Informed Consent* is a complete description and discussion of revised standards and rules governing the acquisition of informed consent from patients who will participate in a clinical trial, effective on July 27, 1981. It also includes revisions of the regulations with regard to approval of clinical studies by Institutional Review Boards (IRBs), and a brief section regarding "expedited procedures" that can be used by a board.

(e) *New Drug, Antibiotic, and Biologic Drug Product Regulations* are final regulations that became effective on June 17, 1987. They concern activities performed in connection with an IND, under CFR parts 312, 314, 511, and 514 (the first two are concerned with IND applications, and the latter two with new animal drugs). The work on a new drug prior to marketing is governed by IND (Investigational New Drug) regulations. When that work is done, a sponsor files an NDA (New Drug Application) in order to obtain permission to market the drug. This document (*item (e)*), together with item (c), the next one, (f), and item (h), are essential reading for anyone planning to begin a clinical trial for a new drug, needing approval for an IND, and expecting eventually to apply for an NDA so that a drug can finally be marketed with relevant claims. This document discusses all aspects of the necessary procedures for compliance, summarizes them, and provides opportunities for certain conferences to be held between sponsors and the FDA following Phase II, just preceding the NDA, and a final "end-of-review" meeting. Of course, other meetings may also be requested by either party. Much of the document comprises a review of many comments and questions about the new regulations that were posed by interested parties when the new rules were proposed. This is followed by a section discussing the new regulations, as implemented, and finally by an actual copy of them.

(f) Item (e) just described final rules for the relevant regulations, issued 3-19-87. This notice, (f), entitled *Investigational New Drug, Antibiotic, and Biological Drug Product Regulations; Treatment Use and Sale; Final Rule,* from the *Federal Register* of 5-22-87, describes some amendments of Part 312 of that rule, which is entitled, as before, *Investigational New Drug Application.*

(g) The *Guideline for the Monitoring of Clinical Investigations* is a short (six-page) document issued for the purpose of assisting a sponsor of an IND in performing or arranging for the performance of monitoring of the necessary procedures, such as the planning, execution, analysis, and submission of results to FDA. The guideline points out that the principles described are not legal requirements but "represent a standard of practice that is acceptable to [the] FDA." It suggests that a sponsor using other procedures may, if desired, submit descriptions of them to FDA for comment" to avoid the possibility of employing monitoring procedures that [the] FDA might later determine to be inadequate." The guideline includes discussion of *Selection of a Monitor*, standardized *Written Monitoring Procedures*, *Preinvestigation Visits* to each investigator chosen for a trial, *Periodic Visits* during the progress of a trial, *Review of Subject Records* maintained by each investigator, and the maintenance of a detailed *Record of On-Site Visits*.

(h) This notice, *Investigational New Drug, Antibiotic, and Biological Drug Product Regulations* ... describes additions to 21 CFR Parts 312 and 314, issued as interim rules for the purpose of further implementing the rules described in items (e) and (f). The principal concern in this case was to further expedite the marketing and use of certain drugs designed to treat "life-threatening and severely-debilitating illnesses," such as AIDS and cancer. As is commonly done, these rules were issued as interim rules to allow time for submission by the public and consideration by the FDA of comments before they are issued as final rules in the forms described or in modified form. They took effect at the time this notice appeared in the *Federal Register*, but allowed 60 days for the submission of comments and promised to consider modifications of the rules after reviewing the comments.

(i) The item listed here as *FDA IRB Information Sheets* consists of a set of documents describing the purposes of IRBs and how sponsors planning clinical trials should deal with them. The principal purpose for IRBs is to ensure protection of human patients and subjects in the implementation of clinical studies. These boards are concerned with medical devices as well as drugs. You should note that devices are regulated by a different division of FDA than that concerned with new drugs. Twenty-two documents are included, on topics, to cite a few, such as advertising for subjects, FDA inspections of IRBs, IRBs and medical devices, informed consent, and payments to subjects.

(j) The next item, *FDA Clinical Investigator Information Sheets*, is intended primarily for investigators, but may also be of interest to IRBs. It contains six documents concerning drug evaluation. They concern record keeping, informed consent, FDA inspections of investigators, regulatory sanctions (disqualifying of investigators), use of investigatory drugs for treatment of life-threatening and other serious conditions, and the use of several kinds of controls in clinical studies.

(k) Dr. Lisook's paper, "FDA Audits of Clinical Studies: Policy and Procedure," is concerned with FDA investigations of studies related to the approval of drug claims. The major concern is with the validity of data. Many irregularities have been found, including nonadherence to protocols, inadequate and inaccurate records, incorrect consent procedures, and others.

(l) This notice from the *Federal Register*, *Federal Policy for the Protection of Human Subjects*, is part of a larger notice from a number of U.S. Government agencies, and describes current regulations administered by the FDA. The relevant regulatory information is contained in 21 CFR, Parts 50 and 56, amendments to which are cited and given in the notice. Part 50 is entitled *Protection of Human Subjects*, and Part 56, *Institutional Review Boards*.

(m) This *FDA Compliance Program Guidance Manual* is concerned with clinical investigators and comprises part of the implementation of an investigator compliance program that was established in the late 1970s and is still extant. The relevant regulations were instituted on June 17, 1987 (21 CFR Parts 312, 314, 511, and 514). The programs concerned with human drugs and biologics are part of a larger program also covering food additives, veterinary drugs, and medical devices. The purposes of the programs are "to (1) assess adherence to guidelines and assure adherence to the regulations and (2) to determine the validity of specific studies in support of products pending approval by the FDA, and (3) to determine that the rights and safety of subjects used in clinical studies have been properly protected." The manual appears to be directed principally to the guidance of FDA inspectors charged with investigating compliance to the regulations. The manual gives details of the activities expected of the inspectors.

(n) The *FDA Compliance Program Guidance Manual* covering sponsors, contract research organizations, and monitors has purposes and implementation analogous to the previous item. FDA inspectors and/or inspection teams are to gather and report certain information regarding the compliance of sponsors, research organizations and monitors to the regulations. This manual, like the one just described, appears to be principally concerned with the guidance of such inspectors and teams. As for the previous item, this manual is intended to guide inspections in all of the five areas mentioned—"food additives, biologics, human drugs, veterinary drugs, and, in this case, medical devices and radiological health."

3.6 SUMMARY OF THE CHAPTER

This chapter is devoted exclusively to a discussion of the procedures necessary or desirable for sponsors, monitors, contract research organizations, and monitors of clinical trials to secure compliance with FDA regulations and the Food and Drug laws. Although the regulations are broad and cover a number of related areas ("food additives, biologics, human drugs, veterinary drugs and medical devices and radiological health"), our focus is concerned particularly with the subject of this book—the regulatory matters of concern to the pharmaceutical industry in connection with clinical trials. Although we have not stressed the development of medical devices and related issues, and although the examples in this book are not concerned with any such items, the experimental design and statistical principles required in their development are completely analogous to those described for the development of drugs for human use, and are covered by analogous FDA regulations.

The role of the FDA in the development of a new drug is described briefly. A summary of the current requirements for approval of a drug, and of postapproval activities, is given. Information is included to help those running or planning clinical trials to procure up-to-date regulatory information to help ensure a successful series of trials leading to approval to market a new drug. It should be noted that the FDA material reviewed in this chapter is current as of mid-1992, but is subject to change. Therefore, sponsors, monitors, investigators, and others concerned with clinical drug and/or device trials should establish procedures for keeping current with new FDA regulations and information regarding compliance.

3.7 LITERATURE REFERENCES

(1) Student (William Sealy Gosset), *Biometrika*, 6, (1908): 1–25.
(2) Kotz, Samuel, and Norman L. Johnson, *Encyclopedia of Statistical Sciences*, Vol. 3, John Wiley, New York, 1982–1988, pp. 461–463.

PART II

Planning Your Trial

CHAPTER 4

Planning Your Trial: I

4.1 INTRODUCTION: CLINICAL TRIALS AND MEDICAL PRACTICE

4.1.1 Aversion to the Idea of Clinical Trials

I have been fortunate in knowing many knowledgeable physicians employed in the pharmaceutical industry who devote their professional time exclusively to clinical studies, and many competent investigators working on trials who are also engaged in medical practice in various specialties. In addition, as a patient, I have known and become friendly with a number of physicians who are exclusively in private practice.

As a result of my sojourn in this environment, I have come to note certain differences in points of view among these three groups. From my standpoint as an observer, these differences seem to be the basis for difficulties some physicians have in accepting and practicing the procedures needed in clinical trials, in contrast to dealing with individual patients. These difficulties seemed more common 10 or 20 years ago than today, but they are still noticeable.

Medical training obviously inculcates the viewpoint that the welfare of the patient is all-important—"*First, do no harm.*" Although the purpose of a clinical trial is and should always be to find or verify some beneficial treatment, whether it is an industry project or is sponsored by a government, a foundation, or an academic organization, I have noted that some physicians tend to look upon any trials, but particularly those run by industry, as cold-blooded commercial exercises, having less concern for the individual patient than would be true in private practice. This seems more common among physicians in practice than among those whose activities are totally devoted to clinical trial work.

Perhaps this problem is rooted in one or both of two aspects of clinical studies. First, there can be a feeling that the adoption of a scientific attitude when carrying out a clinical trial precludes the particular concern for the patients that must also be exercised. Private practice is usually concerned with the diagnosis and treatment of one patient at a time. Clinical studies require *groups* of patients, considered together. There is no reason why patients in a group cannot be dealt with with as much concern as individuals, but the idea persists, although it is less common than in earlier years, that this may not be done generally. Another problem could be that some of the

59

terms used in discussing clinical work, such as *experimental units* for *patients*, convey a sense of impersonality and a loss of concern for the individual, perhaps reinforcing an impression that clinical studies somehow involve abandoning some of the ethical principles governing the practice of medicine.

We all realize that without clinical studies, our present enormous pharma-copeia, upon which every practicing physician depends for the safe and effective treatment of patients, would be vastly reduced. It is true that there are still some trials that may put patients to nontrivial degrees of risk and/or discomfort for the development of products of secondary benefit. Moreover, whether we need a large number of different drugs for treating the same condition is very much a moot point. If there is serious risk to prospective patients with little to be gained from a trial, an investigator or monitor may well feel that he or she should not be associated with its development. On the other hand, there have been and will be many potential drugs that, when shown to be safe and effective in well-run clinical trials, have resulted and will result in a substantial gain in public health.

4.1.2 Why Are Clinical Trials Necessary?

You cannot measure an experimental error, judge the magnitude of a population average, or compare two treatments effectively or at all if you try to do these things with one patient. This is a characteristic of nature that cannot be changed. As you will soon see, one of the most important activities in preparing for a clinical trial—and one that is very often ignored—is the determination (or rather, estimation) of the appropriate sample size, or number of patients needed. A trial can be rendered useless if there are too few or *too many* patients. When there are too few, the risk of missing an important treatment effect can be very greatly increased. And when there are too many, you may detect clinically unimportant differences.

In addition to the careful estimation of the sample size needed, there is no other method as adequate and satisfactory for evaluating a new drug or other medical treatment as the scientific approach discussed in Chapter 2, involving the use of the scientific method and the practice of clinical studies, including randomized assignment of treatments to patients, the use of concurrent controls, and, usually, double blinding. Omitting any of these leaves conclusions open to unnecessary argument and differing opinions.

4.2 BEGINNING TO PLAN

4.2.1 The Planning Steps

This chapter and the other three in this section (Chapters 4 through 7) describe in some detail a number of activities in which you will usually be engaged during the planning stages of a trial. The purpose is twofold: first, to outline and discuss, in a preliminary way, the principal technical and statisti-cal matters that should be considered during the planning (design) of a study, and, second, to introduce some of the more common **experimental designs** used in clinical work through the medium of examples. Many of these topics will be discussed later at more length, but they need to be introduced as early as possible, because in many cases, we must refer to many of them before full clarification would be understandable. These matters include some of the more important points mentioned in Chapters 1 and 2, such as controls, blinding, and randomization, as well as others not yet mentioned. The issues discussed include problems and their solutions, and ways in which you could go astray during the design stages.

We will try to consider each step in the order in which you would normally undertake it when planning a trial. Many of these operations can be done simultaneously, of course. Some of you may already be aware of the issues we bring up in this and the next three chapters, but they must be clarified for the benefit of those to whom they are less familiar. Several examples of industrial drug trials will be introduced to illustrate important points in planning and experimental design. The examples are intentionally simple and somewhat unrealistic in size and concept so that the issues being emphasized will stand out clearly.

4.2.2   The Protocol and Operations Manual

It is advisable to prepare at least a first draft of your protocol and your clinical report forms (CRFs) at the time that you progress through the planning steps. It may be written by you or someone else in your organization who can work closely with you. It may contain sections such as a preamble, a review of the literature, and a discussion of previous work at your company, which will not be discussed in this book. The protocol and CRFs, and the operations manual mentioned in the next paragraph, are discussed briefly further on in this chapter, and more extensively in Chapter 7.

A most useful tool for moderate to large trials, especially multicenter studies, is an operations manual. In many trials, you may find it helpful to prepare one for use by the investigators, CRAs (clinical research associates), and other concerned with the execution of the trial. It can give details, assembled in one place, of the diverse activities that must be performed during the execution of the trial, such as test procedures, record keeping, and other operations. These will help ensure that all concerned use the same procedures, which, as you probably know, is essential in trials employing more than one investigator, such as multicenter studies. Even for small trials, however, an operations manual is useful. Although it will duplicate much information already contained in the sections of the protocol devoted to execution, it can give more detail, be better adapted to the daily use of the investigators and their delegates, and serve as a convenient and rapid reference to all procedures. A useful device is to prepare it with a fairly elaborate table of contents to facilitate and encourage reference. It is best written when the protocol is in the final draft, so that the sections of that document concerned with the execution of the trial can be used as guides. It should not include information about the background and objectives of the trial, the planning, or the data analyses. Rather, it should be a detailed "cookbook" for all operations to be carried out during execution, even, perhaps, those that you may feel are obvious to the people involved. Copies should be available to everyone concerned.

4.3 DEFINING OBJECTIVES

4.3.1 Clarity of Objectives

What are the principal and subsidiary questions that the trial will address? A surprising number of protocols do not clearly or explicitly define these. Others begin with a statement such as, "This trial is designed to show that epizootic acid, given in quantities of 10 milligrams b.i.d., is effective in relieving pain due to misplaced renal tissue." Such a statement makes it appear that the principal reasons for running the trial is to "prove" to others (the FDA?) something that is already accepted as obvious by the writer. This is nonsense, of course, because an experiment can merely provide evidence for a hypothesis. Unfortunately, perhaps, proving things is not the business of science. Furthermore, such a statement carries an odor of propaganda, which conveys a poor impression of the organization sponsoring the trial.

In scientific research, there is very little information that is really obvious, particularly before it has been obtained in an experiment. Despite data from earlier trials in a series, if any, nothing is certain. It is more likely that the sponsor *hopes* to obtain evidence about the efficacy and safety of the drug. It is unlikely that the outcome of the trial will be clearly predictable. If it is predictable to you but not to others, you might as well assume that it is not predictable at all. And if the trial constitutes an example of scientific research, as it should, again there can be no "proof" of efficacy or safety. The best that can be hoped for in this imperfect world is the acquisition of evidence that *indicates* that the drug works satisfactorily and is safe to use. Usually, even this requires further trials to obtain more precise and better-supported information.

A better way to describe the objectives of a trial, then, might be something like: "As described in earlier sections of this protocol, preclinical evidence has indicated that hair growth may be initiated by treatment with a new compound, hereafter referred to as CD-72. To date, the safety data have not suggested any serious toxic effects associated with its use. This trial is the first of a series of clinical investigations that are planned, if evidence that CD-72 is safe and effective in human beings continues to accumulate." Don't assume that you already know the answer to the problem you are investigating. And state the objectives of the trial as clearly and specifically as possible.

4.3.2 Multiple Objectives

If there are primary and secondary objectives, say so, and list them in the appropriate section of the protocol. Arrange them in the order of their importance. But if you list more than one or two principal goals and three or four subsidiary ones, you may have listed too many. This will result in the specification of too many responses. As a result, none of your objectives may be dealt with thoroughly enough, and your hapless investigators may frantically struggle to measure everything but the kitchen sink in unproductive attempts to obtain all of your specified information. Busy clinicians may then perforce provide less time and care for each measurement than is really necessary for satisfactory results. And here are three more points to consider: (a) Several of the responses may be strongly correlated with each other, which means that you will be uselessly measuring nearly the same thing more than once. (b) For probabilistic reasons, the use of multiple-response measurements can seriously affect the validity of the conclusions drawn from the data analysis. (c) If point (b) is taken into account during planning or analysis (as it must be for valid statistical hypothesis tests during the data analysis), this must be done by increasing the size of the trial[1] or reducing the power of the analysis[2] (an important statistical aspect of trial design, explained later). Furthermore, the use of multiple-response measurements resulting from vague and manifold objectives will increase the cost and time required to complete the program, because you will lengthen the time that must be devoted to each patient. Thus, there are altogether too many disadvantages to this whole approach. It is important to keep your objectives simple.

To summarize, large numbers of required responses usually contribute little to the fundamental objective, may be detrimental to careful and precise work, and will introduce needless statistical problems even when they produce positive results. It is not worth trying to do too much in one experiment.

4.3.3 Defining Objectives during Planning

You should set up all of your objectives and their associated questions before the trial begins, and try not to change or add to them later. It is common for unanticipated questions to arise and to be tested with unplanned statistical procedures after a trial is over, often upon the basis of an examination of the data. To answer such new questions, special statistical tests are needed, and even then many statisticians do not endorse such "fishing" or "data dredging." Of course, it is always a statistically valid procedure to note such differences or trends and decide to test them in another trial, but you cannot legitimately

---

[1] It is recognized that you will often legitimately require more than one or two responses. But when this is the case, to maintain the validity of the probabilities associated with the hypothesis tests that will be needed during the data analysis, you must compensate by increasing the sample size (number of patients). If you do not do this, your "p values" will be smaller than the true probabilities, and you will be likely to be misled in your conclusions. Using more than one response is one kind of *multiplicity*. This is discussed, with methods of compensating for it, later in this chapter and in more detail further on.

[2] The power of a statistical hypothesis test is the probability of detecting a difference between treatments, if one exists, in the population of patients sampled. The power will vary depending upon a number of factors, including the sample size (number of patients), the kind of experimental design used, the experimental error of the data, the significance probability adopted as a test criterion, and others, such as the kind of response used.

perform your tests using the current data, on the basis of what you see in those data. This is another **multiplicity** problem, and is related to the one just dealt with.

This problem and similar ones are discussed in detail in later chapters. However, you can obtain an idea of its nature now from the following: The statistical hypothesis tests that the statistician must run while trying to provide evidence that the treatment is safe and effective are based upon certain rules and assumptions. These rules are designed to protect an experimenter from mistaking chance differences between treatment group response averages for actual treatment differences. When the data are available, treatments are compared by performing a statistical test, usually on the difference between the average responses of the two groups receiving different treatments.

One of the usual assumptions upon which such a test is based specifies that if there are more than two treatments, the particular pairs of treatment group means to be compared must be prespecified. Unfortunately, when there is more than one possible comparison, this is usually not done or is implicit only. *If there is any uncertainty at all as to what comparisons are to be prespecified, or if there could be subsequent decision to make more pairwise comparisons than were originally intended, as is also frequently the case, the safe course is to assume that a condition of multiplicity will exist. If so, this can be compensated for by increasing the sample size during the planning stages.* Suppose, for example, that this is done, or that there are only two treatment groups, that you carry out statistical hypothesis ("significance") tests, and that a significance level of 0.050 is used. You and the statistician can then be assured that you would be wrong, on the average, in only 5% of such trials, if repeated, if you conclude that the means of two patient populations represented by the samples (i.e., two patient groups) are different. This is equivalent to stating that there is a probability of 0.05 of being wrong if significance is claimed.[3] If there is multiplicity (more than one comparison) and it is ignored, the probability of being wrong when claiming a population difference between treatments will be greater than 0.050, often very much greater.

4.4   EXAMPLE 4.1: A TENSION HEADACHE TRIAL

Let's suppose that you are planning a single-center Phase II trial to evaluate a new drug for the treatment of tension headaches. Such headaches may last for hours or days, and can produce very severe pain. Tension headache trials can be more complex to arrange than some others, because the times of onset and duration of symptoms are unpredictable. You wish to compare the new drug with currently available materials.

---

[3]"On the average" means that the probability of being wrong varies from experiment to experiment; it can be higher or lower than the stated probability, but the latter is the most likely value.

Your first task is to put the objectives of the trial into plain and specific terms. A fair and reasonably concise statement of objectives might be "The purpose of this trial is to attempt to determine whether the new material is safe and effective in relieving the pain of tension headache." The goal is now to try to obtain evidence regarding whether the material to be tested is more or less effective, with more or fewer adverse effects, than appropriate doses of codeine or codeine with acetaminophen, which is commonly prescribed for tension headache. This statement may be broken down into the following list of "subobjectives":

1. Determine the safety of the treatment.
2. Determine its effectiveness in relieving the pain of the headache.
3. Compare its efficacy with that of codeine.
4. Compare its efficacy with that of codeine plus acetaminophen.
5. Compare its adverse effects with those of codeine.
6. Compare its adverse effects with those of codeine plus acetaminophen.

There are really two major objectives here. They are (a) to determine the safety and efficacy of the new drug per se by the two comparisons with placebo (items 1 and 2), and (b) to compare its safety and effectiveness with those of the two standards (items 3 through 6). There really are no minor objectives; the two major goals are implemented by the six items.

Listing and analyzing your objectives in this way will establish a concise beginning for your protocol. It will help you to realize exactly what is to be done, and will make it easy to select the appropriate responses, statistical analyses, and experimental design.

4.4.1 The Factors in Example 4.1

The Objectives Determine the Factors
In a trial, the **factors** are the **controlled variables** that you will specify as the central feature of your experimental design. In this example, there is just one factor. This will be called *drugs* for want of a better name, and its four **levels** are

$$A = \text{test drug}$$

$$B = \text{placebo}[4]$$

$$C = \text{codeine}$$

$$D = \text{codeine plus acetaminophen}$$

---

[4]It will be possible to specify placebo only if all patients agree to use it if it is assigned. Of course, we are assuming that the test is double blind, so that no patient or investigator will know which treatment is being used. As soon as each examination is complete, each patient who needs further relief should be given his or her customary remedy. In some trials, of course, placebos cannot be used at all because of ethical and safety considerations.

The doses of the standards or commercial controls (the codeine and the codeine plus acetaminophen) should be chosen to correspond to those normally prescribed. The dose of the test drug will depend upon the judgment of the sponsor, based upon early preclinical work and perhaps Phase I dose-response studies. If further dose information were desired or needed, a more complex experiment could have been designed, in which there would be two factors, **drugs** and **doses**.

As you will see later, in this **single-factor** trial, each of the four levels of the factor "drugs" will be given in appropriate doses to all members of one of four particular groups of patients, who will receive no other treatment.

Note that we defined the placebo treatment as a "drug," just like the other three. This was done for convenience. We could have called the drugs factor "treatments," but that would have reduced its specificity. Of course, the placebo is really a material having no active component. Note also that in this example, for simplicity, we do not discuss provision for cases in which a patient receives no relief (either one on placebo or one for whom his or her assigned treatment is ineffective). Obviously, in a real study, provision must be made for the prompt removal of such a patient from the trial and the resumption of his or her regular treatment.

4.4.2 Factors and Responses

A **factor** is an **independent variable.** The term *independent* is used in the algebraic sense; it is a variable that influences the value of a **dependent variable.** In a clinical trial when the statistical analysis planned is to be **univariate,** *factors* (such as *drugs* in this example) are the independent variables. They are those you introduce and *control*, in order to observe their effects upon the **response** or measurement, which is the **dependent variable.** A univariate analysis is one in which only a single set of data for one particular response is used. A **multivariate analysis** is one in which two or more responses are used in the same analysis.[5] Such analyses are very rare in clinical trial work and are not discussed further in this book.

A factor must have two or more **levels,** such as two or more drugs, in order to be used as a variable. If there is only one level, its effect cannot be measured, and to all intents and purposes, it is not a factor at all. The levels of the factor or independent variable can be qualitative, like the drugs factor, or quantitative, such as "doses." One group of patients, formed by random selection of a number of individuals, is assigned to each of the treatments.[6]

---

[5]An analysis is univariate as long as only one *response* (dependent variable) is used. It is common in clinical work, but completely incorrect, to refer to the analysis of a multifactor design with a single response as multivariate, even when there are several separate univariate analyses, each using a different response.

[6]There are some factors for which the levels are inherent in the patients. For example, age, sex, or the presence of a disease can be used as factors, but unlike the levels of the factor, "drugs," their levels (old, middle-aged, young; male, female; ill, healthy) obviously cannot be controlled by the experimenter (e.g., assigned at will to any randomly selected patient).

Note also that there are some designs in which each patient receives two or more of the treatments; some of these are discussed in Part IV.

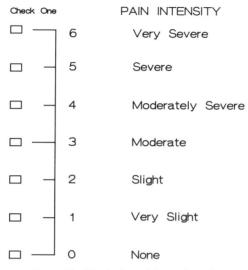

Figure 4.1 Headache pain intensity scale.

In the example, there are four such groups, one for each of the four levels of the factor. When the study is carried out, you measure one or more attributes of the patients in each group. In this book, such measurements are called **responses.** The responses are the dependent variables in the design.

In Example 4.1, one of the responses will be pain intensity of the headaches on a seven-point numerical judgment scale (0 for "no pain," 2 for "slight pain," up to 6 for "very severe pain"). This scale is illustrated in Figure 4.1, and could be used as shown in your clinical report forms. Each group of patients in the trial will receive a different treatment, so differences in analgesic effectiveness among the treatments would be expected to result in different average values among the groups. The experimenter will usually attribute such observed differences to variation among the treatments plus a component due to experimental error. The statistical hypothesis (significance) tests to be done when the experiment is complete will yield the probability that a given observed difference is likely to be due to chance alone.

Despite the fact that you can use several factors in a single experimental design, very few trials use more than three, and most use only one or two. If a trial is multicenter, "centers" becomes a factor, with a number of levels equal to the number of centers. In this chapter, however, we consider one-factor designs only, as typified by this example.

4.4.3 Planning the Comparisons

There are particular **pairwise** comparisons of treatment group averages that can be used to try to answer the questions posed by the objectives in this example. For convenience, let's again examine the numbered list of "subobjectives," listed near the beginning of Section 4.4, in a more organized fashion. The subobjectives are sorted in what follows according to whether they are concerned with safety or efficacy, but maintaining the original item numbers:

Safety "determinations":
1. The test drug vs. placebo: treatment A vs. B
5. The test drug vs. codeine: A vs. C
6. The test drug vs. codeine plus acetaminophen: A vs. D

Efficacy "determinations":
2. The test drug vs. placebo: A vs. B
3. The test drug vs. codeine: A vs. C
4. The test drug vs. codeine plus acetaminophen: A vs. D

For the safety tests, to implement item 1, which reflects subobjective 1 in Section 4.4, you would compare the responses obtained for treatments A and B (adverse effects found in the test drug group with those in the placebo group). For item 5, to compare the test drug with codeine, you would compare those for treatments A and C. For item 6, treatment A would be compared with D. For the efficacy tests, you would make the same comparisons, but this time you would use group mean values of the pain-scale response, as well as those of any other response(s) you may have chosen.

When, as in the present case, there are four treatments, there are six possible pairwise comparisons. These are the following:

1. A vs. B; test drug vs. placebo
2. A vs. C; test drug vs. codeine
3. A vs. D; test drug vs. codeine plus acetaminophen
4. B vs. C; placebo vs. codeine
5. B vs. D; placebo vs. codeine plus acetaminophen
6. C vs. D; codeine vs. codeine plus acetaminophen

In the present case, you will have used the first three of these once for the comparisons of adverse effects and once for each efficacy response. Ordinarily, there would be no need to make the last three comparisons at all unless, perhaps, you wanted to be sure the experiment had worked, by testing the results for a known efficacious drug against placebo (B vs. C or B vs. D). There would certainly be no need to do the C vs. D comparison, because contrasting the two standards is not called for by any of the six subobjectives. To summarize, you might plan to make the first three of the six comparisons for each of your efficacy and adverse effects responses, and perhaps one more to ensure that the trial was detecting known differences correctly.

In making these multiple simultaneous comparisons, the multiplicity problem arises again. If this problem is ignored, the conclusions drawn from the tests can be wrong, doubtful, or weak. Some specific problems of multiplicity, and how to avoid them, are discussed at length in Chapter 13, and, briefly, later in this chapter.

4.5 RESPONSES

4.5.1 Responses for Evaluating Safety

The responses you will need to record for the evaluation of safety in any trial will usually be any adverse effects themselves. Usually, you will want to classify and count these, and carry out comparative tests between treatment groups at the time of the data analysis, using the numbers and kinds of effects found. Sometimes, if there are only a few adverse effects, or if they are mild, you may decide to simply list them and count their incidence by treatment groups.

4.5.2 Responses for Evaluating Efficacy

The kind of responses you use for efficacy will depend upon the objectives that you defined, the factors you selected, and the design. The nature of the responses will affect the type of analysis that should be used. Your choice within this framework will be governed, in turn, by other criteria that, although not essential, are highly desirable.

For Example 4.1, we needed to measure, as well as possible, the degree of pain caused by the headache. If you were running such a trial, you might well use two or more headaches per patient—two separate incidents—and add or average the two responses; we are using one here merely to reduce the complexity of the example so that the basic ideas will be clear. The principal response must somehow evaluate the degree of pain the patient experiences during a headache. It is an unfortunate fact that, like many responses in clinical trial work, this measurement must perforce be subjective. Worse, it may be doubly subjective, because it may be based upon an evaluation by the investigator, which is in turn based upon questioning the patient. But we have no choice.

In Example 4.1, a common kind of subjective response—a pain-intensity scale—was chosen (Figure 4.1). We adopted a seven-point scale rather than a shorter one because such scales have more information-carrying ability than shorter ones. We chose a scale with an odd number of points because it has a center point representing the median, which makes it easier to use. Scales of this kind, in which integers represent the degree of a condition, are called **multinomial scales**. A **binomial scale** is a multinomial with only two points.

Unfortunately, many investigators feel that multinomial scales with more than five points are difficult to use, and you may either have to restrict your scales to this size or have an unhappy investigator. Your investigator(s) should have as much as possible to say about how the trial is run, as long as you have the final decision on the designs and analyses (with your statistician's advice in mind, of course). Some investigators prefer scales with even fewer than five points, such as the popular three-point scale: 1 = "mild," 2 = "moderate," and 3 = "severe," or even a binomial (dichotomous) scale. If there is no reason for using such short scales except an investigator's preference, you should protest strongly. Very short response scales require substantially larger sample sizes than scales having more points.

In this connection, there is one more very important issue. A trial can become disastrously small, in effect, even when an adequately long multinomial scale is used. For example, suppose you reluctantly agree upon a five-point pain scale, but in the trial, the extreme points (such as point 5, very severe pain, and 1, no pain), are never used. You will then, in reality, have a three-point response scale, not the five-point scale you planned to use. Your prior estimate of sample size will likely be too small. In turn, this means that the probability that you will be able to detect an existing difference large enough to be important will be substantially reduced, that is, the statistical power of the hypothesis test done on the data will be lower than you planned. The remedy for this, of course, is to be sure that the labeled points on the judgment scale represent magnitudes of measurements that you expect to be reasonably frequent. Points that are never used are equivalent to no points at all.

These considerations apply not only to multinomial scales, but to continuous responses as well. In the latter case, a problem can arise if a measurement is made to too low a degree of precision. To use a rather absurd example for clarity, if your sphygmomanometer reads to the nearest millimeter (as it probably does), but you read it only to the nearest 10 millimeters, your measurements will lack reasonable precision, and important treatment differences will be likely to escape detection when the data are analyzed.

To summarize, the shorter a response scale, the less information it can convey. If any single measurement provides less information per patient than another, more patients will be needed to obtain the same degree of precision. As you will see when sample size estimation is discussed, this idea can be easily quantified. The use of a five-point pain scale enforces the choice of a larger sample size than a longer scale would require, all other things being equal, but the increase will be much less severe than it would be with a two- or three-point scale. And, if there is a practical choice, use a continuous scale rather than a multinomial judgment scale, because, with a given sample size, smaller differences than those possible with a multinomial scale will be detectable, and, conversely, a given difference will be detectable with a smaller sample. This latter suggestion has a possible exception—the use of rank tests for the hypothesis tests of the data. Ranks comprise a kind of integer scale, but the statistical efficiency of some common rank tests is only minimally less than that of common methods based upon continuous-scale measurements.[7]

4.5.3   Using More Than One Response

Multiplicity in the Analysis of Safety Responses
When you are planning for the safety responses (adverse effects recording and possible analysis), it is obviously important that you provide for reporting as many different effects as appear. You may not know all of the categories that may turn up, and you may have to estimate their number and identity. You should consider them as several series of responses within categories (number of patients on treatment 1 reporting GI symptoms, number with rash, with nervous symptoms, etc.). Each of these symptom categories can then be considered as a different kind of response, like the various kinds of efficacy measurements discussed in what follows.

When data for more than one response from a single trial are analyzed in this way, **multiplicity** problems are introduced, just as mentioned earlier. However, the analyses of safety data can be regarded differently than those of efficacy responses. Because of the multiplicity introduced as a result of the repetition of treatment comparisons, the greater the number of different kinds of response elicited from each patient, the greater is the number of false positives (i.e., significant results even when the null hypothesis is true) that will occur in statistical hypothesis tests of the data.

But the situation and the viewpoint for safety testing is different than it is for efficacy tests. First, you will not always need to test adverse-effects categories between groups. Many times, simple visual comparisons of the numbers of patients in each category by treatment groups may suffice.[8] But, second, if you do use such a hypothesis test, you may, if you wish, ignore the multiplicity, keeping in mind that some of the significances found will be false. Because this is a conservative attitude, you may be willing, in some studies, to allow the safety data to appear worse than it really is, placing additional emphasis upon caution. And if in the past you reported adverse effects without considering the multiplicity, you will be doing nothing different. And because most or all of your tests will consist of counts of adverse effects, therefore requiring statistical procedures that are not very sensitive (see the discussion of contingency tables in Chapter 14), you may be almost forced to allow this to happen, because you will often find that the sample

---

[7]For example, the Wilcoxon Signed-Ranks and Rank Sum tests have a long-run efficiency of about 95.5%. That is, if an ordinary t test (described later, and very common in clinical work) requires, say, 95 patients per treatment, a rank test with about 100 patients per treatment will have equal ability to detect a given treatment difference.

[8]The visual comparison of adverse-effect counts can also be considered to be subject to multiplicity, because such an "eyeball" test can be regarded as an informal hypothesis test in which the assumptions and hypotheses are implicit.

sizes needed to compensate for the multiplicity will be quite large. Of course, you can minimize the numbers of false significances by using as few categories of adverse effects as practical.

Multiplicity in the Analysis of Efficacy Responses

You should limit the kinds of responses to be used for efficacy to a very small number, such as one to three or four. If there are more than one, designate one of them as the response of principal interest. See Friedman et al. [2], pp. 167–8. In addition, when you use more than one response, for statistical validity, you must increase the sample size in compensation. You then should see that the number of different responses to be tested, as well as the number of comparisons to be made, is taken into account a priori. Methods for doing this are described later in this book. It is a good idea, in the protocol, to describe and account for the sample sizes to be used.

Unfortunately, this rule is ignored more often than not in commercial drug trials. The feeling may be that the use of more responses helps ensure that if it doesn't look good with measurement A, perhaps measurement B will show significance. But even if the drug is really ineffective, the chance that the additional significances found ("low p values") are false positives increases very rapidly with the number of comparisons used. This will be true whether the comparisons are of the same pairs of treatments using different responses, pairwise comparisons of more than two treatments using a given response, a combination of both, or other multiple-comparison possibilities.

It is much more practical to give a lot of thought to the choice of response(s) than to use the shotgun approach. I once saw a trial in which over 70 different responses were used. There were more than two treatments, so the number of significance tests made was 70 multiplied by the number of comparisons. In any analysis of those data, none of the many hypothesis tests that would be expected to show significance would be reliable.

Very often, insufficient time and discussion are given to the choice of the kind and number of responses. If the statistician is aware of the problem at the time of analysis, as he or she should be, the appropriate compensatory procedure will then be used. But unless the sample size has been adjusted during the planning stage to compensate for the multiplicity, there will be a severe loss of power (defined later). Taking my own advice, therefore, in the present case, we will limit the number of responses for measuring efficacy to two, and will calculate the sample sizes while taking the multiplicity introduced into account.

The second response we will use will measure the same phenomenon as the seven-point pain scale. It is introduced because it can be made by the patient alone without involving the investigator or his or her delegate, except as observers, and therefore may be more reliable than the first one. For this purpose, we will employ a well-known measurement that patients easily learn, called a **visual analogue scale (VAS).** Its data can be analyzed parametrically (sometimes a "transformation" of scale is needed) and it is useful and

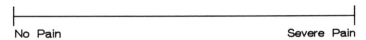

Figure 4.2   Visual analogue scale (VAS).

informative. There are many varieties of VAS responses. One of the simplest and best, which we will use in our example, is shown in Figure 4.2.

Figure 4.2 represents a scale that, in the data sheets to be used, is 100 mm long. The reproduction in Figure 4.2 may not be that length. One hundred millimeters is convenient to use and makes subsequent data management easier. But even if the length is more or less than that, be certain that all copies of the scale used during the actual trial are equal in length. This is not always as simple as it may seem. I recall a trial for a client in which the lengths of the VAS lines on the case report forms varied by as much as plus or minus 7 mm. Before analysis of the data, it was necessary to measure the length of the scale on each individual form and to correct the results accordingly (there were hundreds of them). Without the corrections, there would have been a substantial increase in the experimental error, resulting in reduced statistical power when the data were tested, and introducing the possibility of overlooking some important results. The extra measurements and computations increased the time required to complete the data entry and, of course, increased the cost to the sponsor.

As you can see in the figure, the left end of the scale is marked "no pain," and the right is labeled "very severe pain." Numbered points on the scale, such as 0 and 100, are not used, as many patients find them confusing. The patients should be rehearsed in the procedure to follow. After they mark the scale, the results should be examined carefully while the patients are still at the clinic.

If there is no pain or very severe pain, the patient circles the vertical "stop" at either end of the scale. If the degree of pain experienced lies within those two extremes, the patient should mark the scale with a *vertical* pencil line (a slanted line is difficult to measure). The mark should *cross* the VAS line. If the patient feels moderate pain, this mark will be in the approximate center. If the pain is less than moderate but there nevertheless is some, the VAS is marked accordingly, between the left end and the middle. If it is greater than moderate, the mark is made across some point on the right half of the line.

Patients quickly learn to use such a scale, and the results from trials using VAS scales appear at least as reliable and useful as other measurements, and probably more so than most judgment scales, perhaps because there is no communication problem between patients and the person who administers the test. VAS scales can and have been used not only for pain intensity measurements, but also for recording the strengths of odors, the intensity of light, and other subjective phenomena.

In deciding how many different response measurements to use, you should be sure that each of the objectives or questions is matched to a response capable of fulfilling or answering it. This may appear contrary to the cautions expressed earlier about limiting the number of responses, but limiting the objectives is the place to start. We are using two responses to answer each of the same group of questions (treatment comparisons), but this multiplicity is not extreme, and can be compensated for without greatly increasing the sample size. Many believe that only one measurement should generally be used in a case such as this, but it is important for you to use those you feel necessary, as long as the number you choose is not large and suitable provisions for the multiplicity have been made. Both Pocock [4] and Shapiro and Louis [5] provide interesting discussions of these points. Their opinions are somewhat less rigorous than those of Friedman et al. [2].

4.5.4   Baseline Measurements

For most designs—except for the two-period crossover, a troublemaker in this and many other ways—see Fleiss, Wallenstein, and Rosenfeld (1) and Willan and Peter (2)—using **baseline measurements** is an excellent idea. A baseline measurement is a response taken for each patient at the beginning of a trial, after the patient has been accepted into the study, but before any treatments have been given.[9] If possible, exactly the same kind of response should be used as after dosage. The existence of baseline measurements often allows comparisons of treatments in terms of their changes from baseline. For instance, each pain intensity score in the example may be subtracted from its baseline and the resulting difference used for the comparisons among treatments. This is not the same thing as comparing a treatment with its own baseline to determine whether there has been a change. Instead, here, if two treatments are to be contrasted, the comparison is made by first calculating differences from baseline for each of them and then comparing the two differences. Of course, these observations are of means (averages) of the differences, not of individual patient differences.

Although the use of the baseline in this way is quite popular and can be helpful in correcting for any differences in inherent responses among the patients, there can be some problems in making such comparisons. Two assumptions are implicit when differences from baseline instead of posttreatment data alone are used in the data analyses. The first assumption is that there is a linear rather than a curvilinear relationship between the baseline and posttreatment measurements. This is often not an extremely critical assumption, because a nonlinear relationship is rarer than a linear one, and, furthermore, a moderate degree of nonlinearity may be tolerable. The second assumption is one that is usually not strictly correct, and, at times, can be

---

[9]If the measurements are made before the patients have been accepted, some of them may need to be repeated if the patients are rejected or decide not to take part in the trial.

quite wrong. This is the assumption that the magnitude of the difference between measurements for any two patients at baseline, ruling out random variation, and the same two measurements made later (exclusive of any treatment effect) will remain the same. For example, if you plot the baseline readings against the posttreatment measurements, and this assumption is true, the slope of the line will be 1, that is, the difference between any two patients at baseline will remain the same after treatment. But the slope of the line may not necessarily be 1. If it is not, a difference between two patients of two response-scale units in terms of the measurement at baseline may correspond to a difference of only one unit, or of three units, later, when the posttreatment measurements are made. However, to a moderate degree, violation of this assumption can also be tolerated. Additionally, if you have a moderate amount of data, they can be tested to see whether this idea is reasonable.

To avoid some of these difficulties, when the data are available, including baseline as well as posttreatment results, the biostatistician can carry out a procedure called an analysis of covariance (ACOVA), using the baseline measurements as covariates. This procedure will "adjust" the posttreatment measurements according to the magnitude of the effect of the baseline measurements upon the subsequent measurements, so that the previous second assumption is no longer necessary. Of course, in this imperfect world, the ACOVA also has its disadvantages. The assumption of linearity (the first assumption mentioned earlier) must still be made, although if there are enough data to obtain a reliable test and the relationship is found to be curvilinear, some possible remedies are available. Another, new assumption applies even when the assumption of linearity is true. We might call it the **homogeneity of slopes.** If the slopes are homogeneous, the linear relationships between the baseline data and the posttreatment measurements have the same slope for all treatments.

Thus, whether to use posttreatment data, differences from baseline, or an analysis of covariance using baseline data as the single covariate depends principally upon a statistician's experienced judgment. When the ACOVA can be used, it will possess greater power than the use of differences, sometimes much greater. This means that sample sizes can be smaller, or, conversely, that smaller treatment differences can be detected if the same sample sizes are used.

To sum up, the use of differences from baseline implies a one-to-one relationship between baseline and posttreatment measurements. When this assumed relationship is not true, a trial will *not* be invalidated, but more experimental variation will be introduced, thus reducing the power of the statistical tests. Like many other decisions, whether or not to use simple differences from baseline, an ACOVA, or neither will therefore probably depend upon the judgment of the biostatistician working with you.

In Example 4.1, let us use differences from baseline for each of the two kinds of response measurement. To do so, each patient must be asked to report to the clinic as soon as possible after a headache begins, and, if possible, without taking any medication.[10] At the clinic, with the investigator or a delegate available, each should first self-administer the VAS, be interviewed, and then be given the assigned medication. In most trials conducted at a clinic, each patient would then remain at the clinic for 3 or 4 hours, with both measurements being repeated every hour or half-hour. In this example, however, for simplicity, we will specify a single measurement session at 1 hour after dosage. Each patient will then receive supplies of the assigned drug and of the regular medication (for use if the assigned material is not effective) and may then leave. When these procedures have been completed for all patients, the execution of the trial will be complete. Of course, this will require several sessions, because it is unlikely that large numbers of patients will be seen on a given day.

4.5.5   Types of Measurement Scales

The following classification system is one of several that might be used. The several types of measurement systems are discussed in descending order of information-carrying ability.

Continuous Scales

The quantity of information contained in a measurement used as a response in a clinical study depends upon the kind of measurement scale that is used. A measurement on a **continuous scale** can convey a larger amount of information than any other kind. "Continuous" means that any values between the integer (whole-number) values on the scale can exist, at least theoretically. Examples are a weight or mass, such as 54.3125 or 7.1 grams; a volume, such as 45.63 or 2.0 milliliters, or 3.01 or $25\frac{1}{4}$ ounces; or a velocity, such as 63.25 or 4.0 miles per hour. In practice, the number of points on a measurement scale that can be used is limited by the nature of the measuring process.

Many measurement data are **normally distributed** and form so-called "bell-shaped curves," but there are many others whose distributions are not normal. However, there is a larger body of statistical procedures available based upon the normal distribution than upon any other. Fortunately, these methods often can be used satisfactorily for the analysis of nonnormal data because many of them are **robust** to nonnormality, that is, they can be used even when the data being analyzed depart somewhat from normality. The **normal distribution** and others are discussed in some detail in Chapter 5. For the moment, we are concerned with just one of the properties of some

---

[10]Of course, patients must be allowed to take the medication before testing if they feel it necessary. Should a patient do so, however, he or she should be disqualified from further participation in the study.

distributions, including the normal—the fact that they use a continuous scale.[11]

Continuous measurements are frequently classified into **ratio** and **interval** scales (see Siegel [45]).[12] Although these distinctions are not needed to understand experimental design, they can affect your selection of responses during planning and your interpretation of results after an analysis is done. Ratio scales comprise a class of continuous measurements that has a true zero, such as scales of mass in grams or volume in ounces. With such scales, the ratios of one value to another on the scale does not depend upon the measurement units used. For example, 4 grams represents twice as much mass as 2 (the ratio $\frac{4}{2} = 2$); 8 ounces represents four times as much volume as 2 ($\frac{8}{2} = 4$). Interval scales do not have this property, although their values do convey the size of the intervals between any two points. For example, temperature in Fahrenheit degrees uses an interval scale.[13] But to say that if the temperature today is 30° Fahrenheit and that yesterday it was 15° certainly does not imply that it is twice as hot today as yesterday. The Fahrenheit measure is not a ratio scale. Nevertheless, one *can* say that 101° Fahrenheit is exactly as much greater than 100° as 51° is than 50°, that is, $101 - 100 = 1°$, and $51 - 50 = 1°$. *Differences* on an interval scale are constant in terms of the unit of measurement of the scale regardless of where on the scale they are taken, but multiplicative comparisons, like *ratios*, are not meaningful.

Semicontinuous Scales

Semicontinuous scales is my phrase for a kind of measurement scale that cannot really be classified as continuous, such as judgment scores. Such scores are *not* ranks (see the next section), although they are sometimes carelessly called by that name. They may possess fractional points between integers, although usually to a limited degree, unlike continuous scales, which, by definition, can theoretically take on any value whatsoever between integral values. The "in-between" values are (or should be) set by definition; for example, a judgment scale may be defined to use all the integers between specified limits, and all of the halfway points between integers. Such scales are quite different from continuous scales. They can really be regarded as integer scales, because by expansion, they can be converted exactly to series of integers. For example, a three-point scale to describe degrees of erythema with halfway points allowable $(1, 1\frac{1}{2}, 2, 2\frac{1}{2}, 3)$ is a five-point scale in disguise. It can be completely converted, without any change of meaning or precision, to integers such as 1, 2, 3, 4, and 5. The same can be shown to be true for any

---

[11]A continuous measurement does not necessarily comprise a normal measurement (i.e., made up of data with normally distributed errors).

[12]This classification apparently did not originate with Siegel, but he describes it well, and I have been unable to find any earlier description.

[13]The Kelvin (absolute) temperature scale is a ratio scale.

scale for which a limited number of intermediate values are allowed. On the other hand, there are judgment scales that are theoretically continuous except for the limits imposed at either end; the VAS is one of these.

The important point to remember is that, because semicontinuous scales possess a more limited number of possible points than continuous scales, they are unable to convey as much information. In other words, the power of the eventual statistical test can be less than it would be if a continuous scale were used.

Ranks and Order Statistics

The term **rank** has many meanings. In statistics, a rank is an integer whose value represents the position of an object or quantity in an ordered series. For instance, you might measure the heights of six patients and then rank them in ascending order using the rank numbers 1 through 6, as illustrated in Figure 4.3. The numbers shown on the representations of the patients above their designations (A through F) are rank numbers corresponding to their relative heights. As you can see, there will always be exactly the same number of ranks as there are data being ranked. Furthermore, unless there are ties in

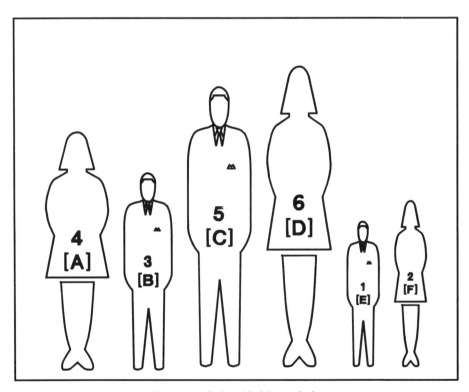

Figure 4.3 Patients' heights ranked.

the data,[14] *every* rank number between 1 and N (where N is the number of data) will be present in the set of ranks. This is in contrast to scores, where one or more numbers in a scoring scale may not necessarily appear in a set of scores representing the responses or measurements of some patient characteristic or treatment effect.

Ranks carry less information than continuous measurements, but not as much less as might at first be supposed. It is well known, for example, that the kind of test exemplified by the Wilcoxon Rank Sum or Signed Ranks procedures (see Part IV) has a long-run efficiency, for data with normally distributed errors, of about 95.5% of that of a t test of the same data. Efficiency (more exactly, **asymptotic efficiency**) can be explained as follows: The t test is the most efficient hypothesis test (treatment comparison method) known when its assumptions are satisfied. The efficiency figure means that if a Wilcoxon test using data from 100 patients is run, it will possess the same statistical power in the long run as that of a t test using between 95 and 96 patients. In Figure 4.3, the heights of the six patients were converted to ranks. The original values of the heights supplied a little more information than the ranks, because the magnitudes of the differences between adjacent values are lost when ranks are used. This minor deficiency is frequently compensated for, however, because, under some common circumstances such as the nonnormality of scores, a rank test can provide some important advantages over other kinds of statistical tests.

Order Statistics and Percentiles
This topic is not directly connected to the classification of measurements into various kinds of scales, but you may run into the term frequently in discussing scales and data when you talk with the company statistician. **Order statistics,** in a way, are related to the use of ranks. If you arrange the heights of the patients shown in Figure 4.3 in the order of their magnitudes (e.g., in centimeters) before you rank them, the set of numbers you obtain is called a set of order statistics. In fact, that designation applies to any set of values of a variable, including ranks themselves, if they are arranged in ascending or descending order. Also, summary statistics based upon order statistics are also sometimes called by that name; for example, the **median,** which is the value of a set of measurements that lies just at the halfway point, can be called an order statistic.

If there is an *odd* number of items in a series of values, the median is the *middle* value of the series. For example, in the set of numbers from 1 to 9, the median is 5. However, if there is an *even* number of values, the median is a value that lies halfway between the lower and upper halves of the set. For example, for the set of numbers 1 through 10, the median is $5\frac{1}{2}$. Unless a sequence with an odd number of values happens to possess a value exactly at the halfway point, the median is a number that does not occur in the series

---

[14]The use of ties in ranking data is exemplified in Part IV.

itself, like $5\frac{1}{2}$ in the example. In such a case, it is the *average* of the middle two values.

Percentiles can be called order statistics. The tenth percentile of a set of numbers is a number equal to or below which 10% of the data lie. For example, a percentile value of 90 is a value that is equal to or greater than 90% of the values in the set. The median is the fiftieth percentile.

Integer Scales

The seven-point pain intensity scale in our example is an integer scale. These are sometimes confused with ranks, but the numbers are **scores,** *not* ranks. Like ranks, they are integers, but their meaning is quite different. The magnitude of an integer score conveys an estimate of a variable, such as the degree of pain, a height, or similar information. For example, instead of measuring the heights of the group of patients in Figure 4.3 in centimeters, or ranking them, you could *independently* estimate the height of each on a seven-point scale ranging from small to tall. The key word is *independence*. When you use ranks, the value of each rank depends upon those previously assigned. But when you *score* a datum, such as a height, the score you choose

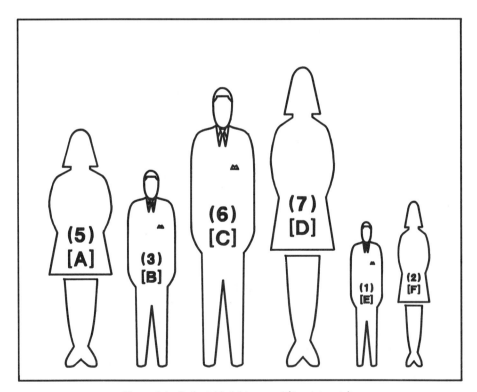

Figure 4.4 Patients' heights scored (7-point scale).

Table 4.1. Heights, Ranks and Scores for Patients Shown in Figures 4.3 and 4.4

Patient	Height Centimeters	Rank	Score*
A	173	4	5
B	168	3	3
C	178	5	6
D	183	6	7
E	157	1	1
F	163	2	2

*Scoring scale: 1 = very short; 2 = short; 3 = moderately short; 4 = average; 5 = moderately tall; 6 = tall; and 7 = very tall.

depends upon nothing but your individual judgment, and is unrelated (or should be) to the scores given to any of the other data. Figure 4.4 represents the same six patients as those in Figure 4.3, but now with their heights represented by scores on a seven-point scale.[15] This scale is an exact analogue of the pain intensity scale of Figure 4.1. The scores for the patients' heights are shown in parentheses above their letters of identification, which are in brackets. A scoring scale can theoretically be any length, but for ranks, there must be exactly the same number of values as there are objects or people ranked. Ranks are not *independent* of the number of items in the sample being measured; scores are. Scoring scales, unless they are long, generally convey less information than ranks, and usually much less than objective measurements, such as height in inches or centimeters.

Table 4.1 shows the heights of the six patients of Figures 4.3 and 4.4, together with the ranks, scores, and the scoring scale previously discussed.

Two-Valued Scales
Two-valued scales are variously called **yes / no, dichotomous,** or **binomial** scales, among other names. They are almost the least efficient kind of measurement you can use, in terms of the amount of information conveyed by each observation. They should be used in clinical trials only if (a) there is no alternative, as when a response is perforce dichotomous, as for mortality; (b) they are a subsidiary response, supported by other. more informative measurements; (c) the trial is extremely large, so that their extremely low efficiency is unimportant; or (d) it would be very difficult or costly to make a more informative measurement.

This is worth emphasizing: A dichotomous measurement scale should not be chosen as a response in a clinical trial when there is any reasonable

[15]As implied later, a judgment scale should not be substituted for a measurement on a continuous scale unless absolutely necessary. Figure 4.4 is included only to clarify the difference between ranks and scores.

alternative. A survey of the clinical trial literature will disclose that there is a widely used practice that effectively causes the loss of much of the information already obtained from a study. This practice would be much less prevalent if their users fully realized its cost. It is the compression of continuous responses into two-valued scales. Doing this amounts to the deliberate rejection of expensive and presumably important information. It could be called unethical in the sense that its usage causes information gained at the risk or inconvenience of the patients to be unnecessarily lost.

At the risk of beating a dead horse a bit more, an example of the degree of damage that can be done in the most extreme case may be enlightening. I once encountered an instance of converting a continuous measurement (a continuously distributed weight) to a two-valued response. The sample size using the continuous measurement was 36 subjects, and had been well-established as adequate not only by means of statistical calculations, but by the experience of its use in many trials in a screening procedure. It was proposed seriously by a responsible organization that the response be changed to a binomial. The required sample size, for the same power, would then have become several hundred subjects!

Classification or Categorical Scales
These scales are the simplest of all, and, as you will guess, usually convey the least amount of information. They were called **nominal** scales by Siegel [45]. Many sciences, in their earlier stages of development, use classification scales as their principal methods of measurement. For example, not long ago, the major measurement system in biology was classification. Using this well-known system, for example, you would be classified as genus *homo*, family *hominidae*, order *primate*, class *mammalia*, phylum *chordata*, and kingdom *animalia*.[16] This scale is still familiar, but, today, biology is more mature, and although a classification system is still necessary, as in most sciences, more sophisticated measurements are also needed. In a sense, the two-valued scales discussed earlier can be considered as classified scales.

In a nominal scale, ratios and differences are meaningless, and the ordering is hierarchical, that is, the classes are arranged from the general to the particular, as just illustrated, or from large to small, or from long to short, etc. But many classifications cannot even be ordered in this way. For example, if you sorted a number of different objects by color (such as a child's crayons), ignoring considerations like the wavelength of the light reflected by each, there would be no numbers involved, and no characteristic to which numbers could be assigned in any order, hence no ratios or differences, nor any orders or hierarchies. Lord Kelvin once remarked, "When you can measure what you are speaking about, and express it in numbers, you know something about it; but when you cannot measure it,

---

[16]Attributed to Carolus Linneaus (Karl von Linné), 1707–1778, famous Swedish Botanist and physician.

Table 4.2. Six Types of Responses

Response	Description
Continuous scales	Theoretically, these can assume any values between integer points, and may be (in theory) infinitely long. Example: weights in grams.
Semicontinuous scales	These use limited fractional values between pairs of integers.
Ranks	Whole numbers assigned to responses in the order of their magnitudes.
Integer scores	Whole-number scales expressing a quantitative characteristic of the response. Example: pain scores.
Two-valued scales	Binary scales (yes/no, black/white, improved/not improved, etc.). These may be thought of as a type of the classification scales.
Classification systems	Categorization by some characteristic or group of characteristics. Cannot necessarily be arranged in any kind of order.

when you cannot express it in numbers, your knowledge is of a meagre and unsatisfactory kind: it may be the beginning of knowledge, but you have scarcely, in your thoughts, advanced to the stage of *science.*"[17]

Summary: Measurement Scales

All of the measurement scales just discussed can be and are used in clinical trials as responses. The reasons for our extended discussion is that (a) response measurements are central to your trial planning and design, and (b) it is important to think about their nature, so that you may choose the most effective possible.

To summarize the choices we have discussed, Table 4.2 lists the several types of measurement, with a brief characterization of each. Measurements could be classified in several other ways, but this classification is one that is useful and convenient in clinical work. Furthermore, the list is not exhaustive; there are other scales that have not been included because they are rarely used in medical work.

As Table 4.2 shows, and as was discussed earlier, the important types of measurement may be classified into six basic kinds. The list is arranged in the order of the efficiency of the measurements: from continuous measurements, which convey the greatest amount of information, to classification scales, which convey the least. A good way to think of response measurements is in terms of the *statistical power* each kind confers. The power of a statistical

[17]From John Bartlett, *Familiar Quotations*, Emily Morison Beck, Ed., Little Brown and Company, Boston, Fourteenth Edition, 1968 (with permission).

hypothesis test is the probability that it will detect a difference of a specified size between two treatment groups if such a difference exists. Many factors contribute to the power of a test. The kind of experimental design used, the nature of the statistical test, the kind of response, and the sample size are among the more important. The six types of measurement in Table 4.2 are arranged, roughly, in the order of the amount of information available from a measurement of each patient with respect to the detection of a given treatment difference. Generally speaking, the measurements requiring the smallest sample sizes (i.e., those conveying the most information per patient or per measurement) are at or near the top of the list, and those associated with the greatest sample sizes are at or near the bottom.

A final point: As was noted earlier, unlike applied research in most of the "hard" sciences, a large proportion of the responses used in clinical trials are judgment scales. These include estimates of pain intensity (as in our example), degree of success of a treatment, degree of severity of a symptom, and others. Unfortunately, there are few examples of such responses in most statistics texts, and at least until recently, many, if not most newly graduated statisticians have had little experience with them. The more common kinds of responses are weights, volumes, temperatures, rates, and the like, which use continuous scales. Therefore, some experience in clinical trial work may be required before a statistician becomes acclimated to it. Such scales also make such activities as testing the parametric assumptions more important in the analysis of clinical trial data than in the physical sciences, because judgment scales are more likely to show deviations from the assumptions upon which many statistical procedures are based.

4.6 THE EXPERIMENTAL DESIGN

The **experimental design** is the **structure** of an experiment. This term, as we use it here, includes whether each patient or subject receives one, several, or all the treatments being tested, how various *nuisance variables* are handled, the number of patients to be treated similarly, and analogous items. Other provisions that must be considered during planning, such as the kind of randomization to be used, the sample size needed, and the nature of the response(s), are not actually part of the design but usually either influence it or are consequences of it. These issues will become clearer as you read the material that follows.

In planning a study, you should keep these considerations in mind:

1. Consider all possible practical designs.

2. You should select the design yourself if you are responsible for the overall planning. But you should also discuss it with the statistician from the points of view of the kind of analysis it implies, the sample size necessary, the kind of randomization needed, and similar questions. In Example 4.1, it

was assumed that these steps had already been done, but you will find information in Part III that will help you in your selection. This choice is one of the most important of all of the steps in planning a trial, if not the most important. As indicated earlier and emphasized throughout this volume, the design largely determines the kind of analysis possible, and therefore the power. Furthermore, some designs are much more difficult to administer, in a practical sense, than others. And some are difficult or nearly impossible to analyze properly under certain circumstances. As you will see, there are many reasons why you should give your choice of design a great deal of thought.

3. Whether the design is to be single or multicenter has probably been settled when you began the current phase of the study (I, II or III). All Phase I and many Phase II trials will be single-center, and most Phase III's will be multicenter. If the trial is to be multicenter, decide upon the number of centers you wish to use. This also should be discussed with the statistician, because the number of centers (independently of the total number of patients to be used), in some circumstances, can have an important influence upon the kind and power of the analysis. In the example in this chapter, the design is single-center.

4. If unequal numbers of patients for various treatment combinations in the design are possible (as it usually is) because of patient incompleters or for other reasons, talk to your statistician about whether the design has a structure that can be readily analyzed in such a case without undue losses of data or unduly complex analyses. Some designs can be very effective if all the data are obtained, but can be seriously reduced in power with even moderate or small losses of data. In Example 4.1, the design will be quite simple, because it is single-center and uses only one factor. Table 4.3 shows it; it is a kind called a **completely randomized one-factor design**, in this case consisting of four equal groups of patients, one for each of four treatments. Patient losses resulting in inequality of treatment group sizes may be unavoidable, and you must therefore make provision for them to maintain your planned sample size. You should do your best to allow for them during your planning by providing for additional patients according to your estimate of the

Table 4.3. Design of Example 4.1

Treatment Number and Name			
1 Test Drug	2 Placebo	3 Codeine	4 Cod. + Act.
P_1	P_{33}	P_{65}	P_{97}
P_2	P_{34}	P_{66}	P_{98}
$\vdots$	$\vdots$	$\vdots$	$\vdots$
P_{32}	P_{64}	P_{96}	P_{128}

Notes: The letters and subscripts refer to patient numbers. The patients were randomly assigned to the treatments, but the randomization is not shown.

expected losses. This is suggested to maintain your planned sample size, not to avoid unequal group sizes. For one-factor designs *only*, although equal group sizes will lead to the greatest power, moderate inequalities in size will not have a serious effect.

5. If, unlike the example, the design will be multicenter, you should discuss whether centers will be considered as "fixed" or "random" with your statistician. This matter is mentioned in Part III. For now, the point is that if centers (i.e., investigations) are to be considered as a "random factor," you may need more centers than if centers are fixed, perhaps five or six, compared to as few as two or three.[18]

4.7 SUMMARY OF THE CHAPTER

4.7.1 Objectives

Perhaps the most important preliminary step in the planning of any trial is that of defining your objectives. These should be specific, clear, and simple, because they will dictate many of the procedures in your trial. It is important that the objectives be described in the protocol and operations manual. There should be as few as possible, because each, if adequately specific, is likely to be reflected in increased sample size, additional response measurements, and sometimes more complex experimental designs.

An example is introduced near the beginning of the chapter and continues throughout the chapter. It is intended to illustrate simply many of the steps that are described.

4.7.2 Factorial Structure

Many trial designs have a **factorial** structure, with two or more **independent variables** to be evaluated, such as drugs, doses, and others. In your studies, after defining the objectives, these definitions should be implemented by a selection of one or more factors. For instance, Example 4.1 in this chapter has a single factor, **drugs,** at four **levels** (test drug, placebo, codeine, and codeine plus acetaminophen). Single-factor designs are discussed in more detail in Part III, and factorial designs using more than one factor are also introduced there.

4.7.3 Responses

In planning a clinical trial, you must define two different kinds of variables. The first kind comprises the factors, defined earlier as **independent** or

---

[18]The matter of whether centers are to be considered as random or fixed is not simply one of selecting the total numbers of patients necessary. The number of centers, if they are considered random, can have an important influence upon the power of the statistical tests to be done.

controlled variables,[19] whose effects the trial will try to assess. The second kind consists of **dependent variables.** These are the one or more types of measurement or response that you will specify as means of obtaining information about the behavior of the experimental system. These responses constitute the **data** that will be analyzed when the trial is complete. In Example 4.1, there were two responses, a pain scale of seven points and a visual analog scale (VAS).

In addition, there is a hybrid sort of factor, the adverse effects, which must be measured for the safety evaluations. The different types of such effects, as noted earlier, can be thought of as independent variables—factors. But unlike factors, they cannot be arbitrarily or randomly assigned to patients. Measurements, such as counts or proportions of occurrences, are used as the related responses or dependent variables. The multiplicity introduced when there are several responses, as is the usual case, is mentioned.

4.7.4 Baseline Measurements

The recommended ways to use baseline measurements are discussed briefly. Such measurements, which are made before the patients have received treatment and comprise the same responses used later, are helpful in improving the precision of the data evaluations when properly used.

4.7.5 Types of Measurement Scales

A classification of measurement scales and their characteristics is included, principally to show the great variability in information-carrying capacity that exists, depending upon the type of measurement.

4.7.6 Experimental Design

The chapter concludes with some general advice regarding the choice of a type of design for a given study.

4.8 LITERATURE REFERENCES

(1) Fleiss, Joseph L., Sylvan Wallenstein, and Robert Rosenfeld, *Controlled Clinical Trials*, **6**, 192–197 (1985).
(2) Willan, Andrew R., and Joseph L. Peter, *Controlled Clinical Trials*, **7**, 282–289 (1986).

---

[19]There can be confusion about the meaning of *controlled*. A *controlled clinical trial* usually means that concurrent controls are used. A *controlled variable* has the meaning given in the text, that is, it is an independent variable or factor, the values or categories of the levels of which are controlled by the experimenter.

CHAPTER 5

Planning Your Trial: II

5.1 ESTIMATING THE SAMPLE SIZE

5.1.1 Introduction

In the following sections, the concepts of **distributions (populations), normality**, and **samples** taken from populations will be referred to several times. Distributions were introduced briefly in the discussion on measurement scales in the previous chapter, but a more thorough explanation of that idea, as well as a discussion of the various types of common distributions and the notion of samples taken from a distribution, will be needed to facilitate your understanding of sample size estimation. Section 5.2 in this chapter will provide that explanation. For the present, the following brief remarks will be adequate: A **distribution**, or **population**, of patients is the hypothetical set of all patients who conform and will conform in the future to the conditions your study requires—that is, they suffer from the disease you wish to treat and possess other characteristics (age, sex, etc.) specified in the protocol. This set (population) would include all present and future patients with such attributes. A **sample** from a population is a selection of a specific and relatively small number of patients taken from the population. The number of patients taken is the sample size. A **normal** distribution or population is one having certain mathematical characteristics. Many numerical responses or measurements made on or of the patients, when considered in groups, form approximately normal distributions.

5.1.2 Sample Size Estimation during Planning

It is very probable that only a relatively few readers of this book will find the time and inclination to perform much, if any, statistical work upon their data. As we have indicated, it is not the purpose of this book to teach you to do so. However, to ensure that your studies are adequate for their objectives and statistically valid, I believe that you *must* become familiar with a minimal set of statistical concepts and procedures. These include the more common experimental designs, the theory and mechanisms of the hypothesis tests used for your data, and the knowledge you will need to obtain adequate sample size estimates during planning. If you have no understanding of any of these, you are transferring your responsibilities to the biostatistician, and relying only upon your belief (not knowledge) of his or her competence. In my opinion, based upon observation of many cases of this kind, without this minimal preparation, you cannot guarantee to your employer, FDA, or yourself that everything possible has been done to help ensure success in your studies.

The correct use of sample size estimation requires a good understanding of the other two topics, experimental design and hypothesis testing. In turn, these two are based upon some general principles of applied statistics. Fortunately, you do not need to become a past master in their use. A reasonable degree of knowledge, based upon your reading of this book, should suffice to provide you with enough understanding to allow you to be sure that the work being done for you is adequate and valid. You will also be able to select your own designs with an adequate knowledge of their characteristics and, if you wish and can find the time, to do your own sample size estimates. As you will see, much of the information needed for the latter, in any event, must be based upon estimates that only you can provide.

5.1.3 Scope of Topic

Because of the importance of the subject of sample size estimation in clinical work, several methods of carrying out some common types of sample size estimates are discussed in detail in Part V. This chapter is an introduction to the subject, is limited to estimates for one-way designs, and describes the use of a table to estimate sample size. The table is useful for any one-way design you may use in the future, remembering, however, that it applies only to studies that produce normally or near-normally distributed data when analyzed by a method appropriate to such responses.[1] In addition to the illustration and the description of the use of the table, this chapter will provide you with some basic knowledge of the purposes, requirements, results, specifications, and statistics needed for any sample size estimate. If a design requires computations or tables beyond those referred to in this chapter or later ones, you will need to seek the help of a statistician, even if you do not do so for the simpler procedures. And it is a good idea, even if you use the methods we describe, to ask your statistician to comment on your work.

If you are interested in delving more deeply into the subject of sample size estimation, a fuller knowledge is not difficult to acquire, but will necessitate considerably more statistical background than is provided in this volume.

---

[1]The concepts of distributions (populations) and samples taken from them are explained later in this chapter.

Nevertheless, even if you are a bit rusty, or perhaps have had no courses in undergraduate statistics, don't worry. Assuming that you have a grounding in algebra, such additional knowledge can be easily obtained by attending some courses in probability, statistical analysis, and experimental design. Alternatively, if you prefer self-study, it is possible to obtain the necessary background by studying two or three good books on applied statistics, such as the fine texts by Snedecor and Cochran [38] and Neter, Wasserman, and Kutner [37]. These should be followed by a review of portions of the second edition of Cohen's book on sample size [27]. The last presents a number of sample size and power tables for fairly simple designs and analyses, and explains their use in detail, with many examples. An appendix gives the mathematical basis for the tables. If you already have some statistical background, you should be able to refer directly to Cohen's book, with a moderate amount of study. Do not be concerned because the title and most of the examples are given in terms of psychology and other behavioral sciences. The methods and tables are equally applicable to clinical trial work.

Finally, there is a paper by Bratcher, Moran, and Zimmer (1) that will be of value when you must plan designs like that of Example 4.1 in Chapter 4 (more than two treatments) using a more conventional procedure than the one described here. The data analysis in that case is most easily done using an **analysis of variance** (ANOVA, mentioned only briefly in this book), but the **Bonferroni** multiple comparisons procedure described in this and later chapters can be used. Some of the sample size tables from Bratcher et al. are reprinted in the Appendix, with permission (see Table A.6).

5.1.4   Definitions

The sample size for a single treatment or treatment group for a parallel design (one in which each patient receives only one of the treatments being compared) is equal to the number of patients receiving that treatment. Each group may comprise a different number of patients, or, as is more common, all groups may be designed to be equal in size. Usually, in planning single-factor studies, we estimate the sample size per treatment group. The **total sample size** will then be equal to the sum of the sample sizes for all the groups.

There can be confusion about the word **estimate**. In applied statistics, an estimate is not a guess, arrived at by experience, intuition, or some other poorly defined or understood mental process. Rather, a statistical estimate is the result of a *calculation*. It is called an estimate merely to emphasize that the results cannot be exact, because its basis is necessarily inexact. For example, you might obtain the arithmetic mean or average of the pain scores for the patients on one of the drugs or combinations in the example introduced in Example 4.1 in Chapter 4. The resulting number would not only be the actual mean of those patients' data, but it would also be an *estimate* of the mean of the population of scores for all patients whom you believe are represented by your sample. Perhaps this population might be all of those whom you expect will use the drug eventually if the trial is successful. *Estimates* of population characteristics such as the mean (parameters of a distribution) are called **statistics**. The patients in the example who are assigned to that drug are a sample of that population. You assume that they are a representative sample, although they will probably not be a **random** selection. The mean or average of that population of patients' scores is a **parameter**, and like almost all such parameters, it is commonly represented by a Greek letter, in this case, μ (mu). Parameters usually remain forever unknown, because, like the population of pain scores, their populations are infinite or at least extremely large, and usually extend into the future. In any study you do, however, it is likely that any sample mean score that you calculate, if your group size consists of 20 or more patients (and if the sample is representative of the population), will be a fairly good estimate of mu.

5.1.5 The Need for Sample Size Estimation

Industrial trials with "negative" results—that is, in which significance for a test drug vs. placebo, say, is not found—rarely appear in print. Reports of such trials from noncommercial organizations, however, are more common. But it is not likely that there are fewer negative trials in industry than in academic circles or government. Rather, this lack of reporting is probably a result of the fact that there is less pressure in industry to publish, and normally little incentive to publish "unsuccessful" results. Few reports from either source, whether "negative" or not, indicate that sample sizes based upon clinically significant values of delta or beta risks have been specified during planning.[2]

In fact, the estimation of sample size has often been neglected in industrial clinical trials, especially in smaller, early phase studies. It is possible that many "negative" trials might show significance if their sample sizes were larger. In published papers, there is usually no mention of tests done after the fact to estimate what the risk of missing a clinically important difference might have been. Yet without a priori specifications of delta or beta, or post hoc analyses, you cannot know whether a drug or treatment was merely ineffective or whether the sample size was simply too small to show efficacy.

Because many published reports of noncommercial studies described in medical journals and elsewhere do not mention the use of a sample size estimate, a reader must assume that such estimates have not been done in

---

[2]Delta is the minimum difference it is desired to detect between a test drug and a placebo or other active drug, and beta is the probability of missing differences larger than delta when performing significance tests of the data. The value of delta specified in a clinical trial would be one large enough to be "clinically significant," that is, of a size of practical importance in the judgment of the sponsor or investigator(s). These quantities are discussed later in this chapter.

most such cases or, at best, were not deemed important enough to describe. In the pharmaceutical industry, however, it is a fact that sample sizes very often have been selected without taking beta or delta into account and without knowledge of the consequences of those omissions. It must be assumed that in such cases, a biostatistician has not been consulted during the early planning stages. When (and if) one is subsequently consulted, preparations may have then advanced so far that it is difficult or impractical to make changes. The result is that too many or too few patients may have been scheduled.

Too large a sample size can be unethical and is unquestionably a waste of money, but a sample size that is too small can be far worse. Using too few patients can easily result in a trial that is worthless. If such trials are early phase studies, as they usually are (larger studies are often planned more carefully, because they represent greater expenditures), further work with potentially useful drugs is often abandoned, because important differences between treatments have not been detected. Thus, this also wastes money, as well as opportunities to develop new drugs. Even more regrettably, those who design and run the trial may not be aware, even after the work is done and the data analyzed, that clinically significant treatment differences could easily have existed without detection. Finally, such trials, again, should be considered unethical, because the patients will have been put to unnecessary inconvenience or discomfort without benefit to anyone.

5.1.6 Factors That Affect Sample Size

Three issues, the type of response planned, the kind of experimental design (including the kind of randomization) used, and the nature of the statistical analysis planned, must be taken into account in estimating the sample size you need for a given trial. These are discussed, in turn, in what follows.

Type of Response
The required sample size will vary depending upon the *type* and *number* of responses to be used. In the example in Chapter 4, there were two: a seven-point judgment scale (the pain scale to be used by the investigator through interviews with the patients) and the VAS pain scale. From the discussion in Chapter 4, you will realize that because the seven-point scale is an integer scale, it is lower in the hierarchy of response scales than the VAS with regard to the amount of information that a single response can carry. The VAS is capable of recording a greater quantity of information per measurement because it is a continuous scale, although it also is based upon judgment, as any pain evaluation must be.

If you were to use the VAS as your only response, you would probably require fewer patients to obtain a given degree of statistical power than if you used the seven-point scoring scale, because the VAS is a continuous scale. Therefore, unless the use of the scores is really of secondary importance to you, you should base your sample size calculations upon the seven-point scoring scale rather than the VAS. Otherwise, a sample size sufficient for the VAS response might be too small for the scores. Of course, if you plan to use both responses, you must take the resulting multiplicity into account in estimating the sample size. This will provide assurance that you will have adequate ability to detect the differences between treatments of the magnitude you desire with both types of measurement.

On the other hand, you must consider the fact that the selection of the seven-point scale as your principal response depends upon the judgment that it is reasonably important to you. Perhaps you should consider the following, however: It may well be better to assign substantially more importance to the VAS than to the pain scale. When using the latter, the investigator must decide upon the score to record based upon each patient's description of the pain. This process requires acts of judgment by two people, so it could be more **biased** and/or more variable than the VAS. Based upon this reasoning, you may feel it safer to depend upon the VAS results for drawing your final conclusions. This argument seems realistic and convincing, therefore, we will base our calculations upon the use of the VAS response alone and abandon the use of the seven-point scoring scale.

Experimental Design

The kind of experimental design you use, that is, the structure of the study, will also affect the sample size. For example, a parallel design will usually require more patients than a changeover design such as randomized blocks with patients as blocks (sometimes referred to as a "repeated-measures" design). This is true because the experimental error in the parallel design is based upon differences among individual patients, whereas that of the changeover design is based upon differences from one measurement to the next, *within* each patient, and is often smaller.

In addition, the kind of design used largely dictates the kind of data analysis that must be employed. Some designs may force the use of an inefficient method of analysis. Therefore, in choosing the **completely randomized one-way design** of the following Example 5.1, we will assume that its influence upon sample size per se, as well as that of the kind of analysis it requires, has been taken into account.

Analyses of Data

As just implied, the sample size needed is also related to the nature of the statistical analysis that is to be used. The statistical power of an analysis will vary with the type of analysis. You will recall that **power** is the probability that a statistical test will detect differences of a specified magnitude among treatment group means, if such differences exist. Power is also a function of sample size, so the trial should be planned so that the analysis to be used will operate upon sufficient replicate data to ensure adequate power.

For your later reference, we will be using *t*-tests, adjusted for use with multiple comparisons (multiplicity) with a Bonferroni procedure, in our examples of one-way parallel designs, when the data of the example are analyzed. You will need this information when you estimate the sample size you need as described in what follows.

5.1.7   Outline of Estimation Procedure

In the 1960s and 1970s, when statistical procedures were just beginning to be used in industrial clinical trials, more often than not a professional statistician did not take part in the trial planning or analysis, but someone involved in the trial nevertheless felt that statistical procedures should be used. In those days, a sardonic question regarding hypothesis (*significance*) tests was frequently asked by distrustful clinical monitors and others, and frequently went unanswered. The question was, to paraphrase: *If we find significance, we understand that the difference (between two treatments) is* **statistically** *significant, but how do we know whether it is* **clinically** *significant*? The implication was that the difference detected may have really existed in the population, but could have been very small and therefore of no practical importance. The skepticism reflected by this question was warranted, but it arose because the hypothesis-testing method and the earlier sample size estimate (if any) were misunderstood and incorrectly done. The confusion was based upon a common method of significance testing, which we call the **simplistic** procedure in this book, which does not limit the hypothesis test to the detection of meaningful differences only. The methods of estimating sample size describedhere, together with the use of the appropriate hypothesis testing procedure on your data, provide the correct tests in this situation.

In the following section, the quantities alpha and beta, although they are conventionally identified by Greek letters, are not parameters of the normal or any other population, but **probability** values that you must specify in order to obtain an appropriate size estimate. Unfortunately, the use of Greek letters for these as well as for parameters can be confusing, but is traditional. Delta, also discussed in what is to follow, although it, too, is a specification, might also be thought of as a parameter, because it can be considered to be a member of a hypothetical population of differences between treatment mean (values of μ).

As described in more detail in Chapter 13, there are two possible common methods of carrying out hypothesis tests. We call the first the *simplistic* procedure and do not recommend its use with clinical trial data for the comparison of treatments or treatment combinations. The procedure we recommend is called the Neyman-Pearson procedure, and is the one that should normally be used for that purpose. To estimate the sample size, in preparation for the use of that method when you test your data, you will need four quantities, commonly called alpha, beta, delta, and sigma. You can specify the first three, but you must estimate the fourth from previous data or a pilot study. The four are discussed in Steps 3 and 4 in Section 5.1.8. Once they are on hand, you can estimate the approximate required sample size either by calculation (which is short and simple and does not require a computer; a scientific pocket calculator will do) or, often, by using a table. In the following example, after obtaining the four quantities needed, we will use Table A.3 in the Appendix to obtain the sample size. This table is intended for use with simple designs having the following characteristics:

1. A single comparison of two treatments, called a **pairwise comparison** (see Step 1 in Section 5.1.8), is planned, using a t test or the equivalent, or:

2. If you plan more than one comparison, you should provide for it by adjusting the sample size and using a multiple-comparison test rather than a series of t tests.[3] If you use the appropriate test but do not use a larger sample size than would be necessary for only one pairwise comparison, your work will be correct, but there will be a loss of **power** (sensitivity to treatment differences).

3. Each patient receives only one treatment.

4. The data are expected to be samples from populations that are normal or near normal (or can be transformed to such data before testing, without affecting the eventual conclusions).

5. The populations of data sampled (the samples of the several populations are the several treatment groups) have equal or nearly equal variances. Variance is a function of the experimental errors.

6. The measurements associated with each patient are independent of those of the others.

Although conditions 3, 4, and 5 may seem restrictive, many common studies yield data possessing such characteristics (although you should not take this for granted). There are tests that you or your statistician can use to test whether your data comply with the latter three conditions. There is discussion of these in Chapter 13. If there is any doubt at all, you should not take any of these three **assumptions** for granted.

The process of estimating the sample size for a clinical trial can be divided into the following five steps. We illustrate these in the form of an extension of Example 4.1 in Chapter 4, which we will call Example 5.1. It will have the same four treatments and responses as Example 4.1, but its purpose will be

---

[3]Except in the relatively rare cases in which you wish to use a **testwise** rather than an **experimentwise** error rate (see what follows).

to demonstrate the estimation of sample size for a simple trial in which near normality is assumed.

5.1.8   Example 5.1: Sample Size for a One-Way Parallel Design

Step 1: Select Comparisons Needed

Select the comparison(s) between treatments that are to be made during analysis of the data. Many of your trials, like this one, will entail more than two treatments. In such a case, you should be sure to specify how many and what kind of comparisons there will be. For instance, in this example, there are four treatments; therefore, there are six possible pairwise comparisons.[4] It is most important, for the reasons given in what follows, to make this decision during planning, rather than after the data are available.

Usually, the comparisons will be **pairwise comparisons**. These are comparisons of the magnitudes of the differences between the mean responses obtained from two or more treatment groups, taken two at a time. However, there are other possible kinds of treatment comparisons. For instance, in Example 5.1, you might wish to compare the average response for two of the groups taken together with that for a third.

As it happens, in Example 5.1, we plan to make four pairwise treatment comparisons for efficacy out of the six that are possible. It is important to limit the number of comparisons to as few as possible. *The more comparisons you make, the larger the sample size must be, everything else being equal.* Many industrial studies are designed without taking this fact into account, and without specifying the number of treatment comparisons, with unhappy results. In addition, when the data analysis is finished, even if sample size estimations have been done, more treatment comparisons may be requested by the sponsor than were planned originally. If such unplanned interim analyses or additional comparisons at the end of a trial are made, additional problems arise. Even if they are done correctly (by taking the resulting **multiplicity** into account through the use of special **multiple-comparisons tests**, as mentioned in Chapter 14, Section 14.6), there will be a reduction of power in the statistical tests. That is, the tests will lose sensitivity, so that you will be less likely to detect a treatment difference of a given size. Therefore, you should take pains to ensure that all the conditions that would introduce additional multiplicity have been foreseen and compensated for during planning. These include the number of treatment comparisons for each response, the number of different kinds of responses, and any other requirement that would have the effect of increasing the total number of comparisons made.

---

[4]That is, for four treatments A, B, C, and D, there would be the following six possible comparisons: A vs. B, A vs. C, A vs. D, B vs. C, B vs. D, and C vs. D.

The effect of introducing such multiplicities will be to increase the alpha risk described in the next section—that is, the so-called **significance level** of the statistical test. This is the chance of claiming that a significant difference (delta) exists when it really does not. For instance, you or the statistician will undoubtedly plan to use a statistical hypothesis test to compare the means of interest in this example. Let's say that you have set a significance level of 0.05 during planning. Using 0.05 means that for all comparisons considered together, you have specified a maximum probability of 0.05 (a "5% chance") that, on the average, an observed difference between any two treatment sample means will be due to chance rather than to a real population difference. Now, suppose you anticipate making tests of four treatment pairs, using only the VAS in each case. To get an **experimentwise error rate** of 0.050 in each of the four tests (i.e., to get an **effective** 5% significance level *applying to all four tests taken together, as one experiment*, you would need a "working" level in your tests of approximately 0.050/4, or 0.0125. If you were planning to use two responses for each of the four, making eight tests altogether, you would require a working level of 0.050/8, or 0.0063. The alternative, staying with the nominal 5% level, would result in your being unable to distinguish treatment differences as small as those you specified, with the probability of success that you decided upon. Your only recourse, to avoid this loss of power, is to plan ahead of time to increase the sample size to that needed for the "working" alpha levels. Thus, it pays to use as few responses as possible, because the smaller the value of alpha you wish to use, the greater the sample size necessary.

Some of the statistical literature has suggested that multiple-comparisons tests are unnecessary, even when there is more than one comparison, as long as you plan from the beginning which comparisons, exactly, you will use, avoiding such decisions after the data can be viewed. However, in this book, we take the position that this will be true only if you decide that you are concerned with a rather uncommon condition—using **testwise** rather than **experimentwise** comparisons (see footnote 12 in Step 5). In the experiment-wise circumstance, which is much more common in clinical work, we feel that it is safer if the multiplicity is compensated for whether you decide upon extra tests a priori or make unplanned comparisons after the data are in.

There are other multiplicity problems. For example, if you wish to make interim statistical tests during the progress of the trial (and this may some-times be an ethical necessity or be desirable for other reasons), another multiplicity problem arises, because, again, you will be making additional comparisons. The solution, as before, is to plan ahead—to decide during the planning of the study whether to use interim analyses. This will not be a factor in Example 5.1, because this study is small and can be completed rapidly. Even in such cases, however, interim analyses, done before all of the scheduled patients have entered the trial, may seem desirable in some trials for ethical reasons (keeping the number of patients taking part in the trial to a minimum), or to reduce expenses, or to save time.[5] Interim analyses are discussed at a bit more length in the next chapter, and this and similar problems will be discussed at some length in Part V.

Step 2: Choose a Response
The second step in estimating the sample size for your trial is to decide upon the response to be used. This has already been described (see Section 5.1.6, "Type of Response"). You have planned to use the VAS measurement only.

Step 3: Specify Needed Quantities
The third step is to set up the following specifications (the first three of the four quantities referred to earlier):

- Establish the smallest difference (the "critical difference") that you wish to detect between treatments, in terms of the units of the chosen response. This should be the smallest difference that you consider "practically" or "clinically" significant. It is called delta (δ).
- Specify the maximum risk that you are willing to assume of failing to detect a difference of this size or larger, if it exists. This is beta (β). Incidentally, the **power** of a hypothesis test, which we have mentioned earlier, is equal to $1 - \beta$, and is the probability of successfully detecting a specified population difference.
- Specify the maximum risk that you are willing to assume of concluding that a difference of the specified size or larger exists in the population as well as in the sample, when it actually does not. This is the significance level, alpha (α).
- Express the alpha and beta risks as **probabilities**—numbers between 1 (certainty) and 0 (impossibility). In doing this, bear in mind that the smaller the specified probabilities (i.e., the smaller your risks), the larger your sample size will have to be. Values of these probabilities that are commonly used are mentioned in the next paragraph.

You will need to use all three of these specifications when the sample size for the trial is estimated. The critical difference is delta (δ). The risk of failing to detect a difference greater than delta if such a difference exists is called beta (β). The risk of falsely claiming that a difference exists is called alpha (α). Common values, which, of course, you need not necessarily adopt,

---

[5]Interim analyses may be done before all of the patients are enrolled. Alternatively, in a study requiring several visits to the clinic, there may be analyses before all of the visits are completed. Finally, there may be interim analyses at times when a combination of these two circumstances exists. The important thing is to *plan* the number of interim tests so that the increases in sample size necessary can be calculated before the trial begins. Even if you were able to provide for extra patients later, *if* interim analyses were done, such schemes could greatly complicate the randomization and blinding procedures and may lead to regulatory difficulties.

are 0.050 or 0.010 for α and 0.050, 0.100, or 0.200 for β.[6] If the sample size estimates are to be computed by your statistician, you may wish to ask for a range of values for all three quantities, so that you may choose the optimum sample size while balancing the cost and time required for the trial against the degree of assurance and power that you need.

Step 4: Estimate the Expected Experimental Error

The experimental error is the fourth quantity needed. This step involves obtaining an *estimate* (you *cannot* specify it) of the **standard deviation** of the selected measurement (the VAS). The standard deviation (full name: **standard deviation of a single item from the mean**) is the experimental error that will be associated with each individual VAS measurement made during the trial, due to measurement errors and patient characteristics. Like the three previous specifications, the standard deviation is represented by a Greek character, in this case, σ, the Greek lowercase sigma. Unlike the other three, however, that were *specified* and therefore known exactly, sigma is a characteristic of the actual data to be obtained during the study. Consequently, before you have done a trial, it must either be estimated by means of a **pilot trial** (defined in what follows), obtained from one or more previous sets of data, if available, or guessed at.

Sigma is a **parameter** of the distribution of population represented by your sample of patients. An estimate of that parameter is called s or s_{xi}, or sometimes $\hat{\sigma}$ ("sigma hat"). The "hat," or circumflex, above the Greek letter sigma (lowercase) indicates that the quantity shown is a **statistic** (i.e., an estimate of a parameter, calculated from a sample). Parameters are characteristics of probability distributions (populations) and are discussed elsewhere. Sigma is called the standard deviation, and, of course, s is the *estimated* standard deviation, for instance, that calculated from your sample of patients. More exactly, the phrase "standard deviation of a single item from the mean" is used. A "single item" is one measurement, and the mean referred to is the arithmetic mean or average of the data (there are several other kinds of means).

There are several ways to obtain estimates of sigma. The best one is to run a pilot trial. This is a trial similar to the planned study, but with fewer patients and sometimes other simplifications. When the pilot trial is finished,

---

[6]These values are conventional maxima. It is not wise to use greater values. For one thing, the FDA will not usually accept significance tests using alpha values that exceed 0.050 as primary evidence of efficacy or safety. You may well wish to use smaller values. If you are using the Bonferroni inequality (i.e., dividing alpha by the number of comparisons to get a *working* alpha value) to compensate for a multiplicity situation of some kind, you *must* use a smaller value of alpha unless you wish to compensate by increasing beta (not a good idea) or delta (which you will probably be reluctant to do). As for beta, remember that the smaller it is, the better your chance will be of finding the difference that you have judged to be important (but remember that a smaller beta value also means a greater sample size).

the statistician can analyze it to obtain estimates of sigma to use in the sample size calculations.

Because of budgetary considerations as well as the time required, there is frequently reluctance to run a pilot trial. This may be especially true if the study is planned for no other purpose than to estimate sigma, because this will seem a trivial need to some if they do not understand its importance. Yet running a trial for that purpose alone often results in very substantial savings of time and money, because it greatly increases the likelihood that your trial will be neither too large nor too small.

Sometimes a pilot trial can be avoided if you have data from a previous study that you are sure is very similar in all respects to the projected trial.

If it is really impossible to run a pilot trial and no previous data are available, guessing at the value of sigma is the only remaining strategy. Sometimes your statistician will be able to estimate probable values of sigma from experience, even when there are no really similar trials available. If so, a good device is to ask the statistician to select several values covering a probable range, using each to calculate a sample size. If the smallest sample size obtained in this way is not impossibly large, you might then choose it for your study. It sometimes happens, when this is done, that the differences among the several estimates are not large. On the other hand, it can happen that none of your results produces a sample size small enough to be practical or economical. If this happens, you really should consider postponing the study until such time as a pilot trial can be run.

For the example study, let's assume that you have already run a small pilot trial of your test analgesic against a placebo. You believe that the **pooled**[7] value of *s* obtained from the resulting data should furnish an adequate estimate of sigma for your sample size estimate.

Step 5: Find the Sample Size for the Headache Study

You are now ready to carry out the fifth and last step in Example 5.1, that of actually estimating the sample size. As indicated at the beginning of this chapter, we will use Table A.3 in the Appendix for this. This procedure is adequate for moderately simple designs like the present one, but will be unsuitable for other designs, such as those with more than one factor, that you will probably need frequently in your work. In addition, tables for more direct estimation of sample size in studies with one factor, when there are more than two levels, like this example, will be introduced in Chapter 15,

---

[7]The terms **pooled** and **pooling** are explained in Chapter 14. When there are two groups of data, as in the pilot trial just described, or more than two, as in Example 5.1, and if each group contains the same number of data, the pooled standard deviation is derived from the *average* or *mean* values of the variances of the groups. If the groups are of unequal size, their variable influences upon the final result can be compensated for by pooling. A pooled value is a **weighted average** or **weighted mean**. In Chapter 14, we demonstrate a method of calculation that gives the correct result whether the group sizes are equal or not. It is not necessary to be familiar with that method until you encounter it in Chapter 14, as long as you understand its purpose.

when sample size estimation procedures for one-way analyses of variance are described. Furthermore, if you need to estimate sample sizes for binomial responses (yes/no, 0/1, true/false, etc.), you can use the tables given in the Appendix for this purpose (Tables A.7a to A.7r).

Quantities Needed
Assume that you have decided upon values of alpha, beta, and delta, and have calculated a pooled value of s (or $\hat{\sigma}$) from your pilot trial. Let's say that these values are[8]

$$\alpha = 0.050$$
$$\beta = 0.100$$
$$\delta = 15$$
$$\hat{\sigma} = 13.0$$

Delta and sigma have the units of the response upon which we are basing the sample size estimation procedure, that is, the units of the VAS scale, millimeters. Both alpha and beta are probabilities, so we could say that their units are units of probability, if you wish.

Number of Comparisons
We must now get ready to enter Table A.3. In addition to the three specifications, alpha, beta, and delta, and the estimate of sigma, we need to know the number of pairwise comparisons we are going to make (cf. "When and How to Compensate for Multiplicity" in what follows). The number of comparisons needed was mentioned in the last chapter, where it was recognized that there are a minimum of three and a maximum of four comparisons, out of a possible total of six, which will be of interest when the data are analyzed. These are A vs. B, A vs. C, A vs. D, and B vs., say, D, that is, the test drug vs. placebo, the test drug vs. codeine, the test drug vs. codeine plus acetaminophen, and the placebo vs. codeine plus acetaminophen, respectively. The first three will give information about the absolute efficacy of the test drug (test vs. placebo), and its efficacy relative to the two standard drugs. The fourth comparison is not necessary to measure the efficacy of the test drug, but is a check to ensure that nothing has gone wrong in the trial, by comparing one of the two drugs of known efficacy with the placebo. If the trial works as intended, we expect to find a significant difference for this comparison, because it is known that drug D is effective, and we do not expect a strong placebo effect.

---

[8]Like most of the examples in this volume, as explained in the Preface, the headache example was not taken from an actual trial, but was constructed using random normal numbers and values of 25, 75, 55, and 35 for the four treatment group means, A through D. A sigma of 10 was used for all groups. The value of 13 for sigma obtained from the previous trial and used in the sample size calculation is a reasonable small-sample estimate of the true value of 10, and illustrates that estimates of sigma can be quite variable.

Thus, you or the statistician will need to plan on at least three and perhaps four pairwise comparisons[9] using the VAS data. We will plan on four to be conservative. Now, we need to compensate for the multiplicity that will be introduced as a result of making four comparisons rather than one. As mentioned, with this kind of design, if there are more than two treatment groups, an ANOVA may be used as the means of data analysis. The biostatistician will be thoroughly familiar with that procedure. An ANOVA can determine whether there are any significant **contrasts** among the treatment groups (significant differences between treatment means or combinations of means). But if significance is found, further tests must be done to find which comparison(s) brought about the result.[10] Alternatively, we could adopt the strategy of omitting the ANOVA and going directly to the individual tests of interest, in this case, the four just discussed. Because this is the simpler procedure, we are planning to use that in this example. Note, however, that we describe this method at this point principally because it is simple in concept. In terms of convenience and time required, a method that is technically more complex may require less time to carry out.

When and How to Compensate for Multiplicity

In the paragraphs that follow, we describe common circumstances in which you should carry out the required significance tests of your data by some means that compensates for the effect of making more than one comparison. In most such cases, you should use some kind of **multiple-comparisons** test rather than repeated t tests. In a few cases, this is not necessary. But the sample size we will estimate in this example assumes the use of such a procedure. The bases for the decision, as given in the literature, are sometimes hard to understand. However, an excellent discussion is given in a chapter by Dunnett and Goldsmith in the volume edited by Buncher and Tsay, Chapter 16 [19].

---

[9]We are using four comparisons here for simplicity. If we were to allow for the seven-point pain scale response as well as the VAS, there would be seven or more, because at least three of the same four would need to be done using the seven-point scale. Faced with the need to do seven pairwise comparisons, we then might decide to reduce the number of treatments in the study to three rather than four. The larger the number of comparisons to be made, the smaller alpha must be and/or the larger the resulting sample size. Using three treatments would result in three pairwise comparisons for the VAS (A vs. B, A vs. C, and B vs. C, where A would be the test drug, B the placebo, and C the standard). We could then probably get away with using just the first two of these for the seven-point scale data, making a total of five comparisons altogether.

[10]An ANOVA can be used even when there are only two treatments (two levels of a single factor), but it is not necessary in this case, as it is exactly equivalent to performing a t test, which many people find simpler to do. A t test is normally applicable to a single comparison, for example, of two treatment group means. The t test is described in Chapter 14. But there is a related procedure as well, also described there, that allows the use of a series of t tests following an ANOVA **if** the ANOVA shows significance (see references to Carmer and Swanson (8) and Bernhardsen (9), also in Chapter 14).

When there are are only two treatments and the two treatment groups are samples from independent normal distributions with the same standard deviation, Student's independent t test (see Part IV for details)[11] is the appropriate significance test to use. But when a study has more than two treatments, as is true for this example, more than one pairwise comparison will almost always be planned. In such cases, you or the statistician will usually use a **multiple comparisons test**. If you wish your conclusions to apply to the experiment as a whole,[12] you may use a **multiple comparisons** test. If, instead, you use two or more t tests, the true alpha value will not be that specified and can be substantially greater. This distortion can easily be so extreme that any significant differences found may be highly questionable. The use of a multiple comparisons test avoids this problem. The one recommended in this book is the **Bonferroni**. Although this procedure is a bit conservative, it is very simple, and is reliable and easy to interpret. The alpha level in each comparison will now no longer be distorted, but will be equal to that specified during planning. But a second problem now arises.

As we indicated earlier, maintaining the value of alpha at the level specified by the use of a multiple-comparisons test to replace a simple and uncompensated series of t tests will result in a loss of statistical power[13] unless you also compensate for that by increasing the sample size during planning. As will be shown in what follows, the Bonferroni test calls for the use of a "working" alpha value less than that specified, and other multiple comparisons procedures imply such a reduced value. As alpha is reduced, the statistical power is reduced and/or the value of delta is increased. To maintain both of these values as well as alpha at the level originally specified, you must increase the sample size.

Let's apply these ideas to our example. You have prespecified alpha, beta, and delta, and you now wish to plan the procedure to be used after the data are available, and to estimate the sample size needed. We are concerned with obtaining a "working" value of alpha.

---

[11] The t test requires reasonably near-normal errors of the data, and approximately equal sigma values in each pair of treatment groups tested. Groups of data with equal standard deviations are called **homoscedastic.** The usual procedure is then to use a **pooled** error estimate derived from all four groups when doing each test. There are methods of testing normality and comparing group variances (standard deviation squared). Two of these are described in Part IV, and these are described in detail there. In Example 5.1, we are assuming normality and homoscedasticity. In your regular work, however, you should be certain that the statistician verifies these assumptions before doing an analysis.

[12] That is, if you wish to use an **experimentwise,** or **family,** error rate rather than a **per comparison** rate. An experimentwise rate applies to all of the comparisons you will make, taken as a group or family. A per comparison rate applies to each test, considered one at a time. In most clinical studies requiring more than one comparison of treatments (or treatment combinations), an experimentwise rate is the appropriate one.

[13] That is, a larger value of beta, or a smaller value of $1 - \beta$ than that specified. Recall that $1 - \beta$ is the probability of detecting a difference of delta or greater (which you have also specified) in your significance tests.

Because we are assuming that our data from the VAS are approximately normal or will be altered by a transformation to make them so, we would like to use Student's t tests for each of the four treatment group comparisons (as we indicated, this is a statistical significance test; it will be explained in Part IV). The t test will indicate whether the observed difference between any pair of group means is large enough to justify a conclusion that the population difference is greater than delta, with a risk of alpha (5% in this case) of being wrong. Remember that the test is not perfect; even when the population difference really is greater than delta, there nevertheless will be failure to detect it in about 10 out of every 100 repetitions of the test, because beta was specified to be 0.10 (you could have reduced this risk further by additional increases in the sample size).

We are planning more than one comparison and wish to use an experimentwise error rate, so we cannot use the t test at the 0.05 alpha level. We need to arrange for an **experimentwise error rate** equal to alpha to avoid the loss of power. Fortunately, there are several ways to accomplish this. In this example, we use the so-called **Bonferroni inequality**. A "working" alpha value is calculated very simply by dividing the specified alpha probability by the number of comparisons to be made. This smaller value of alpha is used wherever an alpha level is called for in the sample size calculations or tables, remembering that the "true" value is still that originally specified (0.05 in this example), and that the working value is merely a device to make it possible to overcome the multiplicity problem. We must use these ideas and procedures now, even though we are not yet analyzing data, because we need to adjust the sample size now. Note that this is a good example of the need to take the kind of statistical analysis to be used eventually into account during the planning of a clinical study.

To calculate the working value of alpha for Example 5.1, you divide the specified alpha value of 0.050 by the number of comparisons planned, that is, 4:

$$\alpha_w = \frac{\alpha}{4}$$

$$= 0.0125$$

where α_w is the working value of alpha, α is the specified value, and 4 is the number of comparisons planned. Because 0.0125 is an awkward value to handle, we will be a little more conservative and reduce it to 0.010. This will increase the sample size estimate a little more than is needed, but not excessively. We will now use this value of alpha as a working value instead of 0.050 wherever alpha is called for when estimating the sample size, remembering that the "true" alpha value (the experimentwise error rate) will still be 0.050.

To find the required estimate of sample size for each treatment group, we will now use Appendix Table A.3a. Table A.3 consists of four subtables for different values of alpha. Table A.3a is the one intended for a specified alpha value of 0.01 (our working value). To enter the table, in addition to the value of 0.01 for alpha, we will need beta, and a statistic that we will call delta sub *s*. This is equal to delta in terms of the number of estimated sigmas it represents, and we symbolize it by δ_s. It is calculated by dividing the specified delta value (which, you will remember, is 15) by the estimated value of sigma ($\hat{\sigma}$, or *s*), which we found to be 13:

$$\delta_s = \frac{\delta}{\hat{\sigma}}$$

$$= \frac{15}{13}$$

$$= 1.15$$

Table A.3a gives sample sizes required for data for which independent *t* tests are to be run. It assumes both normality and equal standard deviations in the treatment groups to be compared, but the results will not be greatly in error if there are moderate departures from these assumptions, especially when the sample sizes are equal in the pairs of groups in each test and amount to 10 to 20 or more patients. We will be concerned with the table for a two-tailed alpha value of 0.010 in finding the sample size for our present study. In each subtable, the left-hand column, labeled "Delta/Sigma" is the quantity just described (1.15 in this case). The other column labels are values of beta. To use the table for Example 5.1, we follow these steps:

1. Find the table labeled "Alpha = 0.01" (Table A.3a).
2. In the left-hand column, find the delta/sigma value of 1.15 just calculated. As you will see, it cannot be found exactly, but it lies between the two rows labeled 1.1 and 1.2. We therefore have to **interpolate** to use the table. In the present case, this is easy, because 1.15 lies exactly halfway between them.
3. Follow the row labeled 1.1 across to the column labeled "Beta = 0.10." There you will find that this value of delta/sigma requires an estimated sample size of 27 patients per treatment. The entry just below that, 23, corresponds to a delta/sigma value of 1.2. The desired sample size is that which would lie halfway between these values; this is 25, your required sample size per treatment. Because there are four treatments, you will need 100 patients altogether. See the note following point 4 for a more complete description of this process of **linear interpolation**.
4. In some trials, additional patients are planned for to compensate for losses. In this case, however, we are assuming that there will be few

noncompleters, and we will not increase the number just found. This step completes Example 5.1.

Note: The process described in previous step 2 can be used whenever the desired value of delta/sigma lies somewhere between two tabulated values in the table. It is called **linear interpolation**, because in using it you assume that differences between tabulated values are proportional, which is reasonable for small intervals. You will need to use interpolation in the sample size tables whenever your value of delta/sigma does not come out to an exact one-decimal value. When delta/sigma does not lie exactly halfway between two entries, as it does in Example 5.1, you take a proportion. For example, if the value of delta/sigma were 1.12, that would be two-tenths, or 20%, of the distance between 1.1 and 1.2, and therefore also 20% of the distance between 27 and 23. Because 20% of the difference between these two points is 0.2×4, or 0.8, the sample size needed would be $27 - 0.8$, or 26.2. We could drop the 0.2 and call it 26, or, to be more conservative, use the next sample size above 26.2, which is 27.

5.2   FREQUENCY DISTRIBUTIONS

5.2.1   Introduction

We include this section because it treats a fundamental topic in applied as well as theoretical statistics, and will supplement your understanding of the previous sample size section. In this and succeeding chapters, the ideas of **distributions (populations)** will be referred to often.

5.2.2   Theoretical Distributions

The concept of a theoretical **probability distribution** or population is part of the very foundation of applied statistics. The concept of such distributions and the probabilistic notions associated with them are basic to the ideas that form the connection between statistical theory and the applied science of statistics. For example, we calculate elementary quantities, such as averages (e.g., arithmetic means) and standard deviations, from measurements made during a clinical study. These quantities are said to be **estimates** of corresponding characteristics of the larger group from which the sample is assumed to have been taken. The estimates are called **statistics**. A mathematical idea called the principle of least squares supports the relationship between the statistics and the characteristics of larger groups that they estimate—viz., the **parameters** of the distributions. The larger groups are called **distributions, probability distributions**, or **populations**. In our example, the **sample** of patients is thought of as a small set of measurements taken from a very large, sometimes infinite population of patients. In the present case, that population would consists of all possible similar patients, existing in the past, present, and future, who might have used, now use, or will use the new drug we are testing.[14]

The population characteristics estimated by statistics such as means or standard deviations are called **parameters**. They are termed **unbiased** estimates if the statistic is believed to be equal to the parameter in the long run, except for random variation. If there is a consistent "leaning" toward a value not equal to the parameter, a statistic is called **biased**.[15]

A theoretical probability distribution or population may be finite or infinite. A population of measurements such as the VAS is usually considered to be infinite. It could be defined as an unlimited number of measurements done on a single patient or as one measurement for each of an unlimited number of patients. Some populations may be finite, but so large that they can be considered infinite as a practical matter. Of course, an infinite population is theoretical, and cannot be manipulated, although there are ways to simulate such a function. Despite this nebulosity, the idea is basic to all of modern applied experimental design and statistical analysis and is universally accepted.

As we said, sigma (σ) is a parameter of a distribution. Geometrically, in a graph (plot) of a symmetrical distribution, it is the distance between *either* **inflection point** of the curve and a vertical line dropped from the center point.[16] A so-called **normal distribution** is illustrated in Figure 5.4, shown later in this section. It is symmetrical from left to right, with an inflection point one either side. These are the points on the curve where its shape changes from concave to convex. The horizontal distance from either inflection point to the center line is equal to one sigma. Figure 5.4 is a conventional illustration of a standardized normal probability distribution. The curve could be a plot of the relative occurrence of given values of the VAS measurement (on the vertical axis, which is conventionally not shown) versus the VAS measurement itself (on the horizontal axis).

In a so-called **standard normal** or **standardized normal** curve, the parameter mu (μ) (the mean) is zero (it is the center point on the horizontal axis), and the negative and positive distances from the mean are expressed as numbers of sigmas. Because the units of sigma are the units of the test used (VAS in this case), the horizontal axis really shows the VAS scale, transformed so that its center point is zero. Note that we are assuming, for

---

[14]The word "population" is frequently used in the medical literature and in conversation by people concerned with running clinical trials when they really mean "sample."

[15]Biased estimates can nevertheless be useful. The standard deviation, s (discussed in what follows), is a biased estimate of the parameter, sigma. The square of s, s^2, however, which is called the **variance**, σ^2, is unbiased. One way to remember this is to note that if the variance is unbiased, its square root cannot be, since the **transformation** of a number to its square root is not a linear one. Statisticians use the variance rather than the standard deviation in their calculations whenever practical.

[16]The **distribution function** is often, inexactly, called a "bell-shaped curve," or a "bell curve." Of course, there can be (and are) many functions having a similar shape, only one of which is the normal distribution function.

illustration, that the VAS scale produces normally distributed data. This is not necessarily true, although the distribution may be near enough to normal to justify the use of statistical tests, like Student's *t*, which assume that the samples are taken from normal distributions. Incidentally, you should remember also that a separate distribution, each with the same sigma value but a different mean, is postulated for each treatment.

The curve of Figure 5.4 is the basis for the tables of the standardized normal distribution given in most statistics texts (Table A.5 in the Appendix is a shortened example). In the most common form of such a table, the units along the horizontal axis (the number of sigmas) are usually called *Z*, and the body of the table shows the area under the curve. Areas are taken between limits subtended by the portion of the curve between some point along the horizontal axis, at one or the other side of the center line, to the end of that side of the curve at infinity. Because the total area under the standardized normal curve is 1.0, such a "tail area" can be interpreted as the probability that a given measurement belonging to the distribution, taken at random, will lie within that area. These concepts are used in Part V in the formulas given there for estimating sample size.

In Figure 5.4, you can see that if sigmas were smaller, the curve would be narrower, and vice versa. Thus, the width of the distribution curve is a function of sigma. If there were no variation at all among repeated measurements or patients, the diagram would have no width, sigma would be equal to zero, and the entire "curve" could be represented by a line extending downward from the location of the present peak of the curve to the baseline. Note that sigma is not only a *geometric* function of the width of the curve (the distances from the inflection points), but it is also an *analytic* measure of the degree of variation existing among the population of measurements. Our use of it in this book will be analytic, that is, we will calculate it algebraically. The geometric concept has been used because it clarifies the nature of sigma as well as the other characteristics of the distribution.

Finally, as you have probably already guessed, the normal distribution has just two **parameters**—the mean and sigma. If you know the function of the normal curve (its "formula" or equation), it can be completely defined when these two values are known. In the standard normal distribution, the mean is called mu (μ), and is zero (the center point on the horizontal axis). Of course, the distribution could be partially represented with actual values along the bottom, in which case, parameter mu would have a nonzero value, that of the treatment population mean.

5.2.3   Sample Distributions

Unlike theoretical distributions, **sample distributions** are always finite and can therefore be studied. As an example, the VAS data for one of the treatments in the trial of Example 5.1 could be sorted by size and arranged along a horizontal scale, providing for measurement units from 0 to 100, as in our VAS scale. Along this horizontal line, bars of equal width, each representing a narrow range of values, could be arranged. Their heights could be made to represent the frequency of occurrence of sample values within each range, on the vertical axis. This kind of graph is called a **histogram**.[17] If there are a reasonable number of measurements in a histogram, say, the 25 obtained from one of the four groups in the trial of Example 5.1, a pattern will begin to appear. There will tend to be a greater number of values near the center of the diagram, and the heights of the bars will tend to diminish at both sides of the center as their distances from the center increase. In other words, measurements on either side of the mean will become less and less common, and the bars will therefore become progressively shorter.

There is a trick to getting a histogram to display the sample distribution most clearly. The number of ranges (represented by the bars) should usually be between about 7 and 12. Too many will result in a "stretched-out" appearance, will tend to obscure the shape of the curve traced by the outline of the tops of the bars, and will result in too many empty ranges. Too few will make the arrangement of bars too narrow for clarity. As the number of data increases, the number of ranges can be increased toward the maximum of about 12, if desired. You will note, however, that in Figures 5.1 to 5.3 displayed a little further on, all of the figures used the same number of ranges. This was done to simplify the comparisons of the figures.

When Example 5.1 was completed, there were 100 VAS data (four groups of 25 each) available. To illustrate the estimation of the parent distribution characteristics from a sample distribution, any one of the four might have been plotted as just described. But you may wish to compare groups or to plot more than one group on the same graph to observe the changes in shape of the outlines of the bars as the numbers of data increase. In such a case, however, if the means of the groups were different as a result of different degrees of efficacy of the four treatments, the center point of each distribution would lie at different points along the horizontal axis. That is, the so-called **location** of each distribution would be different. You would have four small distributions, each having the same standard deviation but different means. However, it is advantageous to show one large sample population with a single mean and standard deviation, because the larger sample size will more nearly approximate the shape and parameters of the parent distribution or population. One simple way to accomplish this is to use **residuals**.

5.2.4 Calculating Residuals

You can eliminate the differences in location due to the presence of different sample means with a little arithmetic. You do this by calculating and plotting **residuals** (error estimates) and substituting them for the original data. A

---

[17]A histogram is a "bar chart" in which the *area* of each bar represents the frequency of occurrence of values within a certain range, and in which the width symbolizes that range or *class interval*. Remember that the area of a rectangle is its width times its height.

residual is a datum from which the mean has been removed (i.e., made to equal zero), leaving only the variable part—the error of the measurement.

To clarify this, consider the following: A measurement can be thought of as having two parts—the "actual value" of the measurement, usually called the **fitted value**, and the error part, or residual. If the residuals were all zero, what would the values of the measurements be? The answer is that they would all be identical and would be equal to the average (arithmetic mean). Therefore, the mean of each group must equal the fitted value of every measurement in that group. It follows that if we subtract the mean of a group from each datum in that group, we can obtain the residuals, or error estimates for that group.[18] Because all the groups will now have the same mean, and if, as postulated, all groups have about the same standard deviation, we may plot residuals together on a single plot from as many groups as we wish. The sum and therefore the mean of the distribution of the residuals will always add to zero, except for rounding error.

Table 5.1 shows the 100 VAS data obtained when the example was run.

To illustrate the method of calculating the residuals, let's compute the first one. The process described earlier is represented by the formulas

$$Y = \overline{Y} + R \qquad (4.1)$$

$$R = Y - \overline{Y} \qquad (4.2)$$

where Y is an individual VAS value, $\overline{Y}$ is the mean of the group to which Y belongs, and R represents the residual. Equation 4.1 illustrates the two parts of the measurement, Y, just described. These are the fitted value (in this case, the mean of the group) and the error estimate, or residual. Equation 4.2 is a rearrangement of Equation 4.1 to define the residual. Now, apply Equation 4.2 to the first VAS datum (which is 24):

$$R = Y - \overline{Y}$$
$$= 24 - 26.68$$
$$= -2.68$$

Table 5.2 shows the residuals calculated from the VAS data of Table 5.1 in this way. They are grouped by the treatments from which they were derived. Because the sums and thus the means of the residuals are all zero, however (in some cases there may be some difference from zero because of

---

[18] Three points with regard to residuals are the following: (1) For more complex designs than that of Example 5.1, residuals cannot be as easily calculated as just described. (2) The residuals are estimates of the population error values, and the value of s can be calculated from them. (3) Although the population error values are independent of one another (if the data were obtained independently for each subject, and only that subject, as specified), *residuals* (which are statistics, of course, not parameters) are *correlated* with each other. This means that each is related in some way to the others. Fortunately, for reasonably sized groups, say, 10 to 15 or more, this lack of independence does not ordinarily severely distort conclusions drawn using residuals.

Table 5.1. Original VAS Data from Example 5.1

	Treatments		
A	B	C	D
24	72	51	58
13	61	58	25
25	77	53	42
30	82	71	30
27	79	56	28
22	64	38	51
1	68	64	32
29	78	58	26
38	60	56	35
19	69	50	37
36	65	72	37
11	80	63	36
25	84	26	34
28	78	54	26
27	67	62	26
33	97	67	2
25	67	73	29
38	68	60	24
28	85	52	28
29	82	52	24
16	59	37	30
37	72	48	31
31	76	75	26
31	83	46	30
44	81	50	32
Sum 667	1854	1392	779
Mean 26.68	74.16	55.68	31.16
Std. Dev. 9.48	9.33	11.75	10.15

rounding), and because we are assuming that the group standard deviations
—that is, the standard deviations of each of the four sample
distributions—are similar (and reflect equal *population* variation), the grouping
by treatments is done merely for clarity. It is *not* expected that the four
groups would exhibit differences if each were plotted separately.

5.2.5   Plots of Sample Distributions

Figure 5.1 is a histogram of the first 25 residuals from Table 5.2 (those
corresponding to treatment A). If the original VAS data themselves had been

Table 5.2. Residuals Calculated from VAS Responses of Table 5.1

Treatment Group			
A	B	C	D
− 2.68	− 2.16	− 4.68	26.84
− 13.68	− 13.16	2.32	− 6.16
− 1.68	2.84	− 2.68	10.84
3.32	7.84	15.32	− 1.16
0.32	4.84	0.32	− 3.16
− 4.68	− 10.16	− 17.68	19.84
− 25.68	− 6.16	8.32	0.84
2.32	3.84	2.32	− 5.16
11.32	− 14.16	0.32	3.84
− 7.68	− 5.16	− 5.68	5.84
9.32	− 9.16	16.32	5.84
− 15.68	5.84	7.32	4.84
− 1.68	9.84	− 29.68	2.84
1.32	3.84	− 1.68	− 5.16
0.32	− 7.16	6.32	− 5.16
6.32	22.84	11.32	− 29.16
− 1.68	− 7.16	17.32	− 2.16
11.32	− 6.16	4.32	− 7.16
1.32	10.84	− 3.68	− 3.16
2.32	7.84	− 3.68	− 7.16
− 10.68	− 15.16	− 18.68	− 1.16
10.32	− 2.16	− 7.68	− 0.16
4.32	1.84	19.32	− 5.16
4.32	8.84	− 9.68	− 1.16
17.32	6.84	− 5.68	0.84

plotted instead of their residuals, the histogram would have been identical in appearance to Figure 5.1, but the values on the horizontal axis would have been different. These ranges are shown in Table 5.3. They are numbered from 1 to 12. The ranges are identified on the plot by their range numbers rather than the actual values, to avoid a crowded appearance. In Figure 5.1, there is one bar for each of these ranges of VAS values, and its width defines the upper and lower limits of the range. Its height represents the number of measurements in the range. The several bars together include all of the values in treatment group A, grouped into the 12 ranges. The horizontal scale thus represents the values of the residuals from the VAS response values, and the vertical scale represents the frequency of occurrence of the responses. The arithmetic mean of the 25 residuals (it is equal to zero) is at the center of the entire group of bars. The overall width of the plot represents the spread of the data and is a function of the standard deviation.

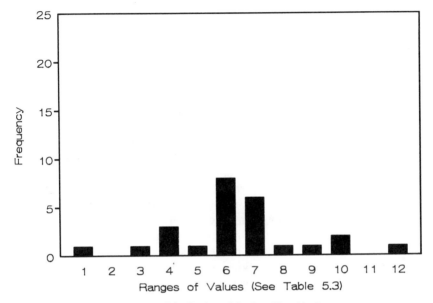

Figure 5.1 Distribution of the first 25 residuals.

Note the rather amazing similarity of Figure 5.1 to a symmetric distribution, roughly the shape of the normal, despite the fact that it was constructed
from only 25 data. If you were to construct similar plots for each of a number
of sets of such samples, but of increasing size (such as the 25 as shown
before, then 50, then 100, then 500, etc.), you would obtain increasingly
smooth curves, on the average. But the increases in smoothness would

**Table 5.3. Ranges Used in the Histograms
of Figures 5.1, 5.2, and 5.3**

Range No.	Range
1	-30.0 to -25.1
2	-25.0 to -20.1
3	-20.0 to -15.1
4	-15.0 to -10.1
5	-10.0 to -5.1
6	-5.0 to -0.1
7	0.0 to 4.9
8	5.0 to 9.9
9	10.0 to 14.9
10	15.0 to 19.9
11	20.0 to 24.9
12	25.0 to 29.9

diminish as the number of data increased, so unless the steps between successive plots were large, the greater smoothness might not be apparent in each successive plot unless the increases in size were successively greater. For certain kinds of distributions, including the **normal** (as these data have been constrained to be), the plots would also become increasingly symmetrical as the sample sizes increased. When the size reached perhaps 200 data or more, they would begin to closely resemble a smooth symmetrical curve.

Figure 5.1 is a **sample distribution** of the 25 residuals. In this graph, you can see the start of the formation of a bell-shaped curve. There are still too few data involved, however, to clearly define the shape of the curve. In studying this and the next three plots, bear in mind that despite any apparent departures of the curves from normality, the original data were deliberately constructed from random normal numbers, and therefore are *known* to be normally distributed and to have a specific standard deviation ($s = 10$). Any departure from normality of the sample distributions, therefore, is due to random variation and will serve to demonstrate the fairly large extent to which sample statistics can sometimes depart from population characteristics.

Figure 5.2 is a plot that was produced in exactly the same way as Figure 5.1, but with 50 instead of 25 residuals—those from both columns 1 and 2 of Table 5.2 (i.e., from treatment groups A and B). Here, the Gaussian (normal) shape is much more apparent, although, by chance, the curve is a bit lopsided (**skewed**). Notice how much difference 25 more residuals made in defining the shape of the curve!

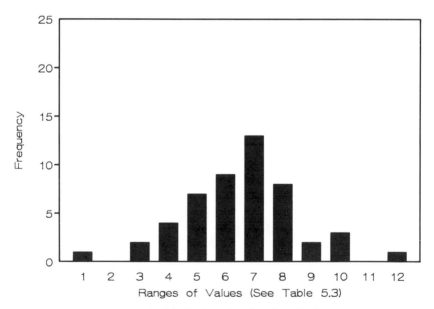

Figure 5.2   Distribution of the first 50 residuals.

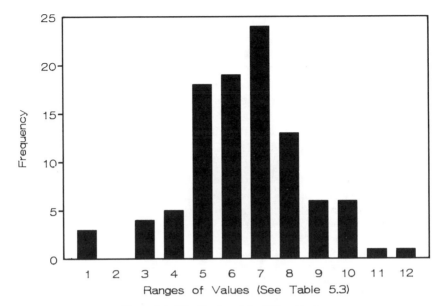

Figure 5.3   Distribution of the 100 residuals.

Figure 5.3 is a plot of 100 residuals from Table 5.2. The appearance of this graph approaches most nearly the ideal Gaussian shape, although because ranges 5 and 6 contain a few more residuals than the ideal numbers, the curve still looks a bit lopsided. If we had 200 or 300 more data, the resulting curve would be likely to appear quite symmetrical and much smoother.

Figures 5.1, 5.2, and 5.3 illustrate very clearly how difficult it can be to show that data are truly normally distributed, although, qualitatively, the plots may strikingly resemble normal distributions. Even when fairly large samples are available, it is often difficult to obtain reasonable assurance that the samples come from a distribution with a shape close to normal, at least without statistical tests of normality more sensitive than the graphical method we have been using here. On the other hand, the requirements of normality in certain statistical tests such as the t test and the analysis of variance (Part IV), which underlie most of the sample size procedures described in this book, are not so rigorous as to preclude their use when the data describe curves as close to normal as those just illustrated by the plots of the residuals in Example 5.1.

Think for a minute about the remarkable resemblance of these small sample distributions to their parent distribution (which we know to have been normal). Perhaps the most remarkable thing about the foregoing exercise is that out of randomness, with simple techniques, we can find order—nearly symmetrical curves from what appear to be confusions of random numbers. In fact, although the random numbers used to construct the data for treatments A through D were random *normal* numbers, normally distributed random numbers can be closely approximated even from *completely* random numbers, that is, from numbers whose distributions (in the long run) show equal frequencies at every range between their maximum and minimum values ("flat" distributions). Such approximately normal distributions can be constructed by using **arithmetic means** (*averages*) of as few as four or five ordinary random numbers from a flat distribution. These form quite good approximations of the normal. This demonstrates a fundamental fact of statistics—arithmetic means tend more and more to be distributed normally as the number of data used to calculate each mean increases. This occurs regardless of the nature of the original distribution. This characteristic is a principal reason for the fact that statistical procedures based upon the normal distribution have such wide applicability.

5.2.6 Plot of the Standardized Normal Distribution

The ultimate normal or Gaussian distribution curve is the one you would obtain if you had the patience and longevity necessary to construct it from an infinite number of normally distributed data. Figure 5.4 is a diagram of that *theoretical* perfect distribution. The measurements could be VAS pain scores, heights of people, blood chemistry, residuals from such data, or any other set of numbers, if normally distributed. The measurements along the horizontal axis are shown as terminating at -3 and 3 sigmas, but, in theory, they extend

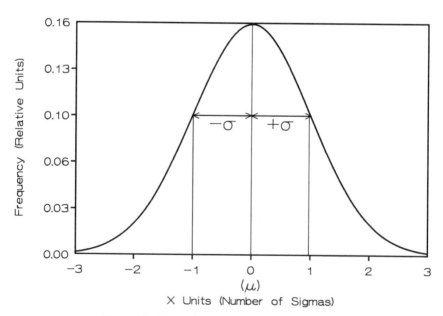

Figure 5.4 Theoretical standard normal distribution.

to infinity in both directions. The curve is perfectly symmetrical, and the heights of the two tails at any point bear a particular relationship to the other dimensions of the curve. Sigma is the horizontal distance from the center line to either inflection point, as shown. The mean of the distribution is a parameter called μ (mu), and is located on the X, or horizontal, axis at the center line. Mu is the parameter that is estimated by the arithmetic mean, a statistic that we represented by $\bar{y}$ (y bar) when calculating our residuals. The normal distribution possesses just these two parameters, sigma and mu.

The VAS is a continuous scale, so it is theoretically possible to have a measurement at *any* point along the line, between the prescribed limits. If the scores were *normally distributed* within these limits, this pattern would be symmetrical and would have the other characteristics of that distribution except for the infinitely long tails (because the VAS scores are limited in extent and cannot be less than zero or greater than 100). Although many kinds of real-life VAS measurements, perhaps most, are not normally distributed, there are statistical processes available to the data analyst (**transformations**) by which many sets of sample data can be made normal or reasonably so. This can be an important step when the analysis is one that is sensitive to nonnormality of the measurements, as many are. But let us continue to assume, in this example, that we are working with four normal distributions.

Distributions that extend for infinite distances in both directions are, of course, impossible mathematical fantasies. Nevertheless, perhaps surprisingly, as already indicated, they are useful in applied as well as theoretical statistics. The properties of an assumed infinite distribution can be determined relatively easily by mathematical means. And it turns out, as in many other fields of science, that real and finite sets of data possess many of the properties conceived mathematically or can be made to do so quite precisely. For example, as you can see, the outline of the tops of the bars in Figure 5.1, although based upon only 25 data, resembles Figure 5.4, the theoretical distribution, to a surprising degree.

5.3 SUMMARY OF THE CHAPTER

This chapter is divided into three major sections. The first is an introduction to the estimation of sample size using a table. In the second, the ideas of theoretical and sample distributions, essential to understanding the material to follow and fundamental to almost all the ideas and procedures of applied statistics, are presented. The third section is this summary.

In Example 5.1, a tabular method of estimating sample size for a study having more than two treatments is given. The meaning and use of the four quantities **alpha**, **beta**, **delta**, and **sigma** in estimating sample size is explained. A sample size adequate to maintain all of these at their specified values is obtained. Other methods of estimation, including other tables or methods of calculation, are shown in Part V.

The section on distributions focuses upon the normal distribution and emphasizes the distinction between a theoretical **distribution**, or **population**, and a sample taken from it. A series of plots is shown, using **residuals** calculated from the data obtained from Example 5.1, to demonstrate the approximation of the shape of the theoretical normal distribution with sample data.

5.4 LITERATURE REFERENCES

(1) Bratcher, T. L., M. A. Moran, and W. J. Zimmer, *Journal of Quality Technology*, **2**, 156–164 (1970).

CHAPTER 6

Planning Your Trial: III

6.1 ABOUT THIS CHAPTER

Most of this chapter is concerned with some general material about randomization. Randomization methods vary with the kind of experimental design used (in fact, the randomization method constitutes the only difference between some designs), so this very important subject is treated again in Part III as each design is introduced and discussed. In addition to the material on randomization, there is some material on blinding in this chapter, as well as a few other topics about planning that should be mentioned.

This book reflects the customary use of the term **randomization**. Unless otherwise stated, it refers to the **random assignment** of treatments to patients (or of patients to treatments). In the domain of clinical trials, it almost never refers to the **random sampling** of a group of patients from a population, such as might be attempted in a poll or other type of survey. If and when we use it in the latter sense, we will so indicate.

6.2 DEVISING A RANDOMIZATION PLAN

6.2.1 Introduction

In this section, in addition to the general coverage of randomization, a description of a random-assignment procedure for specific use in the tension headache study (Example 4.1, Chapter 4, and Example 5.1, Chapter 5) is described. We will present that in the form of a new example, for easy reference. The techniques of this chapter are particularly applicable to "completely randomized" designs, but they will also serve to illustrate a number of the general principles of randomization. We believe that the coverage of randomization and random processes should be very thorough, because it is quite often done improperly.

6.2.2   Topics to Be Covered

The following issues are discussed in this section on randomization:

1. Definitions
2. Why is random assignment essential?
3. Selecting a suitable method of randomization
4. Randomizing in blocks
5. Random assignment and random selection
6. Stratification and matching
7. Example 6.1: Randomizing a One-Factor Design

6.2.3   Definitions

Nature of Randomization

It is easier to describe what is not random than to define randomness, although methods of achieving it are not difficult to explain or understand. However, the **random assignment** of treatments to patients is quite simply explained and described, and is easy to grasp.

An operative definition that describes the nature of random assignment in a parallel clinical study with equal treatment group sizes could be the following: **If the assignment of treatments to patients is done so that there is a known probability of each patient receiving any of the treatments, the assignment has been done randomly**. This defines the *effect* of the process, but not the process itself. Some procedures for achieving this effect are described in this chapter.

Usually, a random-assignment procedure is arranged to give each patient an *equal* probability of receiving a given treatment. This is very simple to do in a completely randomized design. You can choose one of the treatments randomly for assignment to a patient or choose a patient randomly for assignment to one of the treatments. You repeat this step until each treatment group reaches the desired size. You arrange to use group sizes specified by your sample size estimate. The randomization should be done during planning, before any patients are seen. This eliminates one source of bias. When this method is used, you select a group of numbers from 1 to N, where N is the total number of patients required. During the planning process, you randomly assign the treatments to these numbers as if the numbers were the patients. Later, during the trial, the patients are actually numbered by an arbitrary means, such as the order in which they qualify for the test (they should not be numbered until you are sure that they will take part). Once the specified group size for any given treatment is reached, you no longer assign that particular treatment.

One problem that people inexperienced with randomization in experiments often encounter is a difficulty in recognizing a suitable random-selection process, that is, one that is not deterministic. A crude example of a deterministic, nonrandom process is to assign one of two drugs to every other patient accepted into a study, and the other to the alternate patients. Another is to haphazardly decide, as each patient appears, which treatment he or she will get. A third is to assign each of two treatments according to whether a patient's birth date is odd or even. A fourth is to mark patient numbers on slips of paper and draw one from a container as each patient appears. All of these except the last are nonrandom. The last may be a random process, but probably is not, because it is very difficult to make a truly random selection in this way. There are many others. Unhappily, all of them have been used in the "randomization" of clinical trials.

In rare instances, you may need to design a parallel study in which the treatment groups are of unequal sizes (i.e., in which the probability of a treatment being assigned to a given patient is not the same for all treatments). This is easily arranged in the same way as before, by ceasing to assign patients to any group that has reached the desired size.

The foregoing is the usual procedure for **completely randomized** parallel designs, such as that of Examples 4.1 and 5.1, when you wish to provide equal probabilities of assignment. However, it is not a serious disadvantage to let the group sizes vary moderately by *not* suspending assignment when a group reaches a targeted size. This will result in somewhat unequal-sized groups (usually not greatly different percentagewise unless the group sizes are quite small), will complicate the data analysis slightly, and will reduce the power of the subsequent statistical tests a little. However, in this way, you can avoid compromising the randomization at all. On the other hand, the slight departure from pure chance assignment that exists when you control the group sizes is rarely serious.

As you will see later, there are many experimental designs that require randomization procedures more complex than those used in the completely randomized and parallel structure of Examples 4.1 and 5.1. In general, for each type of design, the randomization method will be different. A more detailed description of the *purposes* of randomization appears later, but a major purpose is to ensure that patient differences that might affect the outcome of the test will be distributed as similarly as possible among all treatments. Randomization would not be needed for this purpose if you could sort your patients by *all* the characteristics that *might* affect the outcome of the trial and then ensure the distribution of *each* treatment equally among them. But this is obviously impossible.[1]

Any experimental design except a completely randomized arrangement allows for the identification and compensation of the effects of one or a few of these unplanned-for characteristics (sources of variation). For example, a

---

[1] This is what is attempted by **matching**. But (a) in matching, it is a matter of the experimenter's opinion whether a given characteristic will affect the outcome, and (b) there are likely to be so many characteristics to be matched upon, even in the experimenter's opinion, that the experiment will become impossibly large. This will lead either to the omission of some characteristics that may be critical, abandonment of the experiment, or the use of randomization.

randomized blocks changeover trial in which patients are the blocks eliminates bias due to patient characteristics, because each patient eventually
receives all of the treatments (see Chapter 12). But randomization is necessary even with such designs to take care of variation that is always to be
expected from unidentified sources of variation between and within patients.

The foregoing may sound complex and perhaps vague, and unfortunately
vagueness and complexity are often characteristics of discussions of randomization in the abstract. But you will have no trouble at all in learning how to
arrange for a random assignment of treatments to patients, and in becoming
familiar with some of the properties of the resulting treatment groups. There
are some procedures, such as those mentioned earlier, which must be
avoided; they may seem random, but they are not. **No such system should
ever be substituted for true random assignment**. If any of these are used,
your results will quite likely be wrong or at least not supportable. And the
FDA will most certainly refuse to accept your data as a primary source of
evidence for efficacy. There are one or two quite rare exceptions to this rule.
Such nonrandomization is discussed at more length later in this chapter.

How to actually make the random selections has not yet been shown. We
begin to do so in the following section.

Random Numbers

A series of **random numbers** is one in which each number between defined
limits[2] occurs with equal probability in the long run, and in which each
number has an equal probability of occurring and of preceding or following
any other. The term **random sequence**, implying **random order**, is sometimes
used. In such an array, there could be any number of repetitions of the same
number in groups or distributed throughout the range of numbers. A sample
of such numbers forms what is sometimes called a "flat," or rectangular,
distribution.

Such sets of random numbers can be plotted just as the random normal
numbers were in the preceding chapter. A theoretical frequency distribution
of an infinite number of random numbers (integers) is shown in Figure 6.1.
When such a distribution is created, every time a number is added to the set,
the new number could be any integer within the defined range, with equal
probability. When there is a very large number of values, the graph will have
a smooth rectangular appearance, as represented in Figure 6.1. This is
analogous to the normal curve that was plotted as Figure 5.4 in Chapter 5.
The overall range (maximum and minimum values) is defined by the two
numbers, a and b, on the horizontal axis. As for the normal distribution, the
mean is the midpoint along the horizontal axis, and is called μ (mu).

---

[2]The limits can be any at all, including plus and minus infinity. Usually, however, in our work,
they are definite. For example, you might work with a table, calculator, or computer that
produces random numbers between 0 and 1. There are many ways to obtain random sequences
of numbers in any range.

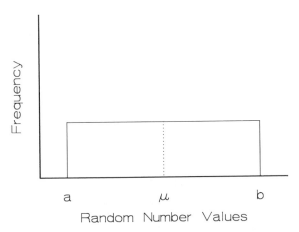

Figure 6.1 Theoretical rectangular distribution.

Table 6.1 contains 100 random whole numbers between 1 and 20, generated with a pocket calculator. This **sample distribution** of 100 is plotted in
Figure 6.2, in the same way as was done with the residuals in Figure 5.3 of
Chapter 5. Ten ranges were set up to plot this set (see the discussion of
histograms in Chapter 5); these are given in Table 6.2. Contrary to the case
of the normally distributed residuals of Figure 5.3, there is no systematic
reduction in the frequencies of values as the extremes (tails) of Figure 6.2 are
approached. The reason, of course, is that when the numbers were being
generated, any number between 1 and 20 was equally likely. Thus, the
long-run tendency was for approximately equal numbers of each value to
appear. This is not true for the normal distribution, or any other in which the
probability of occurrence of a given value becomes smaller as its distance
from the mean increases. Because the distribution in Figure 6.2 is a sample
distribution of a small number of values, like the sample distributions of
residuals in Chapter 5 (as in Figure 5.3), it has an irregular outline.

Table 6.1. One Hundred Random Numbers between 1 and 20

2	11	19	14	2	4	3	17	14	12
5	2	16	12	19	9	13	2	14	2
20	7	14	12	11	19	2	15	9	2
9	9	20	6	7	4	5	9	13	19
14	15	11	19	8	6	14	18	10	12
4	1	17	19	16	13	9	6	11	1
18	13	15	15	9	3	12	4	19	4
9	10	1	11	6	6	15	19	7	17
3	15	9	12	3	6	4	2	16	14
11	16	11	3	19	10	9	2	7	7

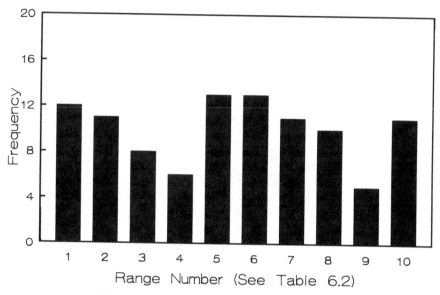

Figure 6.2   Sample distribution of random integers.

Table 6.2. Ranges and Frequencies Used to Plot 100 Random Numbers

Range No.	Range	Frequency
1	1 to 2	12
2	3 to 4	11
3	5 to 6	8
4	7 to 8	6
5	9 to 10	13
6	11 to 12	13
7	13 to 14	11
8	15 to 16	10
9	17 to 18	5
10	19 to 20	11

Random Permutations

A **random permutation** of a string of numbers, letters, or other symbols is an arrangement in which the **order** of each number or symbol is random. In such a case, there would be only one occurrence of each item, but its position in the string would be chosen randomly from all possible positions. Before the permutation was created, each number would have had an equal probability of following any other number. In other words, a *permutation* is one in which each number occurs in a specific *position* in the set. A *random permutation* is one in which that position has been selected randomly.

For example, suppose that in a changeover design[3] you wish to select a set of three treatments in random order. If the treatments were numbered from 1 to 3, there are six possible random permutations or random orders in which they could be administered to each patient in a changeover design, that is, one in which each patient will receive each of the treatments, perhaps one each week. The six possible orders would be 1, 2, 3; 1, 3, 2; 2, 1, 3; 2, 3, 1; 3, 1, 2; and 3, 2, 1. In most cases in such experiments, you would probably arrange for equal numbers of patients to receive the three drugs in each of these six orders. If so, *orders* would be a factor in the design.

When Latin squares are discussed in part III, you will see examples of permutations of sets of letters as well as other symbols.

What Is Not Random

This matter was discussed briefly earlier in this section. In any parallel study design (such as that of Examples 4.1, 5.1, and Example 6.1, described later), one treatment is assigned to each patient. The basic reason for the use of random selection is to make possible valid statistical hypothesis tests of the data (including confidence intervals used as hypothesis tests; see Part IV). That is, to validate the tests, the treatment assigned to any particular patient *must* be a matter of chance. One way to clarify this statement is to consider some methods of assignment that are *not* random. Determining which treatment to assign by the use of any system that does not utilize "chance" (we say, "is not probabilistic") is not random.

For example, "random" assignments have been done in the past by assigning two treatments to alternate patients, or on the basis of the time of day, or by some other systematic (i.e., **deterministic**) procedure. **Such procedures are not random.** As was implied earlier, in some designs, the effects of one or a few specific undesirable sources of variation can be prevented from influencing the responses, so that randomization is not needed to eliminate the effects of those sources. However, some form of randomization must still be used, because any good experimental technique requires the assumption that there can be additional and unknown sources of undesirable variation that the design per se will not eliminate, and that must therefore be spread randomly throughout all observations. Later, you will read about some common designs other than the completely randomized arrangements typified by Examples 4.1 and 5.1, and you will see that as the structure of an experiment becomes more complex, **restriction of randomization** is used increasingly. Thus, it is not necessarily incorrect to limit the randomization of some designs, but it must be done carefully and with understanding.

Characterization of a Randomized Design

Usually, as in this example, the randomization of a completely randomized parallel design is arranged so that each treatment is assigned to the same

---

[3] A changeover design is one in which each patient receives more than one treatment. In common kinds of changeovers, every patient receives each of the treatments used in the trial, one per week, for example. Some of these designs are described in Part III, Chapter 12.

number of patients. That is, before the assignments are made, the procedure is planned so that each patient will have an equal a priori probability of receiving any one of the treatments, and that probability is 1 divided by the number of treatments. In Example 4.1, because there are four treatments, there will be a probability of $1/4$, or 0.25, of any patient receiving a given treatment *before* the assignments are made. In most trials using this kind of design, after the randomization, each treatment group will consist of equal numbers of patients. After a trial is complete, the groups may of course be unequal because of patient noncompleters.

6.2.4   Why Is Random Assignment Essential?

The most important reason for using random assignment in clinical trials is to ensure the validity of the usual statistical hypothesis tests (significance tests) that will be used at the end of almost any industrial drug trial. If an inappropriate randomization is used, the validity of these tests will be unknown, but they will be unlikely to be correct. The FDA recognizes this by generally refusing to approve nonrandomized or incorrectly randomized trials as primary evidence of safety or efficacy.

In the literature, there are many other reasons given for the use of randomization, generally having to do with more obvious matters than the validity of the hypothesis tests used. Most of these are different aspects of the same argument. For example, if the sex of a subject is thought to have an effect on the response in a trial, randomization can make it a matter of chance whether a woman or a man is selected for a given treatment. On the average, with moderate to large sample sizes, the result will be that the number of men and women assigned to each treatment will be approximately equal. As you will see in Part III (experimental designs), it is also a correct procedure to *exactly* balance the numbers of males and females in a trial, and in that way, in the subsequent analysis, completely eliminate any possible sex effect. By the same token, if age or body weight is thought to influence treatment responses, its influence can also be controlled by randomization or balancing. However, there can be many factors beyond those that may be anticipated, and that, consequently, are not "balanced out." Those factors may nevertheless influence results. But such unknown factors need not create any serious problem for you. Even though those factors are not identified, if there are any present, randomization on average will produce a fair assignment of treatments and in most cases will eliminate any serious consequences. And randomization is the only known method by which this can be achieved. A well-designed clinical trial will therefore make provision for the control of such unknown or unforeseen factors by the use of correctly done random assignments.

Successful and Unsuccessful Randomization
No randomization can be expected to provide a guarantee that the assignments will be distributed with perfect equality of patient characteristics. It is

possible to have quite a "bad" randomization, in which there is a serious lack of balance of some patient attributes with respect to the treatment assignments. For example, it could happen, in a two-treatment study, that a large excess of female or male patients is assigned to one of the treatments. If patients are entered into the trial a few at a time, as is often necessary in large trials or when the disease condition is not common, there is little that can be done. If this difficulty is foreseen during planning, and it is believed that such an unbalanced condition may influence the outcome, the sex of the patients could be made one of the factors. If the disturbing factor is unexpected and is not encountered until the trial has been running for a time, there is little that can be done.

If such an unbalanced patient group is obtained in a smaller study, when, in some cases, all the necessary patients may be qualified and available before the treatment starts, the randomization is sometimes repeated. And for a study with patients to be entered sequentially, when the randomization is done during planning, a rare pattern will sometimes emerge (such as a long string of patients sequentially assigned to one of the treatments). In such a case, also, it is perhaps reasonable to repeat the randomization. As long as this is done only in infrequent cases, it probably does no harm; see Neter, Wasserman, and Kutner [37], p. 901, para. 2.

There may be chance unbalances among the treatment groups in a study that remain undetected, and that may affect results. But you have always been aware of that risk. Not every trial can give unbiased results. And almost never will a project rely upon a single trial; the FDA is highly unlikely to approve a drug on such a basis. So if one of your trials was biased, it will be obvious after others have been done.

The use of randomization is the best tool we have for avoiding bias. **Studies done without any randomization are very likely to be seriously biased**. Unfortunately, unrandomized experimental studies are still commonly found in the medical journals, although they are much less frequent in industry, at least after submission of one of them to the FDA.[4]

6.2.5 Selecting a Suitable Method of Randomization

The several components in the design of a clinical trial are interdependent. One of these is the method of randomization. When you specify a randomization method, you must keep the structure of your experimental design in mind. We have shown only one design so far, that used in Examples 4.1 and

---

[4]Nonexperimental studies, such as surveys, cohort studies, and the like, must perforce be done without benefit of random assignment of treatments. In such cases, however, it is often true that no study at all could be run if randomization were required. Interpreting the results of such research should be done very cautiously, and only after more evidence is available than would be usually necessary in a randomized trial. The famous Surgeon General's report on smoking is a case in point. It was not possible to randomly assign smoking to some subjects and nonsmoking to others. Yet, as the evidence accumulated, it finally became obvious that many of the indications were correct.

5.1. However, there are many different kinds of design structures. Almost without exception, each requires a different kind of randomization. In some cases, the randomization procedure is the principal difference you will encounter in setting up two different experimental designs.

As we have said, another of the interdependent components of trial design is the kind of statistical analysis to be used. This is determined to a great extent by three other components: the structure of the design, the nature of the response, and the kind of randomization used. There are also other constituents of your planning activities that must be taken into account in deciding what sort of statistical procedures should be used for the data analyses. For example, the sample size and the method used to estimate it will be factors in determining the type of analysis to use. Another is the kind of response used.

Examples 4.1 and 5.1 use a **one-factor** (or **one-way**) **completely randomized** design. The factor in these examples is "drug treatments," at four levels. The phrase "completely randomized" means that there are no restrictions on the randomization procedure except the limitation that you will usually want to design for equal numbers of patients in each treatment group.

6.2.6   Randomizing in Blocks

The kind of blocks to be discussed here are used solely to prevent treatment group sizes from varying excessively when such variation is considered detrimental. The kind of blocking discussed in Part III, in which the blocks are used to eliminate the influence of nuisance variables or reduce the normal variation in response measurements (**experimental error**), and/or in which each patient forms a block (Chapter 12), is different.

In most clinical studies, except very small ones or special cases, patients will enter the clinic(s) and be qualified for a study at irregular intervals rather than all at once. Sometimes, and in some clinics, they may appear very slowly. If you are running a single-center trial, a decision to abandon the study at that center and start again at another may be made before all the patients planned for have been recruited. In a multicenter trial, because of difficulties of one kind or another, a center may be dropped and a new one substituted. The FDA must be notified if these or any other departures from the protocol are made, and you may often or usually need to submit the data from the old center even if it has been shown that it cannot or should not be used in the data analyses.

If a trial is stopped and it is a single-center trial, it is likely that some or all of the treatment groups will vary in size, possibly seriously. If the differences are large, the power of the eventual statistical tests of treatment group differences may be severely impaired. Thus, if it becomes necessary to abort a trial before all the patients have been entered or have completed the treatments, there will be a loss of power due to two sources, the reduction in sample size and the inequality of the numbers of available patients assigned to each treatment.

A solution to any such problem of unbalance can be provided for ahead of time. You can arrange the randomization in "blocks." To do this for the trial of Examples 4.1 and 5.1, create the blocks by constraining the randomization procedure to assign each of the four treatments to the first four patients, in random order, then repeat with the next four, and so on until the required sample size is reached. To accomplish this, you must increase the initial estimate to the next greater multiple of 4 when you estimate the sample size. Now, if patients are recruited slowly, at least you will have limited the magnitude of the possible discrepancies in size that can exist.

Your blocks in a trial with four treatments need not be limited to four patients. You can use blocks of 8, assigning treatments in random order to each in turn, with the restriction that your blocks, if complete, will contain two patients on each treatment. And you can use other block sizes, remembering that the total number of patients you estimated as needed must be evenly divisible by the block size. In this moderate-sized experiment, a good choice might be blocks of 4 or 8.[5]

With such an arrangement, the randomization is said to be **restricted**. Each block will contain four or eight patients (for example),[6] with one of each of the four treatments randomly assigned to each patient. There will be a guarantee that the patient groups within each block will be equal in size, except, possibly, for the last block. If the trial is stopped before all the planned patients have been enrolled, although the group sizes will probably be unequal, they will be nearly the same, because there will be only one discrepant block. For example, suppose that the trial of Examples 4.1 and 5.1 had been blocked in this way, using blocks of four patients. Now, suppose that the trial must be aborted while the 25th of the expected 25 blocks is in progress, and that the second patient in that block has been interviewed. In this case, we will end up with 24 complete blocks, which means that we will have 24 patients for each of the four treatments, plus two more, each on one of the four treatments. Therefore, there will be 25 patients on two of the treatments and 24 on the remaining two. The experiment will have been quite well balanced despite the early stop. Even if the trial had to be stopped

---

[5]Remember, the larger the blocks, the better the blinding is preserved (see Section 6.3), but the greater the probable discrepancy in group sizes if the trial is discontinued before all of the planned-upon number of patients have taken part. On the other hand, as explained later, there is an advantage, especially in small trials, to making the blocks as large as possible. This is true because the smaller the number of blocks, the smaller the loss of degrees of freedom if a correct analysis is done, and therefore, the smaller the loss of power.

[6]The randomization in this case is done as will be described later for a conventional randomized-blocks parallel design. You randomize the assignments of treatments to patients within each block *independently*. The only difference will be that the blocks in this case will not represent any known "nuisance" variable except the effect (if any) of time, due to the sequential entry of patients into the study.

at any earlier point, there would never be a difference in numbers of patients on each treatment of more than 1.

Blocks of Unequal Sizes
In some trials, the blocks are made unequal in size in a haphazard manner so that if the code must be broken for a given patient because of some adverse effect or any other reason, it will not be possible to make a logical guess as to the identity of the treatments being given to the other patients. Despite that advantage, I do not recommend that arrangement because it will make the analysis of the data less powerful. Concern about breaking the blinding can usually be reduced satisfactorily by using equal-sized but larger blocks.

Analysis of Blocked Designs
Many trials that are blocked as described here are subsequently analyzed without taking the blocking into account at all, either because time is short (as it usually is at the end of a trial), the statistician has not been told of the blocking, or it is thought that accounting for the blocks in the statistical model will not affect the results. This is unnecessary gambling. The blocks may differ from each other due to some variable associated with time or differences in handling each, thus forming an additional factor imposed upon the design. In a correct analysis, any possible block effects must be accounted for. It is easy to do this and will not hurt the analysis in any way beyond the loss of a few "degrees of freedom" for error. This will result in a trivial loss of power if the trial is of reasonable size, as in the example. Such an analysis is therefore strongly advisable if the randomization is blocked.

6.2.7 Random Assignment and Random Selection

The patient population of interest in a drug trial (the target population) is that of present and future patients having the condition or symptoms that the test drug(s) are intended to treat. The broad use of *statistical inference* (statistical induction) to draw conclusions about the entire patient population from the analysis of such a trial is not possible. To make such inferences, a *randomly selected* sample of patients would be needed. This is impossible (you can't sample future patients!). Of course, a random sample from the portion of that population that exists at the time of sampling could be taken, but this also is rarely, if ever, done. There are several good reasons for this.

First, a much larger proportion of the patients in the population of interest always exists in the future, whereas a much smaller proportion exists at the time of a study. In order to secure FDA approval of a drug, several years and a considerable series of individual trials are usually required. A statistical sampling of the current patient population, at best, could only be taken from a population existing at the time of a given trial. As a statistical sample, it could not represent a future population.

Second, if there is reasonable agreement among results from each of the series of trials comprising an entire study, done over a period of years, that would constitute good evidence that the several samples all represented the population of interest. You could call this purely *scientific* inference with no statistical component, used as a substitute for the unavailable, purely statistical inference.

Third, conclusions based upon such scientific inference could be strengthened by taking every feasible step to ensure that the patients selected in every trial of the series were as similar as possible in all relevant aspects to those of the target population.

Finally, it would be almost impossible to attempt to sample any representative population of patients for each trial. Each sample would need to be very large, much larger than that required by any sample size estimate, merely to ensure reasonable representation of all aspects of the population. This would be prohibitively expensive and would require inordinate amounts of time (because it would have to be repeated for each trial in the series). It might also be considered unethical in many cases, because many more patients than necessary for a sound conclusion would be subjected to the bother and possible discomfort and danger of a trial.

For all these reasons, random sampling of a target population of patients for any one industrial trial, let alone for each trial in a series, is essentially out of the question.

Similar reasoning applies to the investigators selected. A random sample cannot be taken, so *statistical* inferences cannot be made to the target population of physicians or centers expected to prescribe the drug(s) if approved. Of course, it is always assumed that the samples of center(s) and/or investigator(s), even in a single-center trial, are *representative* of those who will later use the test drug if it is approved. But, like the patient sample, this sample also cannot be random even in a multicenter trial, because the target population will include physicians not yet in practice. Nor will this factor be "random," because only investigators who are well-qualified, willing, and available can be included.[7]

Accordingly, the only randomization in common use in clinical trials is the random *assignment* of the treatments to the patients. This raises the question of what inferences *can* be drawn.

---

[7]When certain kinds of multifactor data are analyzed, whether the set of levels of each factor is "random" (selected randomly from a large or infinite population) or "fixed" (for which the set of levels comprises all levels of interest or relevance) becomes important. But the sample of investigators is never random, because selection is made on the basis of qualifications and availability. Thus, never, or almost never, are either patients or investigators selected randomly from their populations. There have been one or two very large government-sponsored studies that attempted to achieve random sampling of patients, but whether the results were really random samples from the target populations is debatable.

Fortunately, the problem is not as intransient as it may appear. The solution is based upon the nature of the inference that can be made. Although *statistical* inference cannot be used to draw conclusions based upon patients who are not members of the target population, it is perfectly reasonable to use *logical* or *scientific* inference; see Deming (3) and Nelson (4). Furthermore, the random assignment of treatments to patients in a trial, which, unlike the random selection of patients, is easily done, contributes greatly to the reliability of any particular trial. The patients in a sample usually differ from each other in many respects, any of which can affect the response to a treatment. Random assignment ensures that it is a matter of chance that a patient receives a particular treatment. Therefore, random assignment and the use of adequate sample sizes and other characteristics of a well-done experiment, coupled with careful selection of patients and investigators who are believed to represent the characteristics of the target population, is a reasonable solution that is accepted by essentially all workers.

In addition, as a pragmatic matter, there is overwhelming evidence that statistical design and analysis *work*. Unrandomized or incorrectly randomized studies are much more frequently discovered to have given wrong answers than properly designed trials. There is a most interesting commentary in this connection in a paper by Dr. Alvan Feinstein, Professor of Medicine and Epidemiology and Director of the Clinical Epidemiology unit, Yale University School of Medicine (1).

Thus, you should be assured that, despite this sampling problem, the experimental design and related statistical procedures that we advocate so strongly in this book, and which are used in all well-designed clinical studies, are most important to the success of your trials.

6.2.8   Stratification and Matching

Stratification

In large experiments, the randomization is sometimes **stratified**. Stratification is a procedure for reducing experimental error, thereby increasing the power of the subsequent statistical analyses. Simply put, the patients are divided into two or more subgroups within each treatment group in a particular way so as to ensure that the treatment groups are as uniform as possible. Suppose that in Examples 4.1 and 5.1 it is expected that the sex of the patients may influence the outcome, but that, for whatever reason, you do not wish to use it as an additional factor. In that case, you can stratify during the preparation of the randomization plan. Twenty-five are to be assigned to each treatment in this study; the randomization is therefore restricted to make each group consist of 13 females and 13 males (adding one to the group to make the subgroups equal). In this way, the treatment groups will be balanced with respect to sex, and any differences due to that factor will not affect the results except for the loss of certain information.[8] In addition to the sex of the patients, other variables that may be handled in this way are age, body weight, race, or other demographic or disease characteristics.

This kind of restricted randomization will not be discussed further in this book. More detailed information may be found in Pocock, [4], Chapter 5, pp. 80–87, Shapiro and Louis, [5], Chapter 1, pp. 29–32, and several others among the references listed. As is pointed out in these references, there are simpler ways to accomplish the purposes of stratified randomization. Statistical procedures used during the analysis of the data[9] are easy to do and may save considerable administrative time and expense during the execution of a study.

Matching

Matching is sometimes suggested for medical trials *to avoid* randomizing or in addition to it. For example, in a two-factor study, each patient chosen for the active treatment may be "matched" with another who will receive a placebo. The patients are matched "on" certain characteristics *regarded by the planner* as likely to affect the results, such as severity of disease, demographic factors, and the like. In a sense, matching is a form of stratification, and in another, it is a factorial design. The object is to obtain pairs of patients (or sets of 3 or 4, if there are 3 or 4 treatments) who are as alike as possible with respect to characteristics expected to influence the outcome of a measurement or the action of the treatments. In the past, matching has been frequently used as a substitute for randomization by investigators who mistrusted or disliked the latter and did not understand the dependence of statistical tests upon it. This is very uncommon today in commercial drug work, and any submission of such a study to the FDA would surely be rejected, but it is still sometimes reported in descriptions of noncommercial trials. Sometimes, if available, twins are used for the matched pairs, to ensure that patient characteristics are as alike as possible. Properly randomized, a matched design could be viewed as a randomized-blocks arrangement (Chapter 11).

Another kind of problem existing when matching is used but not otherwise is that important information may be ignored. Although one or more additional factors are introduced, as in stratified sampling, they are typically not

---

[8]In Chapters 10 and 11, however, you will see that this procedure is exactly equivalent to adding an additional factor, sex in this case, to the model, except that it is ignored in the analysis. Because several pieces of valuable information might emerge from such a multifactor analysis (when sex is included as a factor), and because the analysis will not consume any appreciable additional time, it would seem advisable in most cases to do so rather than to stratify in simple cases of this kind. You should keep in mind, however, that this factor and others that are inherent patient characteristics restrict the randomization in another way (see Chapter 10, Section 10.5.7).

[9]Such as the analysis of covariance (ACOVA).

accounted for in the analysis. Whether they have any effects per se upon the response(s) or upon the responses in combination with any of the other factors (interactions) will consequently not be discovered. This problem is avoided when the analysis accounts for all the factors introduced in the design. (See Parts III and IV). It is true that with more than three or at most four factors, a factorial design for a clinical study becomes difficult and unwieldy, but this is also true for matching. Furthermore, if you use a factorial with several factors, it is possible to use a so-called *fractional factorial* design. However, although such designs are widely used in chemical and engineering experimentation, and permit important reductions in the overall numbers of experimental units required, they are almost never used in clinical trials and are not covered in this book. Thus, only a few factors can normally be used in matching, because the increasing subdivision necessary soon requires very large sample sizes. This is not only expensive and unnecessary, but makes the sample size used dependent upon the wrong criteria.

There is no absolute objection to the use of matching if it is used with the appropriate randomization procedure and data analysis. Nevertheless, it can lead to problems. Two negative aspects are the following: (1) As indicated earlier, it is possible that with matching, there will be no randomization of any kind, because the matcher may have chosen it in the first place to avoid that procedure. (2) As the number of characteristics used to match on increases, the number of patients needed rapidly becomes greater, and the difficulty of forming the desired groups also increases very swiftly, because greater numbers of similar individuals must be selected.

With respect to the last point, matching is often a difficult process because of the additional time required to find and qualify the appropriate patients for each subgroup. For example, suppose you wished to match upon four factors: age (young, old), sex (male, female), body weight (heavy, light), and ethnic origin (black, white, Hispanic, yellow). In each subgroup of 32 patients, you would require 16 young and 16 old people. In each of these two groups of 16, eight men and eight women would be needed. Within each of those four groups of eight patients, your study would call for four to be heavy and four light. And in each of the eight groups of 4, one patient of each of the four ethnic origins would be needed. Finally, unless you were satisfied with only one patient in each matching category within each treatment group, with a concomitant risk that normal attrition during the execution of the trial might cause some of the attributes to be unrepresented in some groups, you would have to at least double the originally estimated sample size of 128. But this creates an ethical problem, because you will be using more patients than would be necessary if you did not use matching. There is another problem. Increasing the sample size for such a reason will *increase* the power of the significance tests, thereby making smaller population differences detectable than was intended; such differences may be unimportant from a clinical point of view, causing the trial to give deceptive results. And there are still further difficulties. To match properly, you would need to be sure that all patients selected had the target disease condition, carefully diagnosed and perhaps with a specified severity. And after all this, there would remain the nagging question of whether there might be additional important characteristics that should also have been used to match on.

As you can see, although there may be a large number of desirable attributes that should be used to ensure that the groups are reasonably alike, it becomes almost impossible to match on more than a very few. Also, note that three of the four attributes matched on used only two levels each. You might well have wished that age and body weight could be subdivided further (they could not, because, unless you increased the initial group sizes, further subdivision would be impossible). After trying this once, you might be inclined to say, "Thank goodness for randomization!"

By now it should be clear that in the usual case, randomization, not matching, is the preferred approach to handling the "nuisance" variables. Like the majority of statisticians, I consider any clinical study run without randomization, if randomization is conceivably possible, to be out of the question. On the other hand, stratification (and, to a degree, matching) is often advocated as a means of increasing precision. I do not condemn stratification with randomization, and a moderate amount of matching may also be occasionally useful. But those variables, known or unknown, that are not thus accounted for must then be handled by randomization. It often seems, however, that the effort and cost of such exercises far exceed that of adding additional patients when precision needs to be improved.

6.2.9   Example 6.1: Randomizing a One-Factor Design

The general method for obtaining random assignments in a parallel design is to arrange things so that each patient is assigned to a treatment by a chance mechanism. An easy and acceptable way to do this is to number the patients and then select a group at random from the set of patient numbers to be assigned to one treatment, another group to the next treatment, and so on. More specifically, you begin by choosing one of the treatments to be assigned to a group of patient numbers. The treatment can be designated arbitrarily; a random choice is not necessary. The chance, or **stochastic**, part of the procedure then consists in making a random choice of one patient number at a time, and assigning the chosen treatment to it. This is continued until the desired number of patient numbers has been assigned to that treatment. Still more specifically, one easy method of doing this is to create several columns on a sheet of paper, one column for each treatment in the trial. Head each column with the name of the treatment or a coded identification. Then, using a random-selection procedure, choose a set of patient numbers one at a time, corresponding to the desired group size, and place it in the first column. Repeat this for each of the remaining columns.

Once you have estimated the sample size, you will know how large each of these treatment groups is to be. The most common procedure is to make all of them of equal size. During the randomization, which should be done when you are planning the trial, you will be using patient numbers to which no patients yet correspond. Later, during the actual trial, numbers can be assigned to the actual patients in an arbitrary manner; for example, the patients can be numbered in order as they are accepted into the trial. These numbers then are identified with those chosen during the randomization. You should be sure that each patient is accepted into the trial before assigning a number, or there will be missing numbers and patients in the set. This would create a problem, because new patients should not usually be selected during a trial, unless this has been planned for ahead of time. To summarize, the randomization occurs during the planning stage, when you randomly select a set of patient numbers to be assigned to each treatment. The selected patient numbers are later assigned to real patients in an arbitrary manner.

Note that this procedure restricts the randomization to a degree, as discussed earlier in this chapter, because you will be limiting the size of the set of patient numbers assigned to each treatment so that they will be equal to each other. Of course, a completely random-assignment procedure would avoid this restriction. However, the procedure described here is widely used, guarantees equal group sizes when that is important, and is near enough to complete random assignment to be reasonable as a normal procedure.

It is not advisable to randomize by drawing numbered slips from a box, using numbered or colored balls drawn from a jar, or the like. It is much more difficult than it may appear to thoroughly mix such materials, just as it is to really randomize a pack of cards with a few shuffles; see Weaver (2). Some clinical trials have been "randomized" by mentally producing a series of numbers, but it is virtually impossible to obtain the necessary random permutation in this way.[10] Rather, when you need to randomize the treatment assignments for a study, you should use one of the randomization procedures described in what follows or elsewhere in the literature. There are many methods. The purpose of the following discourse is not to produce an exhaustive catalog, but to try to illustrate some of the principles involved by supplying you with a small sampling of procedures and some practical ideas.

For the randomization of Example 6.1, you will first need a random *permutation* of the numbers 1 through 100, representing the 100 patients. No one of the 100 numbers can be used more than once. A random permutation is a rearrangement of the order of the numbers, done in a random manner. You might think of it as follows: There is a very large number of possible orders (permutations) into which the numbers 1 to 100 may be arranged; a random permutation is any one of these, selected at random, so that all

---

[10] If you wish to try this, try thinking of and writing down a series of numbers, and test the series for randomness with one of the tests in the references (e.g., Siegel [45], pp. 52–60, or Conover [39], p. 189–199).

permutations are equally likely. Once the permutation of the 100 numbers (patients) is obtained, it must be divided arbitrarily into four groups of 25 each, representing the four treatment groups.

In large studies it is desirable to use a computer for the randomization, to save time.[11] This is unnecessary in a small trial, however, as you can probably do the randomization yourself in the time it would take to get your program ready or to wait for the statistician to do the job for you.

You will need to know how the 100 numbers will be associated with the 100 patients when the trial is run. This need not be a random process, as you will have already done your randomization. There are many conceivable methods. The method we recommend is convenient and simple. Ask the investigator to assign a number to each patient, beginning with 1, *after* the patients qualify and are accepted into the trial. It is important that this not be done until then. This or whatever method is used should be described in the protocol and operations manual. Of course, the clinical report form or forms (CRFs) for each patient should provide a space for recording the patient number. CRFs are discussed in Chapter 7.

In some trials, it will be necessary or at least desirable to provide for probable losses due to early dropouts by initially enrolling a somewhat greater number of patients than the sample size calculations have indicated to be necessary. In this example, however, unless you expect heavy losses for some reason, this should not be required.

Methods

We will describe five methods for carrying out the random assignment of patients to treatment groups for Example 5.1. Other designs will require modification of some of these procedures, but most of them will be similar to those described here. One of those we describe requires a computer. If the sample size is large, the use of a computer will save time. And, of course, there are other procedures for which a computer is almost essential. If you use one for randomization procedures or other purposes mentioned in this book, a modern stand-alone desktop machine or a LAN (local area network), using an 80386 or 80486 microprocessor with a reasonably large data storage system, will be completely adequate. There is no operation needed in your work, for your use or that of the statistician, that cannot be handled adequately with such a machine. This includes randomization procedures, the handling of large databases, writing reports and protocols, designing data forms such as CRFs, and any necessary statistical analyses and graphical output. Today, the use of a mainframe machine or even a minicomputer is no longer essential.

---

[11] It is impossible to select a group of truly random numbers or to prepare a group of randomly selected permutations of numbers with a digital computer. The numbers actually obtained are called pseudo-random numbers. They are near enough to true randomness, however, to make them practical for the uses we put them to in experimental designs.

Please note the following: For a trial of any size, the use of a computer program for the randomization is almost essential in order to save time. That method comprises only one of the five procedures listed in what follows. There are at least four important reasons for including the descriptions of the "manual" methods. First, the descriptions provide you with an idea of the basic mechanisms in the random-assignment process. Second, in Part III, when several different kinds of experimental designs are described, different randomization methods are usually necessary for each. These differences are best explained by describing a manual procedure, even if in practice the biostatistician will do the randomization and will use the computer. Third, as with the use of any computer procedure in statistics, it is obviously important that you have a thorough understanding of what the computer is doing. Even if you decide that all the random assignments will be done by the statistician, the same philosophy applies. And, fourth, there are many small studies in which the use of a manual method is actually faster than using a computer, partly because it involves no waiting time or other preparation if the computer is used by more than one person.

Of course, in most cases you will probably wish to use the computer for your regular work. But, again, there is no substitute for a thorough understanding of the random-assignment process. It is true that the principle difference between randomization techniques using a computer and those done manually is that the computer generates the needed (pseudo-) random numbers very rapidly as compared to the manual selection of random numbers from a table, and produces convenient printouts arranged in any way the programmer makes available. But the details of the actual random assignments for various experimental designs are best appreciated by first learning the use of the randomization procedures using a manual method.

First Method: Table of Random Numbers

This method is not recommended for your regular use. It is described here, however, because it is an almost perfect example of the mechanism of randomization, as adapted for a one-factor, completely randomized parallel design. It is an old procedure, and before the days of adequate computer availability, it was very popular. I have been unable to find its origin, but it dates back at least 45 or 50 years, to the early days of applied statistics. It is a basic method and requires no more special facilities than a table of random numbers and some index cards.

Select 100 3 × 5 index cards. In the upper left-hand corner of each, write a patient number, so that you will have cards numbered from 1 to 100. The upper right-hand corner is reserved for a five-digit random number (see what follows). When you employ this or any other randomization method, be sure to use a different randomization each time you need one.

In this description, as a source of uniform random numbers, we use the random number table in Snedecor and Cochran [38], Table A 1, pp. 463–466. Any other statistics text or book of tables, if it contains a table of random numbers, is equally suitable. For example, there are similar tabulations in Beyer [47], Fisher and Yates [48], Owen [50], and in some of the other references in the Bibliography. If you use a different table, be sure that the numbers are called "random numbers," "random units," "random digits," or the like, *not* "random normal numbers," or "random permutations." In many random-number tables, the numbers (i.e., individual digits) are grouped in pairs or by fours or fives. In Snedecor and Cochran, the numbers are arranged in groups of five digits, in numbered rows and columns. The groupings and row/column numbers have no significance except to make it more convenient to read or refer to the table.

Starting on any page of the table and at any row or column, copy a five-digit group to the upper right-hand corner of each of your 100 file cards. For the example, we started at row 50 and the column marked "00–04," [38], p. 465. Note that each column label actually refers to a group of five columns of digits. Proceed vertically, and when the bottom of the page is reached, go to the top of the next column. Continue in this way until you have copied 100 5-digit numbers (this will take you to the bottom of the second column, marked "05–05."[12] If you wish, instead of moving down the columns, you may move across each row. No matter in what direction you proceed (even diagonally), your selected numbers will occur in random order.

The reason for using five instead of fewer digits for each number you select is to avoid ties. In the very unlikely event that you do find a tie or two when sorting the cards as described in what follows, flip a coin to see which of the pair is to come first. If you wish to further reduce the probability of ties, use more than five digits in the groups.

Sort the cards in the order of the random numbers, either ascending or descending. Now divide them into four groups of 25 cards, starting at the top of the pile. Mark the first 25 with the letter "A," signifying treatment A, the next 25 with "B" for treatment B, and so on. Finally, draw up a table with four columns, headed "Treatment A," "Treatment B," etc. Copy the 25 patient numbers from the cards marked "A" to the "A" column, those from the cards marked "B" to the next column, and so on, until you have filled all four columns. Figure 6.3 is an illustration of one of the cards, and Table 6.3 shows the finished randomization.

Second Method: Table of Random Numbers

A second "manual" method of preparing a randomization for the trial of the example is to simply proceed down any column or across any row of Table

---

[12]The starting point was selected arbitrarily. Some texts suggest that it be chosen by a random method, but this is not very important, in my opinion, and was and is often disregarded in practice. Of course, it is important to avoid using the same starting point repeatedly. But a minor departure from exact randomness cannot logically be faulted by anyone willing to bend his or her principles to the small extent needed to use computer-generated randomizations, as is done almost universally today.

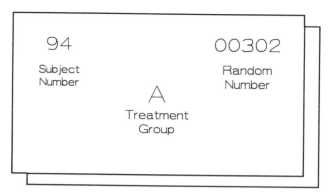

Figure 6.3   Card used in the randomization procedure.

Table 6.3. Randomization of Example 6.1: First Method (Patient Numbers)

	Treatment		
A	B	C	D
94	37	70	65
53	88	76	20
86	38	60	67
24	6	97	44
50	80	58	16
3	82	57	89
47	61	51	15
91	92	18	39
43	23	45	93
71	48	1	95
9	63	27	85
96	26	32	28
35	14	11	59
69	17	81	74
12	8	7	31
25	13	42	87
84	52	66	46
77	36	54	33
62	19	22	30
5	40	72	73
34	78	100	98
21	41	99	56
75	83	68	64
90	10	4	79
2	55	49	29

A-1 in Snedecor and Cochran [38], writing down each *three* digits encountered (including zeros) if they are in the range required and are not duplicates of numbers already obtained. If you proceed across the table, you can ignore the spaces between groups and examine each three digits you encounter. However, it is easier to proceed downward, selecting the first three digits in each group of five and ignoring the remaining two. No matter which of these two methods you use, your sequence will be random. As the numbers are found, copy them to a table with as many columns as there are treatments, as was done in the first method. To avoid duplicates, you will need to prepare a separate list of all of the numbers needed (1 to 100) beforehand, crossing each one off as it is found.

Although this method sounds simpler than the preceding one, it requires considerably more time, unless the total number of patients is much smaller than the 100 of the example. The reason is that you will encounter increasing numbers of ties as you proceed, and will need to discard more and more otherwise suitable numbers. For small problems, however (about 50 or fewer numbers), the method works well, and you can save time compared to the first procedure. If you use it, remember not to use any number or digit more than once.

Remember that when you select 3-digit random numbers, the first digit will be zero except for patient number 100.

Third Method: Pocket Calculator

A third method is to use a pocket calculator, such as the Hewlett-Packard 11c, 15c, 42S, or other scientific calculator, to generate your random numbers. These will be analogous to computer-generated sets of numbers, that is, they will actually be pseudo-random numbers, unlike those you get when you use either of the first two methods. Like method 2, this procedure is not practical for more than about 50 numbers. You can calculate and record 30 numbers in about 15 minutes and 50 in about half an hour, including checks for duplicates. The procedure is not as instructive as the first one in the sense of illustrating principles, but is easy and convenient for small samples.

If you enjoy using programmable calculators, you can program any of several available makes to generate sets of random permutations of the numbers 1 through N, for specified values of N and the set size, thus automating the process.

There are more elaborate modern calculators, which are really small computers. If you have one of these, such as the Hewlett-Packard 28S or 48SX, you can write a routine that will do the job much more rapidly than either of the preceding methods. Both have plenty of memory, so that you can arrange the program to assemble a list of the numbers already selected, checking each new number against the list to avoid duplicates. You can even print the results if you have a printer that is available for these machines, although the printed output will not be suitable for reporting unless it is recopied.

If you use a calculator, and it is not one of the aforementioned HP models, be sure it is one that allows the entry of a new "seed" number for each series of random numbers you generate. If you write a BASIC program for a microcomputer or use one written by someone else, the command "RANDOMIZE" in most BASIC dialects produces a new seed.

Fourth Method: Microcomputer

If you have a desktop computer, you can use that. As indicated before, you can write or purchase a BASIC program to obtain your permutations. Also, most statistical packages include a means of producing random numbers or permutations. The program you use should generate each number, compare it with all those previously obtained to avoid duplication and numbers outside the desired range, divide the final list into k groups of n numbers each, and print out a table similar to that of Table 6.3. Once you have your program, this method is very fast. We encourage you to try this procedure, even though the statistician may do it for you routinely. If you do not have a program available, the statistician can supply one.

Fifth Method: Table of Random Permutations

This method makes use of Moses and Oakford's *Tables of Random Permutations* [49]. It is faster than method 1, and would be as fast as the use of a microcomputer, except that you must prepare your final table by hand. This small book contains sets of permutations of the integers 1 to 9, 16, 20, 30, 50, 100, 200, 500, and 1000. For Example 6.1, you select one of the permutations of 100 and copy all its numbers to your four-column table. Usually, you will not require a set of numbers of exactly the same size as any of those in Moses and Oakford. In such a case, you simply choose a table in the book that has permutations of a size nearest to that you require, but greater, not fewer, of course. You then copy one of the permutations, as before, omitting any numbers larger than the largest you need.

6.3 BLINDING

6.3.1 Nature and Purpose of Blinding

Definition

Blinding (sometimes called masking) means using some procedure that prevents people involved in a clinical trial (patients and/or investigators) from knowing which treatment each patient receives (in a parallel study) or the order of the treatments (in a changeover study). Today, nearly all industrial drug trials are **double blind**. This means that although everyone concerned in a study is told what treatments are being used in the trial (the patients *must* be told), steps are taken to ensure that neither the patients nor the investigators (nor those administering or distributing the dosages) are given specific knowledge of the individual assignments, at least until the trial is over. In many cases, even the statistical analysts who evaluate the data after a trial is completed are blinded. It is a good idea to make blinding as universal as possible.

Purpose of Blinding

The purpose of blinding is to prevent bias, conscious or unconscious, from influencing the results or the interpretation of the results of a trial. The term *bias* in this case refers not to statistical bias, but to recording response measurements that are different from the correct values, often because of an unconscious "mind-set" on the part of a patient or investigator. This is very common, on the part of both parties. In the case of investigators or their delegates, it can occur even in the reading and/or recording of readings of instruments and other so-called "objective" devices. However, it is probably most severe when judgment scales are used. With patients, a knowledge of which drug has been taken often affects the disease condition, either objectively or in a patient's opinion.

In Example 6.1, one of the two responses, the seven-point pain scale, is subject to possible bias by both patients and investigator, because the patients supply verbal judgments about their severity of pain, and the investigator(s) then translate these statements into numerical scores. The other scale, the VAS, when properly used (without prompting after the patient has been trained in its use), is subject only to patient bias. Nevertheless, it is always good scientific practice to use double blinding.

In the past, many investigators have objected vigorously to being blinded, but two circumstances have altered this attitude in recent years. The first is the realization that bias can occur in the inquiries of the most well-intentioned, honest, and careful professionals, as documented repeatedly in the literature of clinical trials, so that blinding is not a reflection upon an investigator's competence; see Meinert [3], Friedman et al. [2], Pocock [4], and Shapiro and Louis [5], to list a few. The second circumstance is based upon a requirement of the FDA. On the basis of its experience, the FDA usually insists upon the use of double blinding in a trial unless there are strong reasons for its omission.

Unlike most topics in this book, blinding is not a statistical matter, and its use is unrelated to whether or not a trial is designed and run in a statistically correct and appropriate manner. Rather, it is simply good science.

6.3.2 Methods of Blinding

In general, blinding is accomplished simply by not revealing treatment assignments to the participants before or during a trial.

Many methods of disguising the identity of treatments have been used. Some are manifestly flawed, such as the use of designations analogous to A,

B, C, and D, that is, specific letters or numbers invariably identified with each treatment. With such a scheme, if the code is broken for one of the patients, because of the occurrence of an adverse effect, by accident, by guesswork, or for any other reason, that treatment is identified for all patients. If the trial has only two treatments, such an event destroys the blinding for the entire trial.

A satisfactory method, widely used today, is the following: The doses are packaged with two-part labels of opaque paper. The visible part of each label is marked only with the patient number and an identification of the trial and sponsor (if a single dose) or with the patient and visit or dose numbers (if dosage is to be repeated) and identification of the study and sponsor. The second part of the label cannot be seen until or unless it is torn off. This identifies the material, and is to be exposed only, if necessary, in an emergency. Furthermore, because there is no relationship between a patient, visit or dose number, and the nature of a treatment, any emergency exposure of the nature of a patient's treatment gives no information about those assigned to other patients. There is always a check on the unauthorized opening of any label. Standard practice, which can be required by the FDA, is for the investigators to return both used and unused packages of drugs after the trial for counting and examination. It is assumed that this procedure will be used in our example.

The basic principles in this system are these: (a) Doses of the same drug given to different patients do not bear the same number or identification. (b) The several treatments use the same dosage form and should be indistinguishable in appearance. (c) There must be some method for rapidly identifying a treatment in an emergency. Some monitors do not use double labels, but mark the doses with patient and visit numbers only. They then arrange for a 24-hour telephone line to be available so that investigators can call a predesignated source at the sponsor's headquarters in an emergency, such as the occurrence of a severe presumed adverse effect, to learn the identity of a treatment.

6.4 PLANNING INTERIM ANALYSES

6.4.1 Dangers of Additional Unplanned Analyses

In some fixed sample size trials there can be important reasons for conducting some data analyses before the study is over. They may be ethical, because time has become short, or because it is believed that the test drug may not be effective. Or you may have planned upon possible early stopping from the beginning, or decided upon it during execution.

However, running iterim tests without allowing for them during planning will result in an increase in the actual alpha risks, assuming that beta and delta remain the same. This often can be a serious increase.[13] This means that the risk of concluding that the difference you are testing is a real population difference, when it really is not,[14] will be higher than the risk that you specified when planning the trial. Putting it another way, by running unplanned interim tests, you will have lost control of your alpha risk and created a shaky basis for your eventual conclusions. To overcome this problem, any interim analyses *must* be planned for *before* the trial begins, when you are estimating the sample size. This allows you to compensate for the repetition of the tests by increasing the planned sample size.

The majority of trial protocols do not provide for preplanned interim analyses, yet studies are frequently interrupted for this purpose. To emphasize the problem again, when this is done, the specified alpha probabilities associated with *all* the statistical tests, both interim and poststudy, become larger. Doing additional unplanned significance tests at the end of a study has the same effect. Of course, the alpha risk is irrelevant *at the time of such tests* if you do not find significance. However, they affect alpha if the experiment is continued.

6.4.2 Compensating for Planned Additional Analyses

Because each unplanned statistical comparison, at whatever stage of the trial it is done, will increase the actual value of alpha beyond that specified, it must be compensated for by modifying the sample size estimate before the patients are selected. To review, one way is to use the principle called the **Bonferroni inequality**. The Bonferroni principle is one of several so-called multiple-comparisons procedures. It can be used as an approximate (somewhat conservative) method of calculating a "working" value of alpha that can then be used to estimate the sample size and will compensate for any multiple-significance testing. It is the simplest of all of the common multiple-comparisons procedures, and is easily adapted to the purpose of estimating sample size a priori when multiple comparisons are expected. Its conservatism is not serious, and keeps you on the "safe side."

---

[13]This also assumes that the sample sizes are constant. Actually, of course, if the trial is still in the recruitment stage, as the experiment proceeds, the sample size will increase. This will partially offset the change in the alpha level, but not completely. In a trial in which there are several or many visits, the sample size may change less rapidly, or even decrease due to dropouts, in the middle and latter stages.

[14]It may be useful to think of a "real" population difference as one that would occur, on the average, in repeated similar trials. In a sense, this definition of a population is really the same as defining it as all of the patients who now have the disease condition or will have it in the future. However, you may find it to be a more concrete and easier concept. Of course, your sampling of this population cannot be random, because any series of trials, real or conceptual, must be taken successively through time. However, despite this, it is realistic to think of your sample of patients as representative.

In using Bonferroni, the calculated value of alpha becomes the new "significance level." This new "working" value of alpha is substituted for the original value when estimating sample size. Doing this maintains the desired **simultaneous** or **experimentwise** value of alpha at that originally specified in all of the tests, when considered as a group. To use Bonferroni, the originally specified value of alpha is divided by the total number of planned comparisons, including those to be done during and at the end of the trial. The result is the simultaneous alpha level. This value is used instead of the originally specified value in the significance tests as well as when estimating the sample size. Using it will guarantee that the original "nominal" level will hold when the tests are considered as a group. In reporting results, you use the originally specified alpha level as the experimentwise error rate.

6.4.3   Example 6.2: Compensating for Additional Significance Tests

Suppose that the value of alpha you specified for the significance tests in Example 5.1 or 6.1 were 0.050. Now suppose, during planning, that you decide that it may be necessary to provide for interim analyses during the trial, in addition to the final tests. If there were to be one interim and one final session, making four pairwise comparisons each time as in the previous examples, there would be a total of eight pairwise comparisons if you were using just the VAS response data each time.

Note that this procedure may be somewhat approximate. If we assume that patients are recruited continually throughout the trial instead of all at the beginning, each succeeding analysis will use a larger sample size, because each hypothesis test will be done at successive times in which the total number of patients providing data will be greater. Of course, it would be possible to take this into account by making separate sample size estimates for each expected test period, but the additional approximation introduced by using the same sample size throughout will result in a conservative, and therefore safer, estimate. However, as is possible in this trial, if all the patients are recruited at the beginning, no such approximation will be introduced unless there are noncompleters.

First, using Bonferroni, calculate the probability level that you will use in the tests to ensure that your desired value of alpha (0.050) prevails:

$$p = \frac{0.050}{8} = 0.0063 \tag{3.1}$$

Now, in estimating the sample size and in doing all the hypothesis tests, you should use an alpha value of 0.006. However, we will use the sample size table, Table A.3 in the Appendix, which was introduced in Chapter 5. The lowest alpha value in that table is the one used for Table A.3a, 0.01. Using this will introduce more approximation, and it would be better to use the exact value, at least to three decimal places, of 0.006. For purposes of illustration, however, we will use 0.01 so that we can use Table A.3a. Later, in Part V, you will be shown a simple equation that will allow you to use any value of alpha in calculating the sample size.

An alpha value of 0.01 now takes the place of your specified alpha value of 0.050 during your tests, but you interpret the outcome of the tests as if you had used 0.050. Because the sample size calculated during planning depends upon alpha as well as delta, beta, and your estimated sigma, it must also be calculated using 0.010 instead of 0.050 for alpha. Doing your two interim comparisons and the final VAS test with an alpha value of 0.010 now gives you an *experimentwise error rate* of 0.050.

Using the Bonferroni procedure will ensure that the specified alpha values hold for all of your comparisons. However, assuming delta is not changed, unlesss you increase the sample size a priori to compensate, the power of the tests will be reduced. You cannot modify alpha, beta, or delta, using a constant sample size, without affecting one or both of the other two. For example, if Bonferroni is used to calculate the reduced alpha value, then, if delta is held constant, beta is increased, reducing the power of the hypothesis test unless the sample size is increased. This is the reason that you must increase the sample size appropriately, thus allowing beta and delta to remain at their specified levels. In discussing Examples 4.1 and 5.1 in Chapters 4 and 5, respectively, the use of Bonferroni was demonstrated to compensate for the four comparisons planned. The same procedure is used to find the appropriate sample size when you plan several treatment comparisons *and* the repeated tests. This procedure will be discussed further in Part V.

6.5 EARLY TERMINATION OF A TRIAL

There will be times when, for any of a variety of reasons, a trial may be cut short before all the patients have been enrolled or all observations completed. Often the reasons are that unexpected and possibly serious side effects have appeared, one of the treatments has exhibited unmistakable efficacy or the reverse at an early stage, or the like. In such cases, a further analysis of the data is often not needed. If it is desirable, however, it may be done, remembering that one or more of the original specifications of alpha, beta, delta, or the sample size may no longer be valid. If an analysis is done, therefore, it is not a bad idea to calculate delta a posteriori, to get an idea of the validity of the reduced database. This can most easily be done for simple designs using the sample-size equations given in Part V.

You should remember that even for a truncated trial, or one that is unsuccessful for some other reason, it is best to inform the FDA of the outcome. If you plan further trials in such a case, such a step is necessary, because the failure of a trial may be expected to have some influence upon the probability of future success.

6.6 WRITING THE PROTOCOL

This topic will be discussed more fully in the next chapter, but we introduce it here, because it is an essential part of your initial planning. In this book, we are concerned principally with the aspects of trial preparation that require or are related to statistical concepts, such as experimental designs, randomization, the relationship of design to analysis, measurements, clinical report forms (CRFs), interim analyses, premature termination of a trial, blinding, sample size estimation, and, to some degree, certain common statistical-analysis (test) procedures. Portions of the protocol concerned with these topics must be presented so that any medical and paramedical people will find it intelligible. But it must also be written so that it will be thoroughly understandable to the various other specialists involved in the trial—pharmacologists, chemists, toxicologists, biologists, CRAs (clinical research associates), nurses, programmers, regulatory affairs people, statisticians, and others. The most effective trial is one in which everyone involved has a thorough understanding of the entire project.

Based upon the foregoing, the following points are particularly important:

(a) The protocol should be written as you go along with the planning steps outlined in this and the previous chapter. It should not be left to the last.

(b) Drafts should be circulated to the monitor, statistician, CRAs, investigators, and others involved in the trial, requesting criticism and suggestions.

(c) The monitor, statistician, CRAs, and others in the sponsoring organization should meet from time to time to review current drafts of the protocol together.

(d) *Every* aspect of the trial should be mentioned in the protocol, at least briefly. For example, the kinds of statistical analyses planned should be described, although not necessarily in great detail (see Section 6.7). It would be adequate to do this in a two- or three-page appendix, for example. If you plan to ask the FDA to review the protocol, as we recommend, it is important that this section be completed beforehand, so that you can request comments from their statistical personnel. If there is disagreement about the projected procedures, they will so indicate, and you will be saved a possible rejection of your work after the final submission.

(e) Some items should be spelled out very carefully. For instance, a detailed example of a patient visit, with every phase of the procedures it entails, should be included. The clinical report forms for recording the test data should also be described and preferably illustrated exactly (see Section 6.8).

(f) The experimental design and sample size calculations should be described fully.

(g) The randomization procedure should also be described fully.

(h) Before finalizing the protocol, if possible, you should meet with the investigator(s) who will carry out the study to obtain their suggestions and criticisms.

6.7 WRITING AN OPERATIONS MANUAL

If the trial is multicenter and fairly large, or if it will require some time to complete, you may wish to prepare an operations manual. Whereas the protocol is intended to provide an overall view of all of the trial procedures and background, the operations manual is written for the use of those actually running the trial. All procedures should be described completely, not only for the record and to allow future repetition, but so that anyone skilled in the necessary techniques may obtain all the guidance necessary from a single source. All the measurement methods (responses) to be used in the clinic(s) should be given in detail. Like the protocol, drafts of this document should be circulated among those planning the trial, as well as among the investigators at the center(s) that will take part, for comment and criticism.

6.8 DESCRIPTIONS OF STATISTICAL PROCEDURES

We emphasize again that the procedures the biostatistician expects to use in analyzing the data should be described in the protocol. The biostatistician should be asked to plan the expected methods of statistical analysis fully, as early as possible during the planning of the trial. This will not only make them available in time to be described in the protocol, but will also make it possible for all involved to discuss them during planning. It should be recognized, of course, that some procedures may need to be changed when the data analysis is done, but it will be expected that any modifications will be as appropriate to the design used as were the original methods.

6.9 CLINICAL REPORT FORMS

Carefully prepared clinical report forms (CRFs) are essential to the execution of any trial. It is important that they be designed early to avoid cutting corners at the last minute. They should be **printed**, not typed, if possible, in a legible and complete format. A small computer, a laser printer, and appropriate software will make possible in-house preparation of easy-to-use and attractive master documents, requiring only final copies for completion.

Photocopy or laser printer reproduction of such masters, if quantities are small, is very practical. For larger runs, the masters can be lithographed in house if equipment is available, or by an outside service. The preparation of well thought out, useful, attractive, and easily readable CRFs is something that is very often neglected in trial preparations. Taking pains to prepare them will reduce errors, incur fewer misunderstandings, and facilitate the work of the investigators, reviewers, and data-transcription staff.

Like the protocol and operations handbook, the CRFs, while in draft, should be circulated to everyone involved in the planning of the trial for comment and criticism. In particular, the investigators should be given a chance to examine them and submit comments.

Full-page optical character readers have become relatively inexpensive. If desired, and if one is available, it is possible to design the CRFs so that, as they arrive at the sponsor's location during the trial, at least some of the data can be read and immediately stored as files in the computer. This will not only save time during the more critical portions of the execution, but will reduce errors.

Complete instructions for the use and performance of each test procedure should be included on each CRF, as well as in the operations manual, whether they are to be used by an investigator, an assistant, or a patient. This, like the printing of the forms, is often neglected, but its omission can lead to serious errors. Separate pages should be used for each response, each patient, and each visit, even if space is "wasted." This simplifies the job of data transcription to the computer and reduces errors. It also allows finished CRFs to be transmitted to the monitor and/or data processing site frequently.

In addition to CRFs for recording measurements such as the pain scores and VAS data in the example, patient demographic data and medical histories, and adverse effects must also be provided for. When preparing these CRFs, try to arrange them with easy transcription of the data in mind.

6.10 DATABASE

In a well-arranged study procedure, clinical report forms are collected from each investigator at very frequent intervals. This reduces the incidence of repetitive misunderstandings by allowing frequent review by the sponsor during execution of a trial, and prevents the accumulation of large amounts of data when the trial is completed.

Unless a study is very small, you will want to store the data in a computer database as they arrive. Your organization may have a separate computer group or department in charge of this activity, or perhaps it will be done in your department. In either case, if at all possible, the database should be prepared during planning, as soon as the necessary information is available (treatment identifications, experimental design, the responses, and the like). Upon receipt of the completed CRFs from the investigator(s), someone familiar with the overall project should read them, checking for numerical and nonnumerical errors, and then pass them along to those in charge of entering them into the database. If the database is ready as soon as the study begins, the results from a trial can be read into the computer as soon as they are generated in the field and can be delivered to the sponsor. If this is done, there will be much less delay later in getting the data ready for analysis, especially for a large trial, and interim analyses will be simplified. Incidentally, data are precious—and expensive. The CRFs should be collected frequently and *personally* from the investigator(s) by CRAs. They should not be mailed unless absolutely necessary. If they must be sent, a reliable overnight service should be used.

An effective error-checking procedure should be in use where the data entry is done. One common method is to have all data entered twice, by two different operators, using a program that will compare the two sets with each other and call human attention to any differences. Such a step may be obviated if your CRFs are designed so that all needed information can be read by an optical character reader. Another method, which I have found very satisfactory for smaller studies, is to have someone enter the data into the database and then print them out. A different person then compares printouts from the database with the original CRFs. This, in effect, gives a double check, exposing any errors of transcription from the CRFs to the computer. The common alternative of directly transcribing the data in the CRFs into the computer by one person, unless by optical reader, usually leads to considerably more errors.

The statistician should approve the methods of setting up the database, and ensure that the data can be electronically transferred to the statistical programs in an effective manner when they are complete and ready for analysis.

6.11 CONCLUSION AND SUMMARY OF EXAMPLE

Many steps were necessarily omitted from the description of Example 6.1 because the relevant procedures have not yet been described in the text. There will be more and fuller examples in later chapters. At least one will be given for each common type of experimental design, following the description of each.

Here is a summary of the principal steps followed in Chapters 4, 5, and 6 and Examples 4.1, 5.1, and 6.1:

1. The objectives of the study were stated.
2. The factors were decided upon—their number and the comparisons to be made.
3. The nature and number of the responses were established.

4. An experimental design (structure) was chosen.

5. The sample size was estimated.

6. A randomization plan was set up.

7. The blinding arrangements were planned.

8. If there were to be interim analyses, they were arranged for.

9. The protocol was written.

10. The operations handbook was prepared.

11. The expected statistical procedures were determined and described in the protocol.

12. The clinical report forms were designed and printed.

13. The database was prepared.

14. Meetings were held with the chosen investigators, the FDA, and others.

15. Arrangements were made to train the investigators, their assistants, and the patients.

6.12 PREVIEW OF REMAINING CHAPTERS

Chapters 1 through this chapter and Chapter 7 are introductory chapters in which we have presented an overall picture of our subject. The remaining chapters treat various aspects of industrial clinical trials in more detail.

The ensuing chapters are intended to review each of the essential steps in planning clinical studies in sufficient detail to enable you to administer the process of planning, designing your studies, and having them analyzed. There is virtually no material in this volume about the execution of your trials, but the Bibliography describes some books on that topic. Furthermore, matters involved in the preparations for a trial that are not somehow related to statistical design and analysis are either not described or at most are briefly touched upon. Most of the material following Chapter 7 (the protocol) will concern the planning and design stages of a study, with the exception of some introductory material on analysis, deemed desirable to provide a fuller understanding of the statistical aspects of any trial. I believe that you should be thoroughly familiar with any common experimental designs that you will be likely to use. This is not the case, however, for the statistical analyses of the data. The availability of an experienced biostatistician from the very first planning session is an absolute necessity for satisfactory trial design and analysis. You will need only sufficient knowledge to understand the interconnection of analysis with design and to enable you to work with the statistician in a knowledgeable manner. You will not need to carry out any data analyses yourself.

However, although you need not become involved in the data analysis, many of the examples in the following chapters will explain the statistical processes in considerable detail. I believe that approach is necessary to foster your understanding of the relationship between design and analysis, a weak point among many nonstatistical department members. Of course, although it is not necessary, you may do the analyses yourself if you desire. If you do, however, unless you have had thorough training in applied statistics as used in clinical studies, you should check all your work with the statistician. Statistical analyses, probability, and their applications are notorious for the existence of subtle traps for the unwary. But in spite of these remarks, merely to develop a good understanding of these processes, I strongly recommend that you actually carry out the procedures and calculations in the examples with your own calculator or computer. Of course, if some of you already have a facility in statistics, you may not require such practice.

Chapter 7 presents a brief set of guidelines intended to help ensure that your protocols are adequate from the point of view of experimental design and statistics. Part III provides a fairly detailed exposition of each design commonly used in industrial clinical trials, with examples of each.

The material on statistics in the two chapters of Part IV is concerned with the statistical analysis of the data resulting from your trials, and also includes examples. Only a few very common and quite simple procedures are described.

Finally, in Part V, some methods for estimating sample size for some common designs are given. Although the material in that chapter is concerned with your planning activities, it was necessary that it follow the two statistics chapters because the material requires some acquaintance with the methods and ideas of analysis. Like the other topics, examples are given for each of the important procedures. Because you must be more familiar with sample size estimation than with some of the more complex methods of analysis, methods of estimating sample size are given for some analytical procedures that are not described in this book, such as the analysis of variance (ANOVA).

6.13 SUMMARY OF THE CHAPTER

This chapter and the two preceding it were intended as an introduction to the major topic of this book—the planning of an industrial clinical trial. A simple but very commonly used kind of experimental design is used so that the major steps in the process would not be obscured by irrelevant details. The bulk of this chapter is concerned with randomization because I feel that procedure to be not only one of the most crucial steps in the design of a trial, but also perhaps one of the least well understood.

Following the material on randomization, there is a section on blinding, giving some information about how it is accomplished and emphasizing its importance. Next, the problems of interim analyses and truncated trials (carrying out statistical analyses on trials before they have been completed, and prematurely terminating a trial) are covered briefly. Suggestions for handling these difficult problems are given.

Finally, there is a brief treatment of several miscellaneous topics. These include (a) some preliminary information on the protocol; (b) a discussion of the uses and advantages of an operations manual, even for smaller studies; (c) the necessity of obtaining a clear description of the intended data-analysis procedures from the biostatistician; (d) a discussion of clinical report forms (CRFs) for recording data during a trial; and (e) some suggestions for the preparation and use of a computer database.

The chapter ends with a summary of the steps recommended in the planning of a trial, with particular reference to Examples 4.1, 5.1, and 6.1, the illustrations used to clarify many of the topics throughout this and the preceding two chapters.

6.14 LITERATURE REFERENCES

(1) Feinstein, Alvan R., *Science*, **242**, (1256–1263) 2 December 1988.

(2) Weaver, Warren, *Lady Luck: The Theory of Probability*, Dover Publications, Inc., Mineola, N.Y., 1989.

(3) Deming, W. Edwards, *The American Statistician*, **29**, 146–152, November 1975.

(4) Nelson, Lloyd S., *Journal of Quality Technology*, **22**, 328–330, October 1990.

CHAPTER 7

The Protocol and Clinical Report Forms

7.1 THE NEED FOR A PROTOCOL

A protocol should be written for every industrial clinical trial. The protocol is the master document that completely describes your trial. It should explain the background of the study, its objective(s), its planning (including the experimental design and sample-size estimates, and how they were obtained), its execution, and the expected methods of analysis of the data, in detail. It may often be the only definitive description of your clinical trial in existence, at least until the study is completed. A detailed and clearly written protocol is needed for submission to the FDA and the relevant Institutional Review Board(s) (IRBs) connected with the center(s) where the trial is to be run.

7.2 PRECISE WRITING AND ATTRACTIVE APPEARANCE

A good and useful protocol should be well-written, clear, very detailed, and complete. With regard to its physical form, it is now easy to produce an attractive, well laid out, and easily read document with presently available and inexpensive equipment (a small computer, a good word processor, and a laser printer). With respect to the writing, a poorly written or sloppy protocol can often lead to mistakes and misunderstandings throughout the execution and analysis of a trial. In the past, before the advent of desktop computers and laser printers, sloppy protocols, hastily copied on the office copier, were common. But today there is no reason to produce unprofessional appearing documents. However, there is still no substitute for the hard work of writing with clarity and of careful editing.

Poorly written or incomplete protocols are not products of an inability to write well and clearly or to produce a neat-looking document. Rather, they usually reflect a failure to provide sufficient time to do a really good job,

155

including editing and rewriting. There is often a subconscious feeling that the protocol, although a necessary component of the trial-planning process, is not one of great consequence. However, the production of a well-written and professional-appearing document should be a matter of pride even in the absence of any other motivation. A poorly written or sloppy-appearing protocol is often the result of an unexpressed feeling that the trial is the thing, not writing about it. The final version (if there are *any* draft versions) is sometimes left to the last minute, and then finished quickly, with a minimum amount of reviewing and editing, so that the writer(s) can get back to "more important" work. But to consider protocols or other written documents related to your studies to be relatively unimportant is a serious error.

So, again: It is necessary to allow time to write the protocol carefully, and to print it attractively. Taking care in these matters will contribute to the success and acceptability of your trial.

7.3 TOPICS THAT SHOULD BE COVERED IN THE PROTOCOL

7.3.1 Range of Topics

This chapter is concerned with the discussion of a number of topics that should appear in the protocol. Of course, it is important that items such as the chemistry of the test drug(s), previous safety testing, descriptions of the handling of unused returned drugs, details of the execution of the trial, recording of patient histories, discussions of the literature, and many other topics be discussed in the protocol. However, many of these issues are not closely related to the province of this book and therefore are covered only briefly here. Emphasis instead will be upon the many items related to statistical design and analysis in one way or another. The protocol topics to which we will devote the greatest attention are the experimental design, the sample size and power, the randomization(s), the kinds of analyses planned, and related matters. However, we show a moderately complete outline of the topics that should be included in any clinical study protocol in Section 7.3.4, for your reference.

7.3.2 The Protocol and the FDA

To the FDA Medical Officer and statistics personnel, your protocol is of critical importance. Whereas a discussion of the provisions of the protocol with FDA during planning is optional, although strongly recommended, that agency must see it before the trial starts. Thereafter, before or during the trial, any changes to the procedures described require early notification of the FDA. These usually take the form of documents called *protocol amendments*.

7.3.3 References

We recommend two fine articles about (a) the preparation of a protocol and (b) case report forms, by Harvey J. Hoyt and Charles C. Leighton, respectively. These comprise two chapters in McMahon's *Importance of Experimental Design and Statistics* [9]. Both authors have had wide experience in major drug companies, and speak with authority.

7.3.4 Checklist of Protocol Topics

Here is a list of the important elements of the protocol. All of them will be mentioned or discussed in the following sections. Items related to important topics covered in this book, including but not limited to statistically related items, will be discussed in greater detail than the others and are given in boldface. Note that any procedures taking place *during* a trial, in addition to some others, are not in boldface. This distinction is not meant to denigrate the importance of any such items, but merely to emphasize those that are related to the principal themes of this book.

1. Background and rationale of the study
2. **Objectives**
3. **Experimental design**
4. **Efficacy and Safety Responses**
5. **Sample size**
6. **Randomization procedure**
7. **Blinding**
8. Selection of patients
9. Estimated duration of study and visit frequency
10. Drug doses and scheduling
11. Drug formulation, packaging, and dispensing
12. Concomitant drugs
13. Statistical analyses
14. **Multicenter trials**
15. **Interim testing and early termination**
16. **Clinical report forms**
17. Regulatory issues

7.3.5 Background and Rationale of the Study (Item 1)

This information should appear in the introduction. A summary of the chemistry of the drug of interest and perhaps of related compounds already in use, the relevant animal pharmacology, the potential uses of the drug, any previous work, and similar issues belong in this section.

7.3.6   Objectives (Item 2)

This very important topic was covered fairly completely in Section 4.3 of Chapter 4, in connection with a discussion of initial planning. You should introduce and describe the objectives of your study early in the protocol. Obviously, a clear and complete statement is crucial to almost every portion of the study, and this section should therefore be written and edited with particular care. The suggestions made and details given in Chapter 4 with regard to defining objectives as a guide to your planning apply equally to the protocol.

7.3.7   Experimental Design (Item 3)

Descriptions of Design

The experimental design may comprise more complex designs than we have described so far. But regardless of its complexity, an unambiguous description of the structure (design) of the experiment should be written in rigorous terms by the statistician and should appear in the protocol, perhaps in an appendix or addendum to the protocol, along with a description of other statistical matters, such as the sample size estimation procedure and the anticipated method(s) of data analysis. References to the literature of statistics and experimental design, where and if pertinent, as well as other appropriate citations, if needed, should be given there. It is usually possible for such descriptions to be reasonably short, perhaps three to five double-spaced pages.

In addition to these items, a brief, unambiguous, and much less technical explanation of the experimental design, without the use of the technical language of statistics, should appear early in the main portion of the document. This section should be presented in terms familiar to scientific and medical readers who are not necessarily experienced in statistics. In general, the approach to this and related topics in the protocol should be similar to that used to prepare a scientific paper for publication, with comparable care and rigor, but with much more explanatory material. You should remember that many readers of the protocol, including, perhaps, company executives, may not be acquainted with the language of statistics and experimental design, nor perhaps with those of medicine and science.

The design may consist of more than one independent variable or factor. The factors should be clearly described, showing how they reflect the objectives of the trial. It should be explained that the mean responses generated by the patient groups treated with each of these factors or independent variables will be compared to determine whether it can be concluded that there are clinically important differences among them. Descriptions of possible interactions between factors may be left to the final report, if any are found, to avoid complexity in this part of the protocol.

7.3.8 Efficacy and Safety Responses (Item 4)

Descriptions of Responses

In the protocol, it is important to list the responses to be used and why they were chosen. These should include not only the one or more measurements for the assessment of efficacy, but, when possible, all the adverse effects that will be used as the safety observations for the trial. If more than one response of either kind is being planned, as is usually the case, a discussion of the methods of compensating for the multiplicity in the calculations used in estimating sample size should appear in the sample-size section of the protocol.

In this section, there should be a detailed description of each response to be measured or recorded, as well as instructions in detail for making the measurement. Complete and explicit instructions should also appear in each individual clinical report form and in the operations manual, if you use one. Of course, you will have chosen investigators who are specialists in the condition being studied. Nevertheless, detailed descriptions in the protocol and manual are important to avoid misunderstanding on the part of any reader. And having the instructions on each page of the CRFs as well will save conscientious investigators and assistants much time spent leafing through the protocol or manual if they have not had patients in the current study for a week or two. In addition, instructions on the CRFs will be useful for the patients in cases where the responses are to be self-elicited, as for the VAS scale. It goes without saying that any instructions included in the CRFs or operations manual should also appear in the protocol, because that is the master document, and includes every item appearing in the other two documents.

Variation in Measurements

The amount of detail in the descriptions of measurement processes in the protocol cannot be too great. Investigators may differ in the way they perform them. Many measurements comprise a number of steps, and it is easy to misinterpret or omit one or more. Even more important, because it may be contrary to intuition, is that when making a series of instrumental measurements, one should introduce as much normal variation as possible among successive repetitions. For example, whenever possible, measurements should be repeated with a moderate time interval between them. Two contiguous blood-pressure readings (not including any taken before the patient has become moderately relaxed) will quite frequently be more similar than two taken over a greater interval. Furthermore, almost *no* measurement should be made only once; with one reading, you cannot know how much variation may occur.[1]

---

[1]Of course, there are some cases, such as clinical laboratory tests, stress tests, and others, in which immediate repetition is impractical.

Blood-pressure measurements are common examples that show a substantial degree of variation. Both systolic and diastolic readings can vary substantially from one measurement to the next. They should always be taken two or three times, loosening or removing the cuff and perhaps even changing arms between readings, leaving an interval of several minutes between them, and averaging the results. The number of readings to be made at each session and the length of the intervals between them should be specified in the protocol, operations manual, and clinical report forms. It is a good idea to provide for the recording of the individual readings, as well as the averages, on the latter forms. If there are only small differences between readings, there may be something wrong. Variation is normal and is to be expected.

When reading the height of a layer of cells in a tube, as in making ESR observations, the tube should be set aside for a moment after the first reading, and then picked up again and reread. When using some kinds of judgment scores, each should be done two or three times with an interval between them. One way to do this is to measure a group of patients, wait a few minutes, and then go back to the beginning and repeat the procedure for each. Of course, this may not always be possible. If you are scoring headaches or other transient symptoms as in Example 5.1, and a treatment has been given, the interval between measurements cannot be great, because the headache may be reduced in severity by the treatment.

If you find repeated physiological measurements or judgment scale scores that show close agreement, you should become skeptical and check them carefully. Were they done without leaving an interval between them? Were they done carelessly? Is it possible that a knowledge of a previous value unconsciously biased the next reading or judgment?

Units of the Measurements

The units of every test measurement should always be given in the protocol and operations manual and shown with the measurements in the CRFs. For example:

Blood pressure (1st reading), systolic _____ mm Hg
Blood pressure (1st reading), diastolic _____ mm Hg

Blood pressure (2nd reading), systolic _____ mm Hg
Blood pressure (2nd reading), diastolic _____ mm Hg

Blood pressure (3rd reading), systolic _____ mm Hg
Blood pressure (3rd reading), diastolic _____ mm Hg

Approximate interval between readings _____ minutes

In this example, you will note that although the three systolic readings will eventually be averaged, as will the three diastolic measurements, they are not arranged for maximum convenience in doing this. Rather, they are arranged for the convenience of the person making the measurements. The averaging can be done later by your biostatistician or data-processing people. Attention to details such as this in planning and writing your protocol, operations manual and CRFs will pay off in greatly reduced errors and misunderstandings.

The units of a test should be specified whenever it is mentioned in the protocol or other documentation of a trial. If the response is a judgment scale, the specific scale to be employed, the method and words used to elicit a description of the pain or other symptom from the patient, the method of recording the data, and any literature references related to the procedure should all be given in the protocol. In the operations manual and CRFs, all these items except the literature references should appear.

Derived Responses

Response data must often be processed in various ways before they are analyzed, as in the averaging of the blood pressures. Other examples might be scores to be combined in assorted ways, nonlinear data transformations, combining pain intensity scores to produce SPID responses,[2] joint-tenderness indices, and others. Details of these procedures should either be given by the statistician in the description of the analyses or in the protocol proper ("Preparation of Data for Analysis"). When appropriate, literature references should appear here also. In the rare cases in which averages or other derived statistics must be entered in the case report form, you should be certain that the protocol requires this.

7.3.9 Sample Size (Item 5)

The sample sizes to be used, as well as the method(s) of estimating them, based upon calculations or the use of tables as described in Chapter 5 and later (in more detail in Chapter 15) should be described in your protocol. Like the description of an experiment in a scientific paper, this should include references and be given in sufficient detail to allow any competent reader to duplicate your procedure at any time. The values of alpha, beta, delta, and sigma employed in making your estimate(s) should be given explicitly. The power, also $1 - \beta$, should be explicitly indicated and probably explained for nonstatistical readers. We devote only a little space here to this topic, despite its importance, but the protocol should give the process used in considerable detail. You may wish to have the statistician give the details in a addendum, but you should present the actual sample sizes, with a reference to the method used, under the heading "Sample Size" in the main part of the document.

---

[2]Sum of Pain Intensity Differences. This is discussed thoroughly in Chapter 10.

7.3.10   Randomization Procedure (Item 6)

As do most practitioners of clinical studies, we consider the **random assignment** of treatments to patients in a clinical trial to be extremely important. The assignments are usually embodied in a **randomization table**. This table, showing the patient groups and their treatments (assignments of treatments to patients or the orders of assignment to each, if the design is a changeover) must **not** appear in the protocol or operations manual if the experiment is blind, as will nearly always be the case. However, the protocol should include a section in which the method of randomization used or to be used is carefully described. The reasons for the choice of a particular randomization procedure (nature of the design, of the analysis, or of the response, etc.) should also be explained.

Some principles of randomization were discussed in Chapter 6. Details for specific designs are given in the chapters on experimental designs (Part III, Chapters 8 to 12).

7.3.11   Blinding (Item 7)

This section should include descriptions of the blinding method in detail, including the method of packaging of the doses that ensures blinding, the procedures for breaking the blinding for any given patient, dose, and visit in case of an emergency, and which participants must be blinded.

7.3.12   Selection of Patients (Item 8)

This section should describe the source of the patients, the method of qualification of each, their numbering, implementation of a provision for informed consent, and the like. Certain cautions should be used when numbering the patients (the numbers will control which dose is assigned to each visit). For example, patients should not be numbered until each has agreed to take part and has been accepted into the trial.

7.3.13   Estimated Duration of Study and Visit Frequency (Item 9)

With the help of your investigators, you should be able to estimate the time required (at each center if the trial is multicenter) to complete the study, taking into account the expected number of patients required and the frequency of their visits to the clinic(s). If there is doubt about the ability of one or more clinics to complete its portion of the study in a reasonable time, you can provide for one or more additional centers to take part. The work at such additional centers should be started as early as possible, treating them like any others in the group, to avoid delay if a center must be eliminated. Be careful not to provide for more such additional clinics than absolutely necessary, however. If the unexpected occurs, and no centers drop out, you would then have a greater sample size than expected if one common method of analysis is used by your statistician, and the study would then possess more power than you planned. This could produce significances for differences too small to be of clinical interest.

7.3.14 Drug Doses and Scheduling (Item 10)

The nature and number of the test drugs and other treatments to be used in a study, the placebos (which we also refer to as treatments or "drugs" in this book), and any standards, such as established drugs of known efficacy, should be described early in the protocol. The frequency and magnitudes of the doses of each must be clearly stated. This information will be used in setting up the factor(s) for the experimental design, and is also necessary for many other purposes.

Some such language as this might be used: "There will be two active treatments: epiphthalic hydrate, supplied as 75-mg capsules, and chlorthalidone as 50-mg capsules (although the latter normally is available as tablets). The remaining treatment will be a placebo, also in capsule form. Each should be taken once a day by the patients to whom they are assigned. All three treatments must be identical in appearance. The placebo capsules will contain a harmless substance having no pharmacological effect (identify)."

If the investigator decides that the dose should be changed or the treatment discontinued for a given patient, that patient should usually be dropped from the study (i.e., the data should not be used in the analysis).[3] Of course, the patient should nevertheless be followed for as long as possible and the relevant records and information included in the final report.

Occasionally, a description of a study appears in which it is stated that the doses or even the drugs were varied irregularly during a trial. There are usually good medical or ethical reasons for such procedures, of course. But if the trial was planned without anticipating such changes, the data from the affected patients should not be used in the analysis.[4] All such omissions, if not planned beforehand, should be described in the final report, and the FDA should be notified immediately, because this is a protocol modification.

7.3.15 Drug Formulation, Packaging, and Dispensing (Item 11)

There should be a section in the protocol describing the composition of the drug treatments and the dosage forms used. If the trial is to be double blind,

---

[3]At times, the protocol will provide a way of altering the dose or dosage without dropping the patient. However, it is better to drop a patient unless that action would result in too small a sample size. If such contingencies are likely, sample sizes should be supplemented during planning, if possible.

[4]There are some trials in which this is expected, and the irregularities are considered an unavoidable part of the regimen. In such cases, the fact that they are likely to occur should be noted in the protocol.

as most will be, and if there is to be a placebo, the preparation of these should be described in detail. There will probably be special packaging procedures needed to allow maintenance of the blinding. Such procedures must allow the code to be broken in emergencies for one or a few patients without endangering the blinding for the others. There may also be details of the preparation of the dosage forms that should be included.

7.3.16   Concomitant Drugs (Item 12)

Any drugs that must be avoided during the trial, as well as others that can be allowed, should be listed in the protocol. If a patient or his or her physician indicates that any interfering drugs must be taken, that patient cannot be accepted into the trial.

7.3.17   Statistical Analyses (Item 13)

We recommend that you include a detailed description of the statistical analyses planned for the data of the study in the protocol, although this is not yet required by the FDA. Nevertheless, it is to everyone's benefit that you do so. If this information appears in the protocol, and if, when a final draft is available, you ask the FDA to comment on it, you may avoid later problems. You can provide for reasonable changes in the methods anticipated by indicating that if it is necessary to make changes, the new procedures will be equally suitable for the design used. If you plan and carry out analyses that the FDA does not favor, but do not ask for comments until the analysis is done, you will risk having to reanalyze the data or, possibly, to repeat the entire trial. To omit details of the proposed data analyses in the protocol, therefore, or to dismiss it with a phrase such as "The data will be analyzed using the analysis of variance," as has been commonly done in the past, is to produce a weak protocol, concerned with only two-thirds of the process of running your study.

Many protocols include almost no details of the analyses to be used. Two common excuses for this are that the usual reader, barring statisticians, will not understand them or that a proposed analysis may be changed when the time comes to analyze the data. Both of these are rationalizations. First, the description may be put in an appendix or addendum to the protocol, signaling the reader that only those interested need read it. Better, it is possible to write it in a way understandable to all. Doing so merely requires a belief that the effort is important. Second, although changes in the planned analyses may well occur, it can be pointed out, as just indicated, that any changes will serve the same purposes as the original procedures, and that the reasons for any changes will be given in the biostatistician's report.

Usually, you will wish to ask the biostatistician(s) to describe the expected analyses for inclusion in the protocol. If you are responsible for the overall project, you may wish to edit this section and then go over it with him or her.

You will usually need no more than about 500 to 1000 words. You should try to ensure that the material is written so that it can be understood by all concerned with the trial, regardless of their specialties.

Unfortunately, it appears to be easier to produce arcane professional jargon, undecipherable to people of callings other than the writers', than to write so that the material is clear to all. Please ask your statistician to write plainly. If he or she does not or cannot write clearly, the only readers who may understand the result may be those who already know what it says. Propagating a mystique may be fun, but it is not helpful. It is rare for a reader to feel insulted by a clear and simple explanation.

On the other hand, it is also common for protocols to contain scientific and medical material other than statistics that has been written with much more care than the statistical items. Poor quality of the statistical material can be easily the result of hasty writing by the statistician, of course. But it can occur for other reasons. I have read many protocols containing descriptions of planned statistical analyses, obviously not written by a statistician, but, not infrequently, by someone with a medical background. I am fairly sure that a study investigator responsible for performing complex medical procedures would object to them being described by a statistician.

If you accept this advice, there will be an adequate description of the proposed analysis in the protocol when it is sent to the FDA for review. At that time, you may want to ask for a meeting with the FDA Medical Officer assigned to your project to review your protocol and CRFs and make suggestions. It will be helpful also for you to ask that an FDA statistician be present—and that the company biostatistician be there also. In granting your request, the FDA will probably ask that the documents be sent early so that they may be studied before the meeting. During the meeting, ask whether the FDA statistician agrees with your choice of an experimental design, sample size, randomization procedure, and proposed statistical analysis. If he or she does not, or seems not to, ask for suggestions. Although, of course, the FDA will reserve the right to criticize or reject your trial when it is done if it feels it to be inadequate, such a meeting will go a long way toward helping to facilitate your project.

7.3.18 Multicenter Trials (Item 14)

In a multicenter study, a single protocol, with copies distributed to each investigator, *must* be used. In large trials, additionally, an operations manual becomes important. It is a good idea during the planning of any trial to hold rehearsals and discussions of the protocol among all personnel who will participate. These things are particularly important for a multicenter trial. A valid data analysis of all centers taken as a group cannot be done if there are major discrepancies among the segments of the data from the several centers because of variations in procedures. It is not true that data can be analyzed effectively regardless of the way they have been obtained. Differences among centers, if important, usually become obvious when attempts are made to analyze the data. If the data cannot be analyzed effectively as a single multicenter trial, as intended, the only recourse will be to try to analyze the results from each center separately, or at least after omitting centers with disparate data. But when that is done, the power of the statistical tests may well be substantially lower than that planned, perhaps too low to detect important treatment differences, because the sample sizes will be reduced below those required.

In planning a multicenter trial, provision should be made for the replacement of any centers that may possibly drop out before completing their part of the work. This is best done during planning by selecting more centers than called for in the original plan. If replacement of missing centers is done only later, after a dropout, the trial will be unnecessarily prolonged, and the cost will be likely to be comparable or greater than that of any additional centers recruited at the start. This kind of preplanning for these problems can be thought of as a contingency or insurance cost. On the other hand, it is important to keep such additional enrollments to a minimum, not only because of the additional cost, but also because, if there are no losses, the inclusion of the additional centers in the data analysis will *increase* the power substantially. Such an increase, if moderate or substantial, could inflate the sensitivity of the tests to a degree where differences of little practical importance may be detected by the analyses.

7.3.19 Interim Testing and Early Termination (Item 15)

The use of interim testing was mentioned briefly in Chapter 5, and methods for estimating the increased sample size necessary to allow for it were described in Chapter 6. The handling of early termination problems was also described in that chapter. If such allowances are made during planning, they should be mentioned in the protocol. A caution about the problem of doing more interim testing than planned for should be included.

If no interim testing is anticipated, and the probability of early termination is expected to be low, this should also be mentioned. The consequences if, contrary to expectations, some interim tests are done, should be mentioned. Frequently, interim tests are done in studies, when they have not been allowed for initially by increasing the sample size. When that happens, the specified risk(s) and/or the value of delta will be increased. This will mean, for instance, that the probability of detecting a treatment difference as small as that planned will be less than the probability you specified, that is, the power of *each* of the hypothesis tests, both interim and final, will be reduced. These facts should appear prominently in the protocol.

As explained in the preceding chapter, because most premature terminations are unexpected (otherwise, the planned sample size of a trial would have been different), little can be done except to calculate the value of delta if a trial *is* cut short, to get an idea of the minimum size of the differences that were detectable.

7.3.20   Clinical Report Forms (Item 16)

Planned Responses

When you plan a trial, you need an efficient system for recording, certifying, and preserving the original records of your study results. The records of the data will be the clinical report forms (CRFs), filled out in multiple copies by the investigators. In the past, many poorly planned, incomplete, and crudely executed CRFs have been produced and used in important industrial trials. It has not been unusual for data-processing people to have difficulty understanding the arrangement of information and interpreting the entries made by some of the investigators. These problems have usually not been the fault of the investigators, but of ambiguous, overcrowded, and poorly reproduced CRFs. Such carelessness is intolerable. CRFs are obviously of central importance. Therefore, they should be prepared with careful and thorough thought.

Copies of the CRFs should be bound with the protocol. As previously indicated, each should contain instructions, in careful detail, for carrying out the response measurements. A caution, such as *PLEASE FOLLOW THESE INSTRUCTIONS EXACTLY* should appear. The protocol, and perhaps the CRFs, should include a caveat against the not unheard-of practice of writing results on scrap paper for later transcription to a CRF. Scrap paper makes a poor and indefensible research record.

In other words, the CRFs, when complete, should constitute the original records of a trial, handled in the same way as properly executed industrial research laboratory notebook records, with entries made at the time the work is done, and with dates and signatures. On a CRF, the space for the investigator's signature should be preceded by a statement such as "I certify that this clinical report form is an original record, and that it is correct and complete to the best of my knowledge."

A separate section of the protocol should be devoted to a description of each of the CRFs to be used, with a sample of each in its final form. Sufficient time should be made available to ensure that all of the needed CRFs have been designed before the protocol is completed as planned and given to the investigators and others needing it.

Figure 7.1 is an illustration of a CRF intentionally made simple and on a single page, to display some of the points discussed here and previously. It is an exact reproduction of an original document produced with a personal computer and a small laser printer. If necessary, more than one page might be used, but such a set should nevertheless cover only one patient, one visit, and one response. The use of a separate CRF page or pages for each visit and patient is important because it will simplify the transcription of the data to the computer when the data are ready. The use of a single response per page is not necessary, although you may find it convenient and simple to do

SUPREMEX DRUG COMPANY, INC.
CLINICAL REPORT FORM

Study of Beta Blocker 741-A	**Study No. 511**	**Page CRF-7**

Blood Pressure Measurements
(Patient Seated)

Patient Number_____   **Visit Number**_____   **Date**_____

Investigator_____   **Name of Clinic**_____

Procedure (Please follow exactly)

Please obtain this response during every visit. Take three sets of measurements, as provided below. Loosen the cuff and allow a two minute interval between sets. Read the sphygmomanometer to the nearest 2 to 5 mm and enter the results *on this form* immediately following each pair of readings. The patient should be seated comfortably at a table, with his or her arm placed horizontally on the surface.

Reading No.	Systolic (mm)	Diastolic (mm)
1	_____	_____
2	_____	_____
3	_____	_____

Comments:_____

_____

_____

Last date sphygmomanometer tested:_____

I certify that the above results were obtained by me or under my supervision on the above date from the patient listed, that they are true and correct, and that they were entered directly and immediately on this CRF.

_____
Investigator

Figure 7.1   Example of a clinical report form (CRF).

so. Note that instructions are given on the form. This should *always* be done, although the same instructions, preferably in a less abbreviated form, should also appear in the operations manual, if any, and in the protocol, because the CRFs will be illustrated there. The preparation time for this sample form was no greater than would have been required for ordinary typing. The greatest amount of time used in its creation was in the planning.

Adverse-Effects Information

In addition to the planned responses, the FDA requires that any adverse effects noted during a trial be reported. If they appear serious in the opinion of the investigator, the blinding must be removed for the affected patients and they must be reported to the sponsor's representative and dropped from the trial. Of course, these noncompleters must continue to be followed thereafter. You may find it desirable to specify in the protocol that the adverse effects be classified, and possibly compared statistically, by treatment groups.

A supply of adverse-effects record sheets should be prepared, along with the other CRFs. Like the CRFs for the planned responses, they should be displayed in the protocol, with instructions for their use. An adequate number should be provided to each investigator before the trial starts. The forms should include space for descriptions of the adverse effects, their frequencies, and their dates of occurrence. Space should be provided for the investigator's opinion as to whether or not the observed effect is drug-related. As for the other CRFs, a set of instructions printed on the forms will help ensure that all investigators tend to act uniformly. Like the other CRFs, these forms should be printed rather than typed and duplicated. The investigator may make copies of these and the other CRFs for his or her files, but the original must be conveyed to the sponsor.

7.3.21 Regulatory Issues (Item 17)

Chapter 3 was devoted to this topic. One way to keep any regulatory information that has particular relevance to the current trial where it can be readily found is to devote a section of the protocol to it. Remember, the protocol exists to provide a *complete* description of the planned trial for all those concerned.

7.4 SUMMARY OF THE CHAPTER

This chapter discusses the major sections that should be included in a protocol. We mention not only the technical and statistical aspects of your proposed trial, but also the more important nontechnical issues. There are 17 important items in this category. After some introductory material, they are listed and then discussed individually.

PART III

Some Experimental Designs, with Examples

CHAPTER 8

One-Factor Parallel Designs

8.1 ABOUT THE DESIGN CHAPTERS

The first three chapters of this book (Part I) were introductory material. Then, Chapters 4 through 7 (Part II) provided a "once over lightly" treatment of the highlights of the process of planning a clinical trial, including examples of simple, **one-factor, completely randomized** experimental designs. In Part III, we present a more detailed treatment of the most common experimental designs used in clinical studies. We will omit some designs that, although used occasionally, are not common in clinical studies and may involve complexities in their relationships to the data-analysis procedures.

As you know, the design establishes the number of factors you must use, their levels, and the nature and arrangement of the experimental units. It also designates the kind and amount of replication used, the randomization called for, and, peripherally, the sample size, the nature and number of the responses, and the kind of analysis to be done. It thus becomes the dominant component of your planning, governs the execution of your trial, and, most important, mandates the nature of the data analysis that must be used when the study is complete. Hence, in this volume, including the chapters in Part II and in this Part III, we devote more space to the experimental design than to any other topic.

This chapter is concerned exclusively with one-factor, completely randomized designs of the kind displayed in the examples in the previous chapters, but treated in greater depth. We believe that a reasonable knowledge of the kinds and properties of experimental designs, like the fundamentals of hypothesis testing presented in Part II, is essential for anyone responsible for the planning, execution, and data analyses of clinical trials. And we believe that this applies equally to those in a supervisory position and those actually carrying out these steps.

We begin with some ideas and definitions that are basic to experimentation. The differences between experiments and surveys are described, some definitions are given, and the idea of diagramming your designs as a planning aid is discussed. After these preliminaries, the remainder of the chapter is

173

devoted to the examination, with examples, of the basic single-factor parallel configuration. Some of this material, including the examples, will be brief, because this design has already been introduced and discussed at some length in Part II. However, because of the importance of the one-factor completely randomized design, we will include further and more complete examples later in Part III.

8.2   EXPERIMENTS AND SURVEYS

Broadly speaking, clinical studies are of three varieties—two major categories and a hybrid of the two. In this book, we call the first kind **experiments** and the second **surveys**. The difference is the following, assuming a parallel trial: In an experiment, it is possible to assign *any* level of an independent variable, such as a drug or other treatment, to *any* patient or subject among those available. For example, if *drugs* is a factor, with three levels (three different drugs), a planner can assign any one of the three to any given patient. In a survey, on the other hand, the levels of some or all of the independent variables or factors cannot be assigned in this way, because they are characteristics of the subjects, or at least they are not in fact assigned freely. For example, suppose that the sex of a patient is to be a factor, with the two levels, male and female. You do not have the freedom to assign the levels male or female to any given patient; unlike *drugs*, one or the other level of *sex* is already "assigned" to any subject you select, and cannot be (easily) changed. You could say that in an experiment, the experimenter possesses complete control over which experimental unit receives a given treatment, whereas in a survey, this kind of control does not exist, or is not used. Of course, even in an experiment, if it is properly designed, the power to control which level of a factor will be used is not applied in an arbitrary or deterministic manner. Rather, almost always, the assignments are done with the use of some randomizing procedure.

The third category, the **hybrids**,[1] are "in-between" studies, in which some variables can be and are assigned randomly, but others are not. These are quite common, but the fact that one or more factors in such a study are not freely assignable to any subject is not always taken into account when the data are analyzed. For survey-type variables, a different kind of analysis is not necessary, but the interpretation of the results will be different.

8.2.1   Experiments

In an **experiment**, treatments are assigned to patients or subjects by an experimenter or planner, and, as just indicated, any treatment may be assigned to any patient who does not already have an assignment. The

---

[1]This term, to my knowledge, is my own, and has not been used generally in the literature.

selection of a patient for each treatment assignment (or the selection of a treatment for a given patient) can be random, although the random allocation is not necessary to qualify a study as an experiment under this definition. Of course, randomization is necessary to ensure that the statistical tests of the data (or even the "eyeballing" of them) will give valid answers without requiring unnecessary assumptions. But the simplest definition of an experiment is that it is a process in which the assignment of any level of any of the factors is not limited by the nature of the experimental unit (the patient, in this case).

8.2.2 Surveys

In a **survey**, an experimenter cannot or does not control whether a specific patient receives a given treatment. An example of a study in which the "treatment" is inseparable from the patient (i.e., in which the selection of a patient also selects a specific treatment) is the comparison of smokers with nonsmokers. "Smoking" or "nonsmoking" cannot be assigned, randomly or otherwise, to a given patient or subject; he or she comes with a ready-made assignment. The patients can be divided into smoking and nonsmoking groups, but *which* patients are put into each group is predetermined. It has not been arrived at according to some procedure employed by the investigator, and is certainly not random. Similarly, sex or any other acquired or inherent trait cannot be assigned to a given patient merely at the will of the experimenter. Instead, treatment groups of subjects or patients who already have the characteristics of interest are formed by the experimenter.

There are some kinds of survey variables for which it is possible to assign any treatment to any patient, as in an experiment, but in which, nevertheless, the patient or investigator chooses not to do so. Such conditions are thus similar in effect to those for a treatment like sex, age, or smoking, because they are not assigned freely to any patient. One kind of variable in this category is a drug treatment (e.g., a steroid treatment for severe arthritis) that, although assignable or deletable in theory, cannot ethically be withdrawn from patients volunteering to take part in a trial.

Thus, in a survey, random assignment is not used either because it is not possible or not practical. A major purpose of randomization is to help ensure, on the average, that patient characteristics that might affect the response are as likely to be present in patients to whom one treatment is assigned as to another. If randomization is not used, the risk that this will *not* be so is increased. In such a case, the experimenter or designer in effect assumes that there is *not* a predominance of particular patient characteristics in a given treatment group that might seriously bias the response measurements relative to those of the other groups. More simply, he or she must assume that if there were no differences among the several treatments, all the groups would be alike in their response measurements or observations, within the limits of normal experimental error. Of course, a careful experimenter, faced with the necessity of running an unrandomized trial, will use whatever precautions are possible.

For example, a planner may wish to measure certain characteristics of heavy drinkers, comparing them with light drinkers, each defined in some explicit way. This sounds like the use of a controlled factor or variable called "drinking," but it is not. In the drinking study, those subjects who habitually drink heavily have already categorized themselves, and the same is true of the light drinkers. That is, the groups have not been formed by the experimenter, but are already defined at the time they are chosen, and cannot be changed. Compare this factor ("drinking") with a factor like "drugs," in an experiment. Here, the experimenter may randomly assign *any* patient or subject to *any* drug. This is an experiment. The drinking study is a survey.

When one treatment instead of another is randomly assigned to a patient, the particular physical and mental characteristics of that patient, some of which may affect the reaction to the treatment, are chosen by chance. This and the other treatments are equally likely to be assigned to similar or dissimilar patients. On the other hand, for example in a smoking study, patients may be smokers because of inherent attributes predisposing them to it. These attributes, rather than (or in addition to) smoking itself, can affect the response measurement. The experimenter must assume that such "lurking variables"[2] will have little or no effect. To put it still another way, the validity of the results of such a study is a matter of opinion. Any conclusions from such a study must depend upon logic and knowledge of the system, that is, they must lose possible statistical support. At worst, they may merely reflect an investigator's opinions or preconceptions.

8.2.3 Hybrids

General
A **hybrid** study is one employing both kinds of independent variables. On the one hand are those already possessed by the patients, which cannot or will not be changed: "survey-type variables." On the other hand, a hybrid study also includes true experimental variables, such as drugs or other medical treatments, that *can* be randomly assigned by the experimenter. Well-designed hybrid studies are necessary and practical. An experimenter can keep the nonassigned variables in mind when drawing conclusions based upon the statistical data analyses, perhaps restricting statistically supported conclusions to the randomly assigned variables.

The Use of Hybrid Studies
When we speak of variables that are not or cannot be assigned at will, and that, when used in a study, make it a survey or a hybrid rather than a "pure" experiment, we are referring to their use as independent variables (treat-

---

[2]Credit for the most expressive term "lurking variable" belongs to a well-known statistician, Professor G. E. P. Box of the University of Wisconsin.

ments). This does not preclude using some subjects or patients with different ages or sexes, for example, in a true experiment, as long as the randomization is properly done. Such characteristics can be used as *nuisance factors*, or their effects, if any, may simply be allowed to add to the error estimate in an analysis, avoiding their influence upon the factors of interest, but perhaps reducing power. For example, in a moderate to large experiment, or in the "long run" in a series of experiments, in most cases the probability of the treatment groups containing nearly the same numbers of males and females or old and young people will be high, unless the investigator intentionally alters it. Thus, if these characteristics have any influence upon the results of an experiment, their effects tend to be "cancelled out," simply by the use of the randomization. When this is true, these effects will not bias the conclusions drawn from the results of a trial, although they may increase the experimental error (the standard deviation or variance of the response data), thereby decreasing the power of the hypothesis tests used.

Even this disadvantage can be eliminated, however. As you will see in a subsequent chapter, the effects, if any, of such "nuisance variables" can be handled by the use of special designs such as randomized blocks, latin squares, or other structures that use special kinds of *blocking*. These arrangements prevent the effects of the nuisance variables from increasing error, thus increasing the power of the eventual statistical tests of the data. The cost of this reduction of error is the greater complexity of such designs, which brings about greater difficulty of administration during the execution of a trial. Some hybrid designs can handle the nonassignable nuisance variables by blocking in this way. But it is also possible to use completely randomized designs, simply remembering that the results of any hypothesis tests involving variables comprising inherent patient characteristics should be viewed with caution.

8.2.4 When Surveys Are Necessary

The paper by Feinstein (1) mentioned previously does an excellent job of discussing the results of dependence upon surveys. It is obvious, of course, that many experiments are impossible or impractical, and surveys must be used instead (e.g., the famous Surgeon-General's report on *Smoking and Health*). But when a study *must* be run as a survey, the investigator or sponsor has a greater responsibility for attempting to avoid ambiguity of the results than for an experiment. Consequently, when there is a choice, a true experiment, rendering less arguable the validity of correctly done statistical hypothesis tests, is substantially preferable.

8.2.5 The Other Side of the Question

In fairness, it must be pointed out that the subject of the use of surveys vs. experiments can be debated, and like all debates, there are two sides to the question. William G. Cochran, one of the greatest and most respected statisticians of our time, was the author of a book on this subject (2). The editors of Cochran's book are also well-known statisticians. No great amount of space is devoted to the argument for the use of surveys; rather, the point of view is that you use them when you really cannot randomize, but must do a study. Surveys should not be used in any new drug submission except as supporting information. Certainly, it would be very difficult for a sponsor to persuade the FDA to accept survey data as primary evidence of efficacy.

8.3   DEFINITIONS

A few common expressions in the language of experimental design will be used frequently in this and succeeding chapters. Although some of them have already been introduced, they are collected here for reference:

- A **factor** is a group or class of treatments, such as "drugs" or "doses." It is an expected "source of variation." That is, the experiment is designed in such a way that if there are differences among the levels of a factor (such as the use of two or more different drugs), the expected response measurement will be affected. There are factors in both experiments and surveys.

- A **treatment** is a substance or procedure administered for medical or study purposes, such as a drug, a placebo, or a medical or surgical procedure. In this book, the word usually refers to a drug or placebo. Generally, a single material that is a member of a group or class is meant. For example, if you are planning a trial to compare a group of drugs with each other, *each one* of those drugs might be called a treatment. The term "treatment" is also used, more loosely, in the sense of "factor." For a survey, we could use the term "treatment" for nonassigned factors, such as sex or age, but that usage could be confusing, because the term conveys the idea of control.

- The **levels** of a factor are the several treatments of which it is composed. For example, the factor, drugs, might have three levels: penicillin V, chloramphenicol, and placebo. The levels can be quantitative, as for "doses," rather than qualitative, as for "drugs." For example, a quantitative factor called "doses" might have three levels: b.i.d., t.i.d, and q.i.d. The levels of a qualitative factor cannot be ordered; one drug cannot be "greater" or "smaller" than another. A nonassignable factor also must have levels; for example, for the factor "age of patient" a planner might specify three levels: 18–35, 36–60, and over 60.

- **Factors** and **levels**: It is important to be sure you fully understand the difference between factors (independent variables, often called "sources of variation"; i.e., variation in the measurement) and their levels. A factor is a major *category* of items, like drugs, doses, characteristics of the patients, chemical classes of drugs, and the like. Every factor must have two or more levels. The levels of factors are subcategories—subsets of types within major categories (*kinds* of drugs within the factor, drugs; i.e., the *components* of a factor). All the examples given in this book will be designs in which it is intended that comparisons among treatments or treatment combinations will be made when the data are analyzed. This being so, although a design can have a single factor, there must be at least two levels of that factor. The examples that follow will make this clear.

- The designs of this chapter and the next are often called **completely randomized designs**. A completely randomized design is one in which the random assignment of patients to treatments is not restricted in any way beyond ensuring that there are one or more patients assigned to each treatment group. Usually, however, we also arrange to obtain equal numbers in each group, but continue to call the design completely randomized. Among other things, randomization helps to ensure that sources of variation not accounted for in the design will tend to affect all of the data equally. In some designs, as you will see later, the randomization procedure is less complete. In these, the designer explicitly accounts for some expected sources of variation in the data and provides for certain limitations in the randomization of the design. This often results in the addition of more factors in lieu of randomizing completely. Such designs will usually provide smaller experimental errors, hence, more power. Unfortunately, for every factor added to a design, its complexity, and therefore the difficulty of administration of the study, increases substantially.

- A **factorial design** (discussed in detail in Chapters 9 through 12) is a design using more than one factor in a single experiment. The designs of this chapter, all of which have only one factor, can be thought of as the simplest members of the class of factorial designs. The term is often not used, however, unless there are two or more factors. Single-factor designs do not possess many of the interesting properties of factorials because of their simplicity.

- **Dependent** and **independent variables**: An **independent variable** in an experiment or survey is another name for a factor. A factor is a variable because it has two or more different levels. It is a variable property, either inherent or assigned, of the experimental units, that is expected to produce some kind of response. For example, if a factor has levels consisting of two different drugs, the two treatment groups (one for each drug) will be expected to produce different mean values of the measurement or response. The dependent variable is the response measurement. One variable (a dependent variable) is a **function** of another (an independent variable) if its value is affected by the level of the latter.

8.4 DIAGRAMS OF EXPERIMENTAL DESIGNS

Throughout this and the following chapters on experimental designs, we will illustrate them with diagrams that show their structure. The diagrams will sometimes resemble data tables lacking data, **table diagrams**, and at other times will be of a sort that we will call **block diagrams**.

The table diagrams will usually be used to illustrate the structures of various parallel designs, and will incorporate rows and columns with particular significances. The block diagrams will be characterized by the use of one or more outlines or "boxes." The boxes will contain information representing experimental units having various treatments.

8.5 TWO-TREATMENT SINGLE-FACTOR DESIGNS

8.5.1 The Usefulness of Single-Factor Designs

The designs of this chapter are all single-factor. Single-factor structures are the simplest and easiest to manage of all experimental designs. They are also the most frequently used of all clinical trial designs, although multifactor designs are much more prevalent in the hard sciences and engineering. The designs described in Chapters 4 through 6 were single-factor arrangements. In general, when a single-factor design will supply all the necessary information, it will practically always be the best choice. However, more than one factor is often needed to satisfy the objectives of a study. At such times, there is sometimes a tendency to use several one-factor designs in separate trials, but this procedure is practically always the wrong choice. When there are several factors, it is almost always better to use multifactor **factorial** designs. Multifactor designs are the subjects of the chapters following this one in Part III.

8.5.2 Example 8.1: Illustration of a Two-Treatment Design

Figure 8.1 is a "table diagram" showing a two-treatment single-factor design with 20 patients in each treatment group. The two columns represent the two treatment groups of patients, corresponding to the two levels of the factor. They were formed by randomly selecting 20 patients for assignment to each of the two drugs, T_1 and T_2. The symbol T_1 represents a test drug, and T_2 may be a placebo or another drug that is expected to be active. Each pair of double hyphens in a column represents a response elicited from one subject. Here, we might use the letter k instead of T, with subscript 1 or 2 to identify the two treatments, K to represent the total *number of treatments*, and N or n to represent numbers of repetitions of an item. Thus, in this design, k_1 or T_1 represents treatment 1 and k_2 or T_2 represents treatment 2. The value of K is 2 ($K = 2$), representing the total number of treatments. Likewise,

Treatments	
T_1	T_2
--	--
--	--
--	--
--	--
--	--
--	--
--	--
--	--
--	--
--	--
--	--
--	--
--	--
--	--
--	--
--	--
--	--
--	--
--	--
--	--
$n_1 = 20$	$n_2 = 20$
$N = 40$	

Note: The clustering into groups of five in the body of the figure was done for ease of reading and counting.

Figure 8.1   Table diagram of two-treatment one-factor design.

$n_1 = 20$, the number of patients who were assigned to treatment 1, $n_2 = 20$, the number on treatment 2, and $N = 40$, the total number of patients taking part.

You may feel that the translation of plain and simple words into this set of symbols unnecessarily complicates the portrayal of the treatments and quantities represented. However, introducing them here for the simplest designs will render these expressions familiar to you at an early stage, and will make it simpler for you to see the relationships among factors, their levels, and their replications for the more complex designs.

The table diagram of Figure 8.1 does not identify the patient numbers assigned to each treatment, but only the response values (represented by the double hyphens) for each patient. However, when the identification of the patients receiving each treatment is necessary or desirable, an additional column for each treatment group, showing patient numbers, can easily be added. Of course, this identification must not be available to patients or team members, who must be blinded until the trial has been completed and analyzed.

In a table diagram of a one-factor design such as that of Figure 8.1, each column represents one level of the factor. The two data in each row have no special relationship to each other, and the data for any patient could be placed anywhere in its column without changing the meaning of the diagram or the outcome of the statistical analysis. That is, in the style of diagram we use in this book to illustrate one-factor designs, the repeated items in each column merely represent **replication** (repetition), using additional patients. On the other hand, as you will see in the next chapter, in a two-factor or multifactor design, both the rows and the columns, rather than the columns alone, represent factor levels.

8.6 ONE-FACTOR DESIGNS WITH MORE THAN TWO TREATMENTS

8.6.1 Description

Examples 4.1, 5.1, and 6.1 in Chapters 4, 5, and 6, respectively, use a design of this kind. In these examples, there is only one factor, "drugs," but that factor possesses four levels, consisting of a placebo and three drugs or drug

Treatments		
T_1	T_2	T_3
--	--	--
--	--	--
--	--	--
--	--	--
--	--	--
--	--	--
--	--	--
--	--	--
--	--	--
--	--	--
--	--	--
--	--	--
--	--	--
--	--	--
--	--	--
--	--	--
--	--	--
--	--	--
--	--	--
--	--	--
$n_1 = 20$	$n_2 = 20$	$n_3 = 20$
	$N = 60$	

Note: The clustering into groups of five in the body of the figure was done for ease of reading and counting.

Figure 8.2 Table diagram of three-treatment one-factor design.

combinations that are expected to be active. A practical matter to keep in mind in this case is that, because there will be more than one comparison to make (because there are more than two treatments), there will be multiplicity problems for which to plan. The resolution of these will require increases in sample size *per treatment* beyond that required for a two-treatment design. The Bratcher, Moran, and Zimmer (3) sample size/power tables discussed in Chapter 15 will solve this problem, however.

8.6.2 Example 8.2: A Three-Treatment Design

Although I am sure that you can visualize this design, it is illustrated for your future reference in Figure 8.2. Here, $K = 3$, that is, the single factor of the design has three levels or treatments rather than two (T_1, T_2, and T_3). The table diagram therefore has three columns instead of two, but is otherwise similar to Figure 8.1.

8.7 DESIGNS WITH UNEQUAL SAMPLE SIZES

8.7.1 Example 8.3: Unequal Group Sizes

A design need not have the same number of patients for each treatment. Although the statistical analysis of designs having unequal sample sizes must

Treatments			
T_1	T_2	T_3	T_4
--	--	--	--
--	--	--	--
--	--	--	--
--	--	--	--
--	--	--	--
--	--	--	--
--	--	--	--
--	--	--	
--	--	--	
--	--	--	
--	--	--	
--		--	
--		--	
		--	
		--	
$n_1 = 13$	$n_2 = 11$	$n_3 = 15$	$n_4 = 7$
	$N = 46$		

Note: The clustering into groups of five in the body of the figure was done for ease of reading and counting.

Figure 8.3 Table diagram of four-treatment one-factor design with unequal group sizes.

take those differences into account, for one-factor designs, the procedure is only trivially more complex than for equal sample size designs. On the other hand, there are advantages (see what follows) to using designs in which each treatment is assigned to the same number of patients. The cases in which it is advantageous to *design* a trial with unequal sample sizes are rare. It is not uncommon, however, to encounter unequal sample sizes among data arriving for analysis after a trial, because of patient noncompleters. Figure 8.3 shows a four-treatment parallel design in which this may have been the reason for the unequal sample sizes shown. Each treatment group contains a different number of patients.

8.8   MORE ABOUT SINGLE-FACTOR DESIGNS

8.8.1   Data for Analysis

When an experiment has been completed and the results are available for statistical analysis, the data from each response in a single-factor design can be assembled into a table that would look like Figures 8.1, 8.2, or 8.3 (with the appropriate number of columns) except that the measurements (usually numbers) would be substituted for the double hyphens in the bodies of the tables. Although it is not essential for the analysis of the data, it is worth some effort to attempt to attain equal sample sizes by trying to minimize the number of noncompleters. This may require unusually careful and attentive administration of the trial by the investigator(s), but could be worthwhile, particularly if the alternative is particularly disparate group sizes. The advantage to be gained is that with equal sample sizes, the statistical power will be at its maximum, because the standard deviation will be minimized. The greater the disparity in group sizes, the greater the standard deviation will tend to be.[3]

8.8.2   Analysis

Although there has been no detailed discussion of statistical methods and related topics in this book so far, a couple of points related to the statistical analysis of your data must be mentioned here. This subject will be discussed and exemplified in more detail in Part IV.

The appropriate analysis for a single-factor study depends principally upon whether the factor has two or more than two levels, and upon the type of response measurement that was used. Some responses require different

---

[3]When using the usual statistical procedures to compare treatments from two or more groups, an estimate of the standard deviation derived from a "pooled" variance (a form of weighted average) is used. For a given total sample size, if the variance of two populations to be compared is the same, it can be shown that, on the average, pooled variances from unequally sized samples taken from them will be larger than otherwise.

statistical techniques for comparing treatments than others. If more than one kind of response measurement is used in the trial, your biostatistician may use several different statistical methods. On the other hand, a specific design or a given response does not always require one particular statistical procedure. There are various kinds of analysis that are roughly equivalent. For example, if there are only two levels of the factor (two drugs, or a test drug and a placebo, for instance), and if the parametric assumptions appear satisfied, either a *t* test or a rank test (explained in Part IV) will give reasonably equivalent results. If there is doubt as to whether the assumption of normality of the populations sampled is reasonable, the rank test is preferable, or, instead, a data transformation followed by a *t* test may be appropriate. Also, unequal variances or lack of additivity among the sampled populations may call for a data transformation before analysis. The most serious problems can arise if the assumption of independence does not appear satisfied. This is quite infrequent, but when it does exist, it can often be traced to poor design or execution of the trial. In such a case, there is often no remedy beyond repeating the entire trial.

If there are more than two treatments, and the parametric assumptions are satisfied reasonably well, there are several equivalent approaches to making the necessary statistical comparisons. These include the use of one of several available multiple-comparisons procedures or the use of an analysis of variance (ANOVA) followed by a series of *t* tests if the ANOVA shows significance. If the assumptions of normality and equal variances in the populations do not appear to be satisfied, there are multiple-treatment rank tests that can be used. Alternatively, a transformation may be found, and, if so, a parametric analysis can then be used.

8.8.3 Factors with Only One Level

You may ask, "What about factors with only one level?" Such experiments are possible, but they usually represent poor science. For example, as mentioned earlier, an experiment can comprise a "before-and-after" test, a favorite of Madison Avenue. In such a procedure, instead of comparing results for the treatment group with a *concurrent* control (i.e., a placebo or standard administered to a patient group that has undergone all the procedures undergone by the treatment group), the experimenter makes the comparison with baseline data gathered before the treatment was administered. This is poor science, because it makes no allowance for possible changes in the potential responses of the subjects after the baseline tests have been done and before the final measurements have been made. When a treatment can be given and its effect observed or measured immediately, such a test may be useful, but this is very rarely the case in clinical studies. When a concurrent control is omitted in a clinical trial, the investigator *assumes* that if the patients had not been given the active treatment, the measurements taken after treatment would be the same as the baseline measurements except for experimental error. This, however, is a matter of opinion. With a concurrent control, there is no need for such an assumption.

Instead of comparing results with baseline data, some papers describe studies in which investigators have gone even further by substituting information from previous experiments described in the literature, mental concepts, "common knowledge," or hearsay. Each of these has at times been called a "historical control." Such studies are common in the medical literature, but, unfortunately, they represent a step backward in the application of the science of experimental design in clinical work.

To summarize, with a few rare exceptions for which no choice exists, *every* well-designed clinical study should be planned so that the results can be based upon *internal, concurrent* comparisons with one or more other treatments, usually including a control or standard. There are many assumptions that an experimenter and a biostatistician must make, but it is important to avoid those that are unnecessary and increase the risk of a wrong conclusion when the trial is done.

8.9   EXAMPLE 8.4: A ONE-FACTOR TWO-LEVEL PARALLEL DESIGN

8.9.1   Objectives of the Study, Treatments, and Response

The illustrations of one-factor parallel designs presented in Chapters 4 to 6 were only partially described, because not all the necessary background was then available to you. We now have sufficient acquaintance with parallel designs, as well as their prerequisites, to provide a more complete description of all the planning steps. This example will be patterned upon the model of the two-treatment one-factor parallel design of Example 8.1, which was diagrammed in Figure 8.1.

This study was a small early phase trial of patients with angina pectoris. Before and during the study, all the patients selected used self-administered sublingual glyceryl trinitrate tablets as needed, but no other treatment. The object of the study was to compare the efficacy of two drugs in reducing the frequency of angina attacks and of providing more rapid relief from them. The two were a beta blocker (T_1), and a calcium-channel blocker (T_2). There was no placebo, as it was strongly suspected by the sponsor that at least one and probably both treatments would show efficacy, and it was felt to be unethical to refuse the patients an opportunity to experience longer and perhaps greater relief than that afforded by the nitroglycerin. Exercise tolerance tests, self-counts of the number of times each patient used the nitroglycerine in each of two 1-month periods, and other measurements were used as responses. The exercise test data only are used in this example because they are measurements on a continuous scale (number of minutes before a response was noted in the EKG). Note that although we have recommended the use of replicate measurements on each patient when practical, this is an example in which repeated measurements would not be realistic.

Safety measurements (adverse effects data) are of course necessary in any trial involving a new drug or one that has not been used for the current purpose before. For simplicity, however, we ignore them here.

One of the two treatments, the particular calcium-channel blocker selected, had not been used for angina before. The principal object of the investigation of which this trial was a part was to evaluate that drug in several ways as a treatment for angina in comparison with a beta blocker, a known angina treatment. A larger single-center trial was expected to follow this one, and, if the results were promising, one or more additional single-center trials followed by two or more very large multicenter trials were planned. A single investigator, a cardiologist, took part in this trial, and all the patients were hers.

8.9.2 Protocol

Throughout the process described here, a protocol was in preparation, following the ideas and principles detailed in Chapter 7.

8.9.3 Sample Size Estimation

Estimation When There Is Information about Sigma

This section treats the subject of sample size estimation briefly and without much detail, as part of this example. A more complete treatment was given in Chapter 5, and still more detail will be presented in Part V.

When you use well-planned and carefully done estimates of sample size in your studies, the dependability of your final conclusions will be increased. You will be able to assume, with adequate confidence, that the trial is neither so small as to prevent dependable detection of a clinically important treatment effect (such as a difference between two treatment population means) nor so large that it will yield statistically significant results even if the effect is too small to be important. You will remember that the actual value of delta (the minimum treatment difference that you wish to detect) depends upon the magnitude of the risks, alpha and beta, that you have specified, upon an estimate of sigma, and upon the sample size of either group. You will undoubtedly *not* wish to change the values of the two risks unless there is no alternative. Therefore, you must estimate the sample size needed per group for the values of delta, alpha, and beta that you have already specified, as well as upon your estimate of sigma. The latter is best derived from a pilot trial, or, if that is not possible, from estimates based upon recent work done under similar conditions.

The sample sizes to be estimated here will be symbolized by the lowercase letter *n*. This will represent *the group size for each treatment* in a parallel trial, assuming that all groups are the same size. We will also use capital *N*, which will represent the *total sample size* for the entire design (all patients).

As we indicated, our response will be exercise time, obtained in an exercise tolerance test. A patient, with EKG electrodes in place, walks a treadmill. There is a schedule of treadmill angles and speed adjustments that is ignored here for simplicity. The response units will be the time in minutes, to the nearest tenth of a minute, from the beginning of the exercise until an S-T segment flat, a depression, or a related end point appears on the EKG plot.

To use the preferred test (Student's *t* test) for the data analysis, we must assume that the data are distributed approximately normally or will be normalizable by the use of a transformation (discussed later), and will therefore fulfill the assumptions underlying the use of a parametric hypothesis test when the data are analyzed. This is reasonable for the response (treadmill time) that has been chosen. Under these circumstances, in addition, when there are only two levels of a single factor in the form of two independent groups of patients, and there is only one set of response data, Table A.3 in the Appendix can be used to estimate the sample size needed for each treatment. If approximate normality of the data cannot be assumed, there are other kinds of hypothesis tests that may be used, including the Wilcoxon Rank Sum test or the Mann-Whitney U test. These rank tests are also accompanied by certain assumptions, however; one that must be made is that the variances are homogeneous or, to use the common term, homoscedastic. This means that for complete validity, the variances in the two groups must be assumed to be equal in the two populations represented by the samples, so that they differ, if at all, only in their **locations**, that is, in having different population means. Table A.3 will give reasonably adequate estimates for these two rank tests, also, if the above assumption is true.

Estimating Sample Size without Information about Sigma
In estimating sample size, you need to use a value of sigma, as you know. Of course, the more dependable your estimate, the better your chances of a successful trial. However, there will be times when you cannot obtain an accurate estimate, and must use a guess. The procedure described here is valid whether your value of sigma is a reliable quantity derived from similar and recent work, a pilot trial, or simply a guess.

Quantities Required
You will usually have *some* information about sigma, either from a pilot trial, a previous study, or some other source. To make this example a "worst case," however, we will assume here that you have no such knowledge.

To review, recall from Chapter 5 that to estimate sample size, you should have the following specifications and information:

Quantity	Description
Alpha (α)	Significance level (risk of claiming an effect such as a treatment difference equal to or greater than delta when there is none; specified)
Beta (β)	Risk of failing to claim a treatment difference equal to or greater than delta when one exists; specified
Delta (δ)	Smallest difference that you wish to detect (specified)
Sigma (σ)	Standard deviation of single observations (statistic from pilot trial, previous data, etc.)[4]

As you would expect, the smaller the value of delta, the larger the sample size must be. The alpha and beta risks work analogously; smaller risks require larger sample sizes. In this case, having no idea of the value of sigma, you will not know how small alpha, beta, or delta can be without requiring an impossibly large sample size.

However, it is likely that you will be unwilling to make the alpha or beta risks much more liberal than you originally planned. The only remaining variable that you are free to specify is delta. Naturally, you will want to make it equal to the smallest treatment difference that you judge to be clinically important, consistent with a reasonable and practical sample size. Sometimes, the following procedure works well, assuming you have little or no reliable information about the magnitude of sigma: Begin by setting the values of alpha and beta to reasonable levels, say, 0.05 for alpha and 0.10 for beta (these can be varied according to your desires, but if you are submitting data under an IND, do not use any larger value than 0.05 for alpha). Next, set the value of delta to the smallest value you wish to consider. Finally, assume perhaps three possible values for sigma, say, 1.0, 2.0, and 5.0. The values you use should reflect the kinds of variation you expect for the

---

[4]If estimated from data, sigma is, of course, not a parameter, but a statistic (s or sigma hat; $\hat{\sigma}$). Nevertheless, you will thereafter *treat* it as a parameter, and we will use plain sigma in this exposition. Calculations similar to those used to estimate the sample size table, Table A.3, take the fact that sigma is actually unknown into account. See Snedecor and Cochran [38], p. 104.

response under consideration. For a VAS ranging from 0 to 100, for example, perhaps 5, 10, and 20 percentage units would be reasonable (remember, sigma, like delta, has the same units as your response). Remember also that if you are using a value of 0.05 for alpha, you are postulating minimum detectable variation between single replicate measurements of about two times sigma. With this alpha value, averages of 2 would vary about 0.707 times that amount, or ± 1.41 sigma, and averages of 4, one-half of the value for a single measurement, or ± 1 sigma.

If you tabulate a set of possible values of combinations of specifications of alpha, beta, and delta, using values of sigma that you and the statistician judge probable based upon general experience, and then find the sample size corresponding to each combination, you may arrive at a practical set of values. Perhaps, more simply, you might start by setting up two tables: one specifying alpha and beta as 0.05 and 0.10, and the other 0.05 and 0.20 (of course, if you wish to be safer when you conclude that there is a difference, you can try a smaller value of alpha than 0.05). Now, create three columns in each table: one for sigma, one for delta, and one for the corresponding sample size. In the sigma column, write 1 minute. In the corresponding delta column, write 5%, meaning that you wish this combination of values to detect differences of 0.5 minutes on the average. Using Table A.3, find the sample size for the postulated combination of alpha, beta, delta, and sigma. For the next line, retain the same sigma value, but increase delta to 1. Next, make a third line for the same sigma, with delta of 1.5. Now, repeat these three lines with a greater value of sigma. Do this perhaps for one more set of three. Now compare the sample sizes you found, and select the largest your budget will tolerate. When you finish the trial, you can calculate delta and sigma using the formulas given in Parts IV and V to see how close to the actual outcome your guesses were.

The above is a "worst-case" procedure. Usually, however, you and your statistician will not be completely in the dark about the probable range of values of sigma, and this procedure will then be more likely to span the value of sigma you finally achieve when the trial is done. The method is more often successful in getting reasonable values of delta than you might at first expect.

Alpha and Beta
Some guidelines for selecting these values are the following: My suggestion is to use 0.05 *or less* for alpha and 0.20 *or less* for beta. If you are submitting your results to FDA, you must expect to be able to show significance with an alpha value of 0.05 *at most*. If you must use different values, think about the relative importance of alpha and beta in your particular study. There are cases in which having a small value of β is more important than a small α. If you feel that alpha must exceed 0.05, however, be prepared to present a valid argument if you are making a submission to the FDA or publishing your work.

Delta and Sigma

For a treadmill stress test, with the end point defined either as a maximum heart rate or a change in the T wave, the usual exercise times will range from 1 or 2 to 7 minutes or so. Therefore, you should tentatively focus upon the detection of differences between perhaps 0.5 and 2 minutes, with possibly 1 minute as optimum (although you may find, of course, that with a delta value that small, the sample size is impractically large).

Let us begin by postulating values of sigma between 1 and 2. For this sample size procedure, you will use the *estimated standard deviation of a single item from the mean.*[5]

Tabulating Trial Values of n

For this purpose, we will use the tables of sample size that appear as Table A.3 in the Appendix.

We will construct a table using alpha, beta, delta, sigma, and *n*, and try to obtain values of *n* that are practical for the trial. This is illustrated in Table 8.1. In this table:

1. Alpha and beta were held constant at 0.05 and 0.20. Of course, changing their values would affect the sample sizes obtained.
2. The first column gives values of delta, and trial values of sigma are shown in the second. The quantity in the third column, delta divided by sigma, need not appear in the table, but it is convenient to record it there. It was calculated from the values in columns 1 and 2, and will be used to enter Table A.3 in the Appendix to obtain the sample size.
3. Please remember that the last quantity, *n*, is the number of patients *per treatment group*, obtained from Table A.3 (see the explanation that follows). In this experiment, because you are using equal sample sizes and there are two groups, you would double it to obtain the total patients required.

How Table A.3 Was Used to Create Table 8.1

All but three of the values of *n* in Table 8.1 were obtained from Table A.3c (the subtable of Table A.3 in the Appendix for an alpha value of 0.05). This table was entered using a beta value of 0.20 as specified—the fifth column in Table A.3c—and delta over sigma (the first column). This located the sample

---

[5]This is not the only kind of standard deviation. Another common and important one is the standard error of a mean. It consists of *the standard deviation of a single mean of n items from its grand mean.* The grand mean is the mean of the individual means. The standard error of a mean is smaller than that of the original individual items, provided that both are derived from the same population. This makes intuitive sense, because a standard deviation is a measure of precision, and a mean of more than one datum is based upon more information than a single datum. It should thus be less uncertain, so it should have a smaller standard deviation.

Table 8.1. Possible Sample Sizes for Example 8.1, Based upon Appendix Table A.3c (Alpha = 0.05, Beta = 0.20)

Delta, Minutes (δ)	Sigma, Minutes (σ)	δ/σ	n (per treatment)
0.50	1.00	0.50	64
1.00	1.00	1.00	17
1.50	1.00	1.50	9
0.50	1.50	0.33	143*
1.00	1.50	0.67	37*
1.50	1.50	1.00	17
0.50	2.00	0.25	252*
1.00	2.00	0.50	64
1.50	2.00	0.75	29

*Calculated values of n; see what follows.

sizes, which were then transferred to Table 8.1. In one case (the value of 37 marked with an asterisk in Table 8.1), the delta/sigma value fell between entries given in Table A.3c. The sample size in this case was therefore calculated. Linear interpolation could have been used, and is adequate for the smaller sample sizes, but gives only a fair estimate for the larger values. The other two asterisked values of n lay outside the range of Table A.3c, and therefore were also calculated, using an equation that appears in Part V of this book. Thus, values not obtainable directly from Table A.3 are best calculated; you can do this easily using a scientific pocket calculator. Of course, if you prefer, you can use the equation in all cases. Remember that any result that is not an integer should be increased to the next whole number, whether you are interpolating or using the equation.

Choosing a Sample Size from Table 8.1
After all the sample sizes are entered in Table 8.1, you should examine the results. Let's say that you decide that you can afford to use $n = 29$ patients per treatment, or a total, N, of 58. As shown, when the data are analyzed, if sigma were found to be 2 minutes and if you obtain significance, you could conclude, with a risk of being wrong of 0.050, that the treatment difference (delta) is 1.5 minutes or more, which we will assume is the smallest difference of interest. If the treatment difference were equal to or greater than this, there would be a probability of 0.20 that significance would *not* be obtained. More clearly, significance *would* be obtained in 80% of such trials. If the actual sigma were smaller, smaller treatment differences would be detectable. In such a case, an a posteriori calculation of delta, which should be done in any event, would give an idea of its actual magnitude.

There were three major reasons for selecting this sample size, all based upon judgment. First, it should provide sufficient data to obtain a satisfactory chance of detecting a clinically important treatment difference, if one exists. Second, you judged that you would obtain a reasonably reliable estimate of sigma from a trial of this size, for use in estimating sample sizes in further trials. Finally, with this size, you expected that the trial would be complete in a reasonable time, allowing an early decision regarding further work.

If the observed difference in this trial is greater than delta, but not significant, you may wish to do a further trial or trials using the more accurate knowledge of sigma gained from this trial. In such a case, this trial will have served the purpose of a pilot trial.

8.9.4 Randomization Plan

The experiment of this example can be randomized by any of several methods, as discussed in Chapter 6. In many cases, you may decide to ask the statistician to obtain a randomization using the computer. Nevertheless, for pedagogical purposes, let's assume that you decide to use the Moses and Oakford tables [49], because they provide a convenient and rapid procedure.

Because there will be 58 patients, you need a table of random permutations of a set of numbers 1 to 58 or greater. The tables for the numbers 1 to 100, on pages 93 to 119 (Table 6), are the nearest greater sized set in Moses and Oakford. You select a page haphazardly (not necessarily at random); see page 99. Each group of four rows in this table consists of 100 randomly ordered numbers, arranged horizontally in four blocks of 25 for convenience. You pick (again haphazardly) the fourth row of blocks; the one beginning with 15 and ending, on the right, with 25. You then prepare a table with two columns, labeled T_1 and T_2, copying the numbers from the selected permutation to the T_1 column, *omitting numbers greater than 58*, until 29 numbers are listed. Twenty-nine numbers will remain, and you place them in the T_2 column.

It is important that the randomization table be checked carefully for duplications, errors in copying, and so on. An easy way to do this is to write down the numbers 1 through 58 and then go through the randomization table, crossing off each number on the new listing as you find it. This will ensure that there are 58 numbers, that there are no duplicates, and that no numbers greater than 58 have been accidentally included.

The resulting table is your randomization plan. It is illustrated as Table 8.2. When the trial is run, the numbers in the table will represent the patient numbers, obtained by assigning a sequential number to each patient as he or she qualifies and is accepted into the trial (*not before that*), beginning with patient number 1. Of course, any patient numbers occurring in the first column are assigned to treatment 1 (the beta blocker), and those in the second column receive the calcium-channel antagonist.

Table 8.2. Randomization Plan for Example 8.1 (Patient Numbers)

Treatment	
T_1	T_2
15	37
49	18
41	34
19	13
23	10
50	11
47	43
40	7
12	1
27	17
16	21
48	9
53	46
33	5
20	55
39	29
28	24
35	58
2	4
38	56
52	8
57	54
14	3
22	42
6	44
26	31
36	51
45	32
30	25
$n_1 = 29$	$n_2 = 29$
$N = 58$	

8.9.5 Blinding Arrangements

Of course, as in most cases, the trial should be double blind. The doses will be contained in capsules sealed in envelopes marked only with the trial identification, the sponsor's name, the date or range of dates for the trial, and the patient number. Because each patient is to be scheduled to visit the clinic only once, only one envelope per patient will be needed. The same scheme may be used for any trial, but more care in avoiding mixups is necessary when patients make more than one visit, receiving additional doses of test products each time.

In this example, instead of the use of double labels, you arrange for the investigator to call to request the identity of a treatment in the event of a severe adverse reaction. A 24-hour emergency line is set up for this purpose.

8.9.6 Interim Analyses

As explained in Chapter 5, if you plan to do interim significance tests during the execution of this trial, without provision for them during the planning of this trial, the alpha value of all of them, as well as of subsequent statistical tests, will be increased. To avoid this, you must use a multiple-comparisons procedure during your analysis.[6] But to preserve the original power, you must also allow for the repetition of the tests by increasing the sample size during planning. This then requires that you restrict the number of interim tests to no more than that planned. If you decide to use fewer analyses than the planned number, there is a possible problem of another kind. You will then have used more patients than necessary, thus increasing the power of the test, reducing delta to a lower value than originally planned, and possibly giving you significance for differences not judged to be clinically significant.

There will be occasions when unplanned interim tests will be necessary, or at least desirable. If any such are done, you should remember to use a multiple-comparisons test. You must also note, however, as just mentioned, that the power of these and any final statistical tests will then be curtailed because you will not have planned the trial with an adequate estimate of the sample size. In some such cases, it is arguable that you may add additional patients by prolonging the trial. There may also be occasions when, for ethical or other reasons, perhaps because of the results of the interim tests, a trial must be cut short before all the patients provided for have taken part, with a similar effect upon power. In either of these cases, the values of delta and sigma can be calculated a posteriori. If you obtain significance in the final test, and the value of delta just calculated is satisfactory, you should then find it possible to state whether the apparent conclusions from the data analyses are adequate for your purposes.

8.9.7 Clinical Report Forms

The CRFs for this example will not be illustrated, but should be similar to Figure 7.1 of the preceding chapter. This trial was designed as a one-visit arrangement, of course, and the exercise tests were run only once for each patient. Even though there may be only one response value per CRF page, we recommend that a separate page be used for each patient. This plan will

---

[6]In addition to the Bonferroni procedure, which has already been described, others are mentioned in Chapter 14.

simplify transcription when the CRFs arrive at the sponsor's data center, and will reduce errors and confusion.

8.9.8   Final Statistical Analyses

At an early stage of the process of planning this trial, you should request that the biostatistician write up a tentative plan for the data analyses for guidance during planning and for inclusion in the protocol. This should be completed in time for any pretrial submission and/or conference with the FDA.

8.10   SUMMARY OF THE CHAPTER

Except for a small amount of more general material, this chapter has been devoted to experimental designs having the simplest structure of all—those with a single factor. In your work, you may find that these simple designs are suitable for a substantial proportion of your small clinical trials.

The idea of diagramming designs is introduced early in the chapter. This is a useful device that can be used whenever you are preparing a design. I believe you will find it helpful, not only for your own guidance, but also when explaining your designs to others. We will continue to use it in later chapters.

Although there are many kinds of statistical analyses of drug trial data, most studies in the pharmaceutical industry are concerned with making pairwise comparisons (comparisons of two treatments) for safety, efficacy or both. When more than two treatments are used in a trial, there will then be more than one such comparison. Thus, there are, in a sense, two categories of one-factor designs—those with two treatments (i.e., two levels of the factor), and those with three or more. The first type can be analyzed by the simplest sorts of analyses. These include Student's t tests (if the error structure of the data conforms reasonably well to the normal or Gaussian assumptions), simple rank tests if the error structures are not normal (although, for large N, this is not very important), and other quite simple methods of statistical analysis. As you have noted, it is impossible to discuss or work with experimental designs without giving some thought to the statistical analyses that will be used when the data are on hand. I hope and expect that your biostatistician's assistance and your reading and reference to the chapters in Part IV will be of help to you in this respect.

Although we have previously presented brief examples of one-factor designs, Example 8.4 in this chapter is intended to supply you with a more complete description of the necessary planning than was given for the earlier examples. The design of one-factor trials with more than two levels of the factor has been discussed. Although the analyses of such designs is slightly more complex than those suitable for one-factor two-level designs, the creation of the designs is almost as simple, and you should now be able to produce them easily. Some of the analyses commonly used for such designs, such as the analysis of variance (ANOVA), regression, and related methods, are not described in this book, but the biostatistician will be very familiar with them. The methods of randomization and the structures of both types of design are almost the same. The major differences that you will encounter during the design phase are slightly more complex estimations of sample size, because of the multiplicity problems introduced when there are more than two treatments.

This chapter has introduced several ideas. First, the idea of *factors* and *levels* was explained. The structures of two-level and multilevel single-factor designs were discussed. Characteristics of one-factor designs in which the treatments may have unequal sample sizes were described.

Following these major fundamental ideas, Example 8.4, a two-level single-factor design, was provided. The steps in its planning were described following roughly this sequence:

1. Writing the protocol
2. Establishing the objective(s) of the study
3. Carrying out the sample size estimation
4. Performing the randomization
5. Planning the blinding
6. Providing for interim analyses if necessary
7. Designing the clinical report forms
8. Planning the data analysis

8.11   LITERATURE REFERENCES

(1) Feinstein, Alvan R., *Science*, 242, 1257–1263 (December 2, 1988).
(2) Cochran, William G., *Planning and Analysis of Observational Studies*, John Wiley, New York, 1983. (Edited and completed by Lincoln E. Moses and Frederick Mosteller after Cochran's death.)
(3) Bratcher, T. L., M. A. Moran, and W. J. Zimmer, *Journal of Quality Technology*, 2, 156–164 (1970).

CHAPTER 9

Multifactor Parallel Designs

9.1 INTRODUCTION

Although there is a great deal of literature about experimental designs, especially factorials, not much has been written for professionals with little or no training in statistics and experimental design, and even less than that for people engaged in clinical studies. For the eventual statistical analysis of the data following your trials, it is very likely that you will rely upon the services of a biostatistician. It is my emphatic belief, however, that the *designs* for your studies must be selected by you, because your training and experience have made you the one most familiar with the subject matter of your studies. I am certain that you will find it easy to become adequately proficient in selecting the designs you will need. Of course, I recommend that you discuss your designs with a biostatistician and ask for comment.

This chapter and the others in Part III constitute an introduction to the broad subject of factorial designs. The discussions in Part III are restricted to the designs most suited to and most often used in clinical trials. As a result, these chapters include only the "bare bones" of the subject. Should you be interested in further reading and information about experimental designs, Cochran and Cox [11], Cox [12], Davies [14], and Fleiss [8] comprise some of the best in the literature.

Almost every experiment you will work with in pharmaceutical clinical trial design can be understood and manipulated in terms of the ideas of factorial structure. We have mentioned the idea of factorial designs previously, of course, but only in the elementary case of single-factor structures. To make it easier for you to use this chapter as a reference after your first reading, as well as to add emphasis (for it is the central theme of this book), the topic will be treated here as if it were quite new to you.

9.2 FACTORIAL STRUCTURE

9.2.1 Background

The designs we will consider in this book are of a type called **crossed**. The structure of a crossed design can be understood by contrasting it to that of a

nested experiment. Although nested designs are almost nonexistent in clinical trial work, we discuss them briefly here as a means of clarifying the nature of the crossed designs.

Nested experimental designs involve configurations in which there are one or more stages of subdivision of factors. Their purpose is usually to estimate what are known as **expected mean squares** or **components of variance**, whereas crossed designs are generally used to estimate **means**.

Nested arrangements often involve the successive subdivision of materials from a hierarchy of sources, with statistics from each stage being calculated. For example, an analytical chemist responsible for determining the acceptability of carloads of coal arriving at a power-generating plant might arrange to have each load sampled before analysis. He might use the following procedure: From each of several randomly selected 100-car trains, two or more cars are selected randomly. From each car, two large samples are taken from random locations.[1] Thus, there will be three stages of sampling—from trains, from cars within trains, and from locations within cars. These can be considered to be factors—trains, cars, and samples. At each stage, a laboratory-sized sample is taken for analysis, grinding and mixing it thoroughly. Each is then analyzed. The chemist uses the data to compare the magnitude of the variation within each stage with that of the others.

The structure of a nested design looks something like a genealogist's "family tree." There must be at least two stages, and there may be any number of stages greater than that. In the earlier example, the object of the successive sampling procedure was to estimate the variability between and within shipments of coal. Note that the sampling is random for all three stages. Of course, this process will continue with more trains, cars, and samples as they arrive at the plant, so that there will be additional checks upon the uniformity of the samples. Should an unusual train, car, or location be encountered, further investigation and perhaps more sampling will be done to try to obtain more information about the source of the problem.

A crossed design does not possess the hierarchical or treelike structure of nested designs. In crossed parallel designs, no factor is subsidiary to any other, and each is independent of the others. (Note, however, that blocked, changeover, and split plot structures, described later, do possess a kind of correlation among factors that, however, is not a hierarchical arrangement such as that possessed by the nested designs.) The word *crossed* comes, perhaps, from the customary arrangement used in the tabulation of the data for a two-factor crossed design, which will be illustrated presently. In such a table, the rows are labeled with the levels of one of the factors and the columns with those of the other. Each intersection of one row and one column may be called a **cell**, and is formed by the "crossing" of one level of

---

[1] The word "sample" is used here in the chemical sense to refer to *one or more* portions taken from a larger supply of a material. As you know, the *statistical* use of the word always refers to a *group* of items taken from a distribution. The meanings of the two words are related, but are not the same.

the row factor and one level of the column factor. In the designs of this chapter and the next, a cell is equivalent to one patient who has been assigned a treatment consisting of a combination of a specific level of each of the two factors. However, there are also designs in which a cell does not always correspond to a patient. These are the **changeover** designs, which will be discussed later.

We will define the terms **factorial structure** and **factorial design** in a rather limited way in this and the next chapter, confining ourselves to what are known as **full factorial designs,** or **full factorials.** In this book, we will not be concerned (beyond a brief mention) with so-called fractional factorial designs, nor with designs such as latin squares[2] (which can also be regarded as fractional factorials), because such structures are only rarely used in clinical studies. However, in a subsequent chapter in Part III, we will discuss some designs that utilize blocking, a form of additional factor.

There is overlap in the classification of experimental designs. For instance, as you will see in later chapters, a randomized blocks design can be a parallel or a changeover design. A multicenter trial can be classified as a randomized-blocks design of a special kind. Nevertheless, we will discuss these in this section to avoid excessive fragmentation in our classification system. The classification of experimental designs, in short, can be quite arbitrary, because what we perceive as the basic nature of a design may depend upon our point of view. It is nevertheless helpful to set up some kind of system.

The ideas of factorial designs and the general concept of randomization as we are using it in this book were introduced by Sir Ronald A. Fisher, the founder of modern experimental design and many techniques of analysis, in the 1920s. For the first time, his factorial patterns made it possible to design and analyze studies using two or more factors simultaneously in the same experiment. Concurrently, the use of randomization enabled the calculation of reliable probabilities when estimating confidence intervals and doing hypothesis tests.

Factorial experiments are arrangements in which more than one independent variable or **source of variation** can be used, such as a factor comprising several drugs and another comprising several doses of each drug. Compared to the older "one factor and level at a time" experimentation, this not only saves much time, but, as you will see, makes it possible to reliably evaluate combination effects, *interactions*, that may often exist between different factors and could not be detected by the older procedure. Thus, the evaluation of interactions produces information that was not directly available at all to experimenters prior to Fisher's work, yet which can be crucial in the interpretation of the results of clinical trials or other experiments. The old way of running successive experiments, each at one level of one factor, made it impossible to learn whether any observed differences were results of the

[2]The use of a lowercase "l" in "Latin" is frequently used in this context.

changed levels or factors, or of some "hidden" factor that existed at the time of one of the experiments but not at the other.

The designs and short examples of this chapter and the more complete examples in the next are meant to supply you with a set of so-called completely randomized, full-factorial parallel designs for your reference. We devote more space to these than to other types because they are the ones likely to be used most frequently in your trials.

9.2.2 Multifactor Designs: General Discussion

Before we illustrate and discuss particular kinds of multifactor parallel designs, we should expand briefly upon some of the points mentioned earlier.

Multiple Factors

In the single-factor designs exemplified in several of the preceding chapters, the independent variable, **drugs**, was the **factor**. Each drug, drug mixture, or placebo in those designs constituted a **level** of that factor.

However, as we have mentioned, a design may have any number of factors, although few clinical studies use more than two or three, or, more rarely, four. For example, each of several drugs could be given at both a low and a high dose, with those amounts defined according to normal practice for the particular drugs used. This experiment would possess a two-factor design, with *drugs* and *doses* as the factors. With two drugs, each at two doses, there would be two levels of each factor. For a parallel design, there would then be four treatment groups: one consisting of patients to whom drug 1 and dose 1 would be assigned, one to which drug 1 and dose 2 were assigned, and two more analogous groups with drug 2. We could symbolize this by using the symbols T_1 and T_2 for the two drug treatments, and D_1 and D_2 for the doses. Then, the assignments to the four groups could be symbolized by $T_1 D_1$, $T_1 D_2$, $T_2 D_1$, and $T_2 D_2$.

To represent this design, we could construct a table diagram with two columns labeled T_1 and T_2 and two rows labeled D_1 and D_2. Of course, that table would provide for only four patients, one for each of the four combinations of drugs and doses. Because we would need some replication, we could provide for that in the table by labeling several rows with the same dose level and then adding rows for the other level.[3] Each entry in such a table is called

---

[3]It is usually desirable to have more than two patients for each combination of levels. The reason is that with two, the loss of a single patient during the trial would leave one of the treatment combinations with no repetition. An important component of the data analysis is a comparison of the effects of the treatments against a calculated estimate of the **experimental error**. This estimate is often obtained by calculations that depend upon the repetition of data for the same treatment combinations; this is sometimes called **within-cell error**. It is an estimate because a **sample** is used to **estimate** a population parameter, sigma. If there is only one (or no) datum in a cell, that cell can contribute no information toward the error estimate.

a **cell**, and represents one patient treated with one of the four drug/dose combinations.[4]

The Use of a Placebo When Doses Are a Factor

If one of the "drugs" used in a design is a placebo, both the low and high doses for that level of the drugs factor will be placebos, although the blinding may be maintained, for example, by using two tablets or other dosage form for the "high" dose, and one for the "low." However, having two groups with the same treatment combination may seem wasteful of resources. There are several possible ways to handle this.

One alternative is to omit a placebo and use two drugs which are expected to be active. In that case, you could still use two levels of dose. However, in this case as well as the original one, it would be better to use three. The reason is that the statistician can then obtain more information about the behavior of each drug, *including* an estimate of curvature as well as one of the rate of change in the drug effect as the dose is increased. With two doses, even if there is curvature, it will not be detectable, and only the slope (the overall rate of change in the drug effect) will be estimable.

Another approach might be to use only one placebo group, eliminating the duplicate placebo. However, the kind of information obtainable with this arrangement would probably be less satisfactory than the original arrangement with the four groups.

All things considered, if you wish to use doses in a two-factor design in which the other factor is drugs, it would probably be better not to use a placebo, but two presumably active drugs. And, in fact, if you were sure, perhaps from previous work, that there would be no interaction between drugs and doses (i.e., that any difference between the doses would be the same for both drugs), it would be advisable to use a one-factor trial, with the two drugs only. In that case, they might both be active drugs, or one could be a placebo.[5]

9.2.3   Example 9.1: A 2^2 Factorial Design

The expression "2^2" is usually read "two to the second," or "two to the second power," or sometimes "two squared." A 2^2 design is one with two levels of each of two factors. The first figure 2 (the **base**) stands for the

---

[4]In a parallel design, the patients are called the **experimental units**. These are the basic units to each of which one of the factor/dose combinations is applied. In a crossover design, however, as discussed later in Part III, each patient receives more than one treatment or treatment combination over a period of time. In such a case, each patient "contains" several experimental units, defined by the several treatment times.

[5]Note that you might well *expect* an interaction between drugs and doses if one of the drugs is a placebo. Unless there were a strong placebo effect, if the "active" drug were really active, and if the doses chosen were both in the middle of the effective range (the "straight-line" portion), this interaction would be evidenced by a smaller mean response difference between drugs at the low than at the high dose. Such an interaction would probably not be of interest, and you could forego the use of a dose factor in such a case.

number of **levels** of each **factor** of the design. The second figure 2 (the **exponent**) stands for the number of factors in the design. Of course, this notation is usable only when all factors have the same number of levels. Mathematically, a base with an exponent, like 2^2, represents a result derived by writing the base as many times as specified by the exponent and multiplying these numbers together. Hence, the expression 2^2 is shorthand for 2×2. When used to describe an experimental design, the number 2^2, 2×2, or 4, represents the *minimum* number of **runs** required. A run is the number of different treatment combinations (and therefore patients) in the design. For a 2^2 design, the notation 2^2 represents the four runs necessary if there is no replication. If there were replication, this number would be multiplied by a number representing the number of times each run is to be repeated. For example, if each of the four possible combinations of levels of the two factors were to be given to three patients, there would be 3×2^2, or 12 runs. In this example, at the moment, we are assuming that no replication is to be used, so that there will be only four runs (this assumption is for illustration only; so small a trial would almost always be highly impractical, of course). The four runs will consist of (a) one patient who receives level 1 of factor A and level 1 of factor B; (b) one who receives level 1 of factor A and level 2 of factor B; (c) a third who receives level 2 of factor A and level 1 of factor B, and, finally, (d) a fourth who receives level 2 of both factors.

If each factor of a design has three levels and there are four factors (this many factors is rare in clinical trials), we can call it a 3^4 or a $3 \times 3 \times 3 \times 3$ design. This, of course, would have 81 runs if the design were not repeated.

Each of the several factors in a factorial design need not have the same number of levels. When they do not, however, exponential notation cannot be used fully or at all. For example, a multicenter clinical trial with three factors represented by three drugs, two dose levels of each, run at each of five centers, and with no replication between centers could be represented by the expression $3 \times 2 \times 5$. A single execution of this trial would consist of 30 runs. Thus, if it were a parallel trial, there would be six patients at each of the five centers. Of course, in practice, you would be likely to use some repetition of each combination of the three factors.

Figure 9.1 shows the simplest possible full factorial design, the one we have just discussed, with two factors at two levels each, or a total of four runs.

With Figure 9.1 before us, we can redefine a factorial design more succinctly as one that uses two or more factors simultaneously. This is

	B_1	B_2
A_1	--	--
A_2	--	--

Figure 9.1 Simplest two-factor factorial design.

accomplished by arranging for each experimental unit to receive one level of *each* of the factors *concurrently*. Let's explain this further.

Suppose that you wish to design a factorial experiment to compare a test drug with a standard drug of known efficacy. Suppose, also, that you want to make the comparison using two doses of each drug—one high and one low. Let's say that you have defined the quantities "high" and "low" according to your knowledge of the properties of the two drugs. There are then two factors in this experiment. We will call them "drugs" and "doses."

Each of the two factors has two levels. The experimental units are patients. A response measurement for each patient is represented by pairs of dashes in the body of the table. The experiment is to be a parallel study; each patient will get only one treatment, but the "treatments" in this case are combinations of one level of each of two factors rather than one level of a single factor, as in the examples in the previous chapters.

In Figure 9.1, the row factor, factor A, represents the kind of drug. A_1, the first drug, identifies the first row of the table. Thus, both patients in that row, represented by the two sets of double dashes, will be given the first drug. The two patients in the second row, labeled A_2, will receive the other drug. The column factor is labeled B. The first column is labeled B_1 because both patients appearing in that column will receive the low dose of their drugs. Those in the second column will receive the high dose, B_2.

Thus, the first of the four patients represented in the upper left-hand cell of the table will receive the first drug at the low dose (A_1B_1). The patient in the upper right-hand cell will receive the first drug at the high dose (A_1B_2). Similarly, the two cells in the lower row represent two patients who will receive A_2B_1, the second drug at the low dose, and A_2B_2, the second drug at the high dose, respectively.

To analyze the structure still further, see Figure 9.2, which shows the same design in the form of a geometric diagram. Now, each of the four runs is labeled to show its treatment combination, and their locations in the diagram form a square. You could draw X- and Y-axes around this figure, with the X-axis (horizontal) representing factor B and the Y-axis representing A. Then A_1 could be regarded as the "low" level of factor A and A_2 as its "high" level.[6] Each of the subsequent figures could have been represented in this way. They are not, only because the diagrams would have become excessively congested and difficult to read.

9.2.4 Example 9.2: Replication in a 2 × 2 Design

The four-run design of Figures 9.1 and 9.2, as we indicated, is quite impractical, because it is too small for any ordinary study. In fact, if an interaction existed, it would not be detectable. To make this design practical

---

[6]When a factor is qualitative, like A (drugs), the subscripts "1" and "2" simply mean that the two levels are different, not that one is somehow greater than the other. When it is quantitative, like B (doses), the subscripts take on this additional meaning as well.

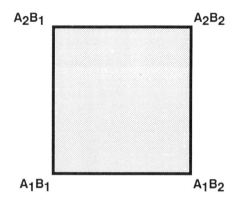

A₂B₁ ... A₂B₂

A₁B₁ ... A₁B₂

Note: This is the same design as that of Figure 9.1, arranged differently.

Figure 9.2 Factorial of Figure 9.1 shown geometrically.

for use in a real clinical drug trial, some repetition must be introduced. This not only increases the sample size so that a smaller difference between factor levels will become detectable, but it also supplies information necessary for estimating the fundamental value of the experimental error (sigma).

Kinds of Replication

Repetition (we will usually use the term **replication** hereafter) can be introduced in one or both of two ways. The first is to repeat, or replicate, each run by using two or more experimental units instead of one in each cell of the design. Because this is a parallel study and the experimental units are patients, to do this you would assign two or more patients to each cell. The second way is to **replicate** the entire design two or more times, for instance, on successive days. The two methods are often used together in the same design. We will illustrate both of these arrangements.

For the first procedure (assigning more than one patient to each cell of the design), we will use equal numbers of patients in each cell of the design of Figure 9.1. We choose 10 in each cell, assuming the sample size estimation procedure so indicated. The resulting design, using 40 patients at a single center, is illustrated in Figure 9.3. This figure represents a trial that is identical to that of Figures 9.1 and 9.2 except that each of the four cells now contains 10 patients instead of one. We will call this method of replication **cell replication**. Note that we are defining the term **cell** as a section of the table within which all entries represent a single treatment combination.

To use the second scheme, the entire design is repeated several times. We will call this arrangement **full replication**. We say that each repetition of the design is a **replicate**; the design is done **in replicates**. You might wish either to run a pilot trial or secure an estimate of sigma from a similar trial before deciding upon the number of replicates to use. Let's assume, however, that

	B_1	B_2
A_1	--	--
	--	--
	--	--
	--	--
	--	--
	--	--
	--	--
	--	--
	--	--
	--	--
A_2	--	--
	--	--
	--	--
	--	--
	--	--
	--	--
	--	--
	--	--
	--	--

Figure 9.3   Factorial of Figure 9.1 with cell replication.

you have done this, plan to label the several replicates as week 1, week 2, etc., and have come up with an estimate of 14 replicates,[7] to be examined a week apart on *separate* groups of four patients each. You should be sure that the patients in each group are *new* patients, none of whom have appeared in any of the other replicates. It is not uncommon for this precaution to be omitted, so that some or all of the patients in each replicate are repeaters. However, this procedure should be carefully avoided, except, possibly, in very special cases. Using it greatly limits the reliability of inferences drawn from the trial, because the sample will then be based upon a smaller number of patients, and the estimate of sigma will probably be smaller than otherwise (because it will use repetitive measurements of the same patients).

Very frequently the use of **full replicates** instead of **cell replicates** has some purpose beyond merely increasing sample size. For example, the replicates may each be identified with a different week, if it is thought that measurements made some time apart will show greater differences than otherwise, as is usually the case. Again, if a multicenter trial is planned, and the entire experiment is repeated in each center, a set of replicates, each identified with a different center, is automatically created. In such cases, the replicates not only provide increased sample size when needed, but also allow investigation of any differences among the responses for different weeks or centers, whether they be caused by temporal, geographical, or other

[7]Estimation methods for sample sizes in factorial designs are different than the procedure illustrated earlier for single-factor designs, and are more complex.

	B_1	B_2		B_1	B_2	$\cdots$		B_1	B_2
A_1	--	--	A_1	--	--	$\cdots$	A_1	--	--
A_2	--	--	A_2	--	--	$\cdots$	A_2	--	--
Week 1 (C_1)			Week 2 (C_2)			$\cdots$ $\cdots$	Week 14 (C_{14})		

Figure 9.4 Factorial of Figure 9.1 in 14 full replicates.

factors. A multiweek or multicenter trial is often used also because the temporal or geographical differences produce a more representative sample of patients, practices, clinics, or hospitals. When you use a multicenter trial, or when you recognize time periods as a possible source of variation, you must perforce use a design with at least two factors, such as centers and drugs or weeks and drugs.

In this example, instead of separating the replicates by a week, you could have chosen another interval, or you might have separated them spatially instead of temporally by making the trial into a multicenter study with 14 investigators. (Of course, the use of 14 as the number of replicates is merely an example; you might use some other number, depending upon your sample size estimate, your feeling about the variability of centers or weeks, or your impressions or knowledge about the ability of certain centers to supply all of the necessary patients.) In both cases, you would also be likely to add some cell replication, if for no reason other than to avoid complete losses of a factor combination in the case of noncompleters. Note again that when you use full replicates, you are really adding a factor to a design. When we introduced the idea of replicating the entire design two or more times, we were really creating a third factor. Figure 9.4 is an example. Factor C, weeks, by its 14 levels, represents 14 full replicates. No cell replication is shown in this case.

9.3 FACTORS WITH THREE LEVELS EACH

9.3.1 Introduction

There is really no difference in the concepts of these designs and those of the previous section. They are merely larger. We are concerned at the moment with designs in which each factor has the same number of levels. The smallest three-level multifactor factorial design of this kind would be one having two factors at three levels each, symbolized by 3^2. If there were no replication, such a design would require nine runs. If the trial being planned was to have a parallel structure, there would be nine patients. Each of the nine would be assigned to a different one of the nine combinations of

	C_1			C_2			C_3		
	D_1	D_2	D_3	D_1	D_2	D_3	D_1	D_2	D_3
A_1B_1	--	--	--	--	--	--	--	--	--
B_2	--	--	--	--	--	--	--	--	--
B_3	--	--	--	--	--	--	--	--	--
A_2B_1	--	--	--	--	--	--	--	--	--
B_2	--	--	--	--	--	--	--	--	--
B_3	--	--	--	--	--	--	--	--	--
A_3B_1	--	--	--	--	--	--	--	--	--
B_2	--	--	--	--	--	--	--	--	--
B_3	--	--	--	--	--	--	--	--	--

Figure 9.5   Factorial design with four factors at three levels each, in one replicate.

the levels of the two factors. Let us call the two factors A and B, and identify the levels with the subscript numbers 1, 2, and 3. The combinations would then be identified as $A_1B_1, A_1B_2, A_1B_3, A_2B_1, \ldots, A_3B_3$.

9.3.2   Example 9.3: The 3^m Factorial Design

Figure 9.5 is an example with four factors at three levels each. Like the preceding figures, the diagram can represent any such design. An example using this design in the next section will employ specific factors and levels.

Figure 9.5 is a table diagram for any 3^4 design (four factors at three levels each), arranged in the same way as the previous two figures. Let us assume that this design is to be done once and in one location, so that there will be one replication only. Also, as the diagram shows, there is only one patient per cell. In a design of this size, the use of more than one patient per cell may not always be strictly necessary. When there are sufficient patients to satisfy your sample size estimate, if you can make certain assumptions, error estimates can be obtained from such factorial data even if there is no cell replication. It is usually a good idea, however, to avoid those assumptions by providing for some replication, if you can afford the extra time and your budget will allow it.

The arrangement in Figure 9.5 is one of several that could be used. All of the factors could have been listed across the top or down the side, and the labels could have been interchanged.

It is common to think of each factor in a multifactor design[8] as occupying one dimension in space, orthogonal (at right angles) to each of the others. In

---

[8]There are multifactor designs that are not factorials. A common type is discussed in Box, Hunter, and Hunter [32] (central composite designs and related structures). These designs, however, have not been used in industrial clinical trials, to the best of my knowledge, although they are very common in engineering and the sciences.

a two-factor design, this requires a square, and the design is two-dimensional, with the treatment combinations occurring at the corners, beginning (arbitrarily) at the lower left, as in Figure 9.2. In a three-factor design, representing the design geometrically in this way would produce a more congested diagram, a bit more difficult to decipher on the two dimensions of a sheet of paper. For the clearest illustration, a solid cubic shape would be needed with, for example, A_i and B_j occupying the rows and columns of the original square, as in Figure 9.3, and the third factor, C_k, occupying the third dimension and forming the cube. In the case of Figure 9.5, however, which displays four factors, the representation cannot be done intelligibly at all, whether on paper or as a solid structure, because it would require the display of a four-dimensional figure in the two dimensions of the paper or the three of the solid. In such cases, we must simply dispense with the assistance of a diagram.

9.3.3 Example 9.4: Four Factors at Three Levels Each

A design with four factors at three levels each is very rare in clinical work, although I have used them in preclinical experiments. This one is included primarily to help clarify the idea of factorials. Assume that you wish to compare the levels of the following four factors:

A_i: Three "drugs": a placebo (A_1), a standard drug (A_2), and a test drug (A_3).

B_j: Three dose levels of the drugs, with the actual quantities of each specified during the planning by an experienced specialist.

C_k: Three patient conditions: patients confined to bed during the entire course of the study (C_1), patients allowed to be out of bed for 4 hours each day (C_2), and patients out of bed daily for 8 hours or more (C_3).

D_m: Three replicates (repetitions of the entire experiment), 1 month apart (D_1, D_2, D_3).

The design of Figure 9.5 can be interpreted as an embodiment of this design. Each of the three replicates is represented by one set of three columns in Figure 9.5. The three D_1 columns can represent the first replicate, the D_2 columns the second, and the D_3 columns, the third. Thus, there would be 27 patients, each treated with one of the combinations of factors A, B, and C, in each replicate. Any difference between replicates would be attributed to some differences in conditions from month to month, and such effects would not affect the estimates of the effects of the other factors. As a practical matter, however, if such a design were used with similar identifications of the treatments, it should normally posess more than three full replicates. The reason is that in the analysis of such an arrangement, it is common to assume a "mixed" analysis of variance model, with factors A, B, and C being considered "fixed" and factor D taken as "random." In this case, certain interactions with factor D will be used as error to test the three fixed main effects when the data are analyzed, under the assumption that any apparent interaction consists solely of experimental error. Under the assumption of a mixed model, this must be done even if there is cell replication. To provide a reliable and reasonably small estimate of the replicate error in such a case, there should usually be at least five or six such replicates.

9.3.4 Replicated Designs

Treating the replicates in this design as a set of three levels of the fourth factor helps to clarify the nature of this kind of replication,[9] as opposed to cell repetition. You can think of the design as a three-factor structure that has been repeated three times.

Trials using more than three factors almost never occur in clinical work, but they are not rare in other fields, such as chemistry, agriculture, animal pharmacology, and engineering. But a design like that of Example 9.3, in which there are four factors (e.g., drugs, doses, and dosage forms, with the subset of these three repeated at each of several centers comprising the fourth factor) is not extremely rare among industrial clinical trials. And three-factor designs in which two factors are replicated in cells (e.g., drugs and doses), with the two run in each of several centers, are common.

For most designs, you will probably wish to use some cell replication, but you may or may not want or need to run full replicates of an entire design, as in the earlier examples. Trial data with losses of some of the replicates from cells resulting because of patient incompleters are common, and can be analyzed readily, although the analyses are more complex than when all cells are the same size; see Bancroft (1). When one or more cells are completely empty, however, the situation is more serious and the information available from the analysis is reduced, because some factor combinations will be absent. Therefore, every effort should be made to avoid this difficulty by using adequate cell replication.

The sample size is likely to be different for each change in the experimental structure. This being so, whether you do the design in complete replicates, use cell replication, or both, all repetition must be planned for and quantified when you do your sample size estimates. This is discussed in Chapter 15.

A final point: When you call a set of replicates a factor, as for factor D in Figure 9.5, it is implied that each additional set represents a different level of that factor and is therefore somehow different than the other(s), perhaps because of temporal or spatial differences. But it may turn out that there is no detectable difference, and that the replicates have simply improved your estimate of the variance (or of sigma, its square root). Usually, however, it is safe and conservative to assume that there *are* differences among the

---

[9]The repetitions of an entire design at successive times, or in several different locations (centers) are usually called **replicates**, or **complete replicates**. The use of more than one experimental unit per cell in a design, on the other hand, is a different kind of replication. We will try to avoid confusion by referring to multiple units per cell as cell repetition, or a similar term.

replicates, and to treat them as another factor during the planning and the data analyses. If the replication is spatial, there are likely to be differences among locations of the several replicates (such as different clinics) that will affect the responses (in addition to the expected effects due to the other factors). If it is temporal, again, differences among replicates will probably occur, due to accumulated changes in patients and other experimental conditions with time.

9.4   FACTORS WITH UNEQUAL NUMBERS OF LEVELS

9.4.1   Background

It is not necessary to use the same number of levels for each factor in a multifactor trial. Any number greater than 1 can be used for any factor. You can easily see, however, that increasing the number of levels of a factor, or the number of factors, whether or not all factors have equal numbers, rapidly increases the size of a study. In the 3^4 design of Figure 9.5, for example, a single replicate consists of 81 runs. If just one of the factors had four instead of three levels, there would instead be $(3 \times 3 \times 3 \times 4)$ 108 runs, 33% more! Thus, it is easy to design experiments that may be much larger than can be run economically or conveniently.

If it is necessary or desirable to use more factors, the fractional factorials mentioned earlier can be used. These consist of fewer runs than are necessary with a full factorial. These, like trials with more than three factors, are very rarely used in clinical studies, although they are very common elsewhere. They can sometimes be quite useful for small exploratory clinical trials. But whereas four-factor full factorials are perhaps rare because of their size, I suspect that fractional factorials, which can overcome that disadvantage, are rare because many practitioners in the pharmaceutical industry are unaware of them. We are not accustomed to thinking of the simultaneous evaluation of more than two or three factors, and therefore if such a need arises, we are more likely to run two or more two-factor experiments.

9.4.2   Example 9.5: A 2 × 2 × 5 Factorial Design

This design can also be called a $2^2 \times 5$ design. As can be shown by multiplying the numbers of levels together, one replicate will require 20 runs. Because it is unlikely that an experiment this small will detect clinically important differences, replication is usually necessary. The structure of such a design, using cell replication, is shown in Figure 9.6. As an example, 10 repetitions are shown in each cell, making a total of 200 runs. We will assume that this number of runs was found necessary when the sample size estimation was done. Because this design is a completely randomized *parallel* design, the 10 repetitions in each cell represent 10 patients.

This example is a comparison of two drugs, a test drug and a standard (factor A_i), in two forms, a salt and the free base (factor B_j), run in each of

	B₁					B₂				
	C_1	C_2	C_3	C_4	C_5	C_1	C_2	C_3	C_4	C_5
A_1	--	--	--	--	--	--	--	--	--	--
	--	--	--	--	--	--	--	--	--	--
	--	--	--	--	--	--	--	--	--	--
	--	--	--	--	--	--	--	--	--	--
	--	--	--	--	--	--	--	--	--	--
	--	--	--	--	--	--	--	--	--	--
	--	--	--	--	--	--	--	--	--	--
	--	--	--	--	--	--	--	--	--	--
	--	--	--	--	--	--	--	--	--	--
	--	--	--	--	--	--	--	--	--	--
A_2	--	--	--	--	--	--	--	--	--	--
	--	--	--	--	--	--	--	--	--	--
	--	--	--	--	--	--	--	--	--	--
	--	--	--	--	--	--	--	--	--	--
	--	--	--	--	--	--	--	--	--	--
	--	--	--	--	--	--	--	--	--	--
	--	--	--	--	--	--	--	--	--	--
	--	--	--	--	--	--	--	--	--	--
	--	--	--	--	--	--	--	--	--	--
	--	--	--	--	--	--	--	--	--	--

Figure 9.6 Factorial design with three factors at 2, 2 and 5 levels ($2 \times 2 \times 5$), with ten repetitions per cell.

five centers, each supervised by a different investigator (factor C_k). It is diagrammed in Figure 9.6. One of the variables is centers (investigators), so in a sense we can think of the design as using five complete replicates of a $2^2 \times 5$ design with 10 replicate measurements per cell; each of these complete replicates is identified with a different center (including a different investigator and patient population). Note that if you ignore the centers factor, and run only one complete replicate (i.e., use only one center), this design is identical to that of Figure 9.3.

9.5 RANDOMIZING SOME FACTORIAL DESIGNS

9.5.1 Random Assignment

As discussed earlier, in clinical trials, we are normally concerned only with the random *assignment* of factor combinations to the patients, not with random *selection* of patients or centers. Unless the target population is finite and very limited in time and space, it is almost never possible to obtain and use a random sample of a patient population for a clinical trial.

9.5.2   Example 9.6: Review of Randomization of One-Factor Designs

For a completely randomized, parallel, full factorial design (two or more factors), you may use any of the methods mentioned in Part II. There is really little difference in the randomization procedure; it is just the composition of the cells in a multifactor design that make it seem more complex. The designs discussed in the earlier chapters were all "one-way" (one-factor) structures, so we did not speak of "cells" in discussing them. Nevertheless, they really do have cells, just as do multifactor designs. The cells are the groups of patients receiving each of the "treatments," or **levels**, of their one factor. Thus, those cells are **one-way** cells, while each cell of a factorial with two or more factors is a **multiway** cell. In the so-called **full factorial**[10] designs we are discussing here, each cell represents a patient or experimental unit *treated with one level of each of the factors in the design*, and every factor-level combination is represented in some cell of the design.

Let's say that you have a three-treatment one-factor design (one factor at three levels), like that illustrated in Figure 8.2 in Chapter 8. You can randomize the assignments to the patients by using a permutation of the numbers 1 to N, where N is the total number of patients for all three treatments. You can use an appropriate permutation set from Moses and Oakford [49]. If you plan to use 20 patients for each treatment, as in Figure 8.2, N would be 60. You would thus need assignments for 60 patients (assuming that you plan to assign equal numbers to each treatment). The nearest permutations greater than this in Moses and Oakford are those for the numbers 1 to 100, so you would choose one of these. Now, you would list the first 20 numbers between 1 and 60 (ignoring any greater than 60 that occur in the permutation) in a column headed "Treatment 1" (treatment T_1 in Figure 8.2) in your table of the randomization, the 20 following under T_2 and 20 more under T_3.

Now, let's assume that you are planning a design with three treatments, and that your sample size estimation procedure indicated that 15 patients were necessary for each treatment.

You need a randomly ordered set (a permutation) of the integers 1 to 45. You can use one of the Moses and Oakford tables if you wish. The set of permutations of the integers 1 through 50 is the most suitable. Of course, you could use any of the larger tables in a similar way. Without bothering to make a random selection of the page number and the particular permutation, you may just select Table 5 on page 87 haphazardly and then the fourth set down in the left-hand column of the page. Using this set and copying the

---

[10]This term refers to designs in which each experimental unit (equal to one patient, in the case under consideration) is associated with a "treatment" consisting of a combination of one of the levels of *every factor* in the design. In these designs, every level of every factor is associated with every other in at least one patient. For example, in a design with two factors, each at two levels (say, two drugs at two doses each), each patient would receive one of the two drugs at one of the two doses. There are other designs, called fractional factorials, in which this is not true.

Table 9.1. Randomization of a Three-Treatment One-Way Design

	Treatment	
T_1	T_2	T_3
40	36	44
38	19	17
28	35	37
14	27	8
13	12	21
25	11	7
4	23	42
18	24	3
6	22	10
5	45	2
33	1	20
26	32	15
16	30	29
31	39	41
34	9	43
$n_1 = 15$	$n_2 = 15$	$n_3 = 15$
	$N = 45$	

numbers line by line from the selected block (and skipping the five integers from 46 through 50, because you need only the first 45), you would come up with the randomization shown in Table 9.1.

9.5.3   Example 9.7: Randomizing a Two-Factor Design

In a similar manner, let's randomize the two-factor cell-replicated design shown in Figure 9.3 earlier. The design calls for 40 patients, 10 assigned to each of the four cells. The designations A_1 and A_2 refer to a test drug and a standard drug, and B_1 and B_2 represent high and low doses, respectively. Thus, for example, the combination A_1B_1 refers to the test drug at the high dose. Specifically, we wish to assign 10 patients each to the combinations A_1B_1, A_1B_2, A_2B_1, and A_2B_2.

Again, let's use the Moses & Oakford tables. Although I do not feel it really necessary, you may wish to select the page number and permutation randomly, as some statisticians recommend. You may then feel certain that your randomization is beyond criticism.

You will need a permutation of the numbers 1 through 40. As before, the nearest appropriate set of tables is that containing the integers 1 through 50. These sets appear on pages 68 through 92 of Moses and Oakford. To select a

Table 9.2. Randomization of a 2 × 2 Design with Cell Replication

	B_1	B_2
A_1	24	1
	36	8
	25	35
	29	10
	7	39
	6	16
	2	37
	11	38
	34	4
	20	19
A_2	15	30
	21	28
	32	40
	9	5
	27	3
	26	31
	14	7
	22	18
	13	33
	23	12

$$n_1 = 10 \quad n_2 = 10$$
$$n_3 = 10 \quad n_4 = 10$$
$$N = 40$$

page at random, you must select one of these numbers by some random or pseudo-random process. The simplest and probably the fastest method (there are many ways, as you can imagine) is to use a table of uniformly distributed random numbers, going through the rows or columns until you find one number within the desired range. I used the table beginning on page 463 of Snedecor and Cochran [38], going down the first column and looking at the first two digits in that column.[11] The first number in the range between 68–92 is 85, the third number down, and you will therefore use one of the permutations on page 85 in Moses and Oakford.

You now repeat the procedure to choose one of the 16 permutations on page 85. Let's assume that they are numbered by columns, starting at the left, so that the first permutation on the page, at the top of the left-hand column, is numbered 1, and the last one in the right-hand column is 16. Let's use a new page in Snedecor and Cochran, turning to page 464, the second page of their random number table. Going down the first column of this table as

[11]When you need a one-digit number, use two-digit numbers in which the first digit is zero.

before, this time looking for an integer between 1 and 16, we find 10, again the third number down. We therefore select the tenth permutation in Moses and Oakford, which is the second one in the right-hand column on page 85, the one beginning with the integers 24, 1, 36, etc., in the first row.

Finally, we draw up a table similar to the diagram of Figure 9.3, with the cells left blank. We then copy the numbers from the Moses and Oakford table, let's say by rows, to the new randomization table, skipping any number greater than 40. The result is shown as Table 9.2.

For practice, you may wish to actually go through the procedure just described. If you do, check yourself by making sure that your numbers agree with Table 9.2.

9.5.4   Trials Designed in Full Replicates

You may wish to use this kind of design for any of several reasons. Sometimes you may feel, for greater generality, that your trial should include a range of time periods (several days, weeks, or months). Or the sample size may be so large that the trial cannot be run over one uninterrupted period of time. Or, even if that can be done, you may believe that there will be differences in response from one day, week, or month to the next that are irrelevant to your system and greater than those that might occur if the trial could have been run over a shorter period. Or, finally, you may need to run a multicenter trial because no single center can obtain the number of patients you need.

If any of these circumstances prevail, you can prevent such differences from increasing your experimental error by running a set of complete replicates and identifying each with a specific segment of time. If the "nuisance variable" is not temporal but spatial (or both), of course, you would virtually always do exactly this. A multicenter trial in which all the factors of interest would occur at each center (the centers would then be an additional factor with each center comprising one level) is an example. The full or complete replicates would be the segments of the trial at each center. Depending upon certain statistical assumptions and the kind of statistical analysis that would consequently be done, the effects of the centers in adding to the total error could be isolated from the evaluation of the treatment effects. Exactly this kind of design is illustrated in Figure 9.4 in Section 9.2.4, although in an actual trial, it would be wise to use at least two or three patients per cell in each center.

In doing your sample size estimates, use the nearest number greater than that which results in an integral number of replicates with no patients left over. For example, if you had calculated that you needed 54 patients for the trial illustrated by the design of Figure 9.4, use the nearest multiple of four patients that is greater than 54. In this case, you would therefore need 56 patients (14 full replicates).

This kind of trial should be randomized separately at each location or time period one at a time, following the procedure described in the last section for each. As mentioned earlier, if such designs, like the one illustrated in Figure 9.4, have only one patient in each cell, and even one patient turns out to be a noncompleter, there will be no direct information at all available in that replicate for the treatment combination corresponding to that cell. For this reason, it is a good idea to arrange for some cell replication, even if the sample size estimate does not require it.

To further clarify, in a design done in full replicates, whether or not there is cell replication, the randomization is done by assigning patients to the cells in each replicate separately and independently, just as if each replicate were a complete experiment. Of course, as mentioned previously, you should use a different set of patients for each repetition of the design. For example, suppose the replicates were a set of hospitals and clinics in various parts of the country, and that you are planning a 2^2 design (two factors, A and B, each at two levels, with cell replication at each hospital or clinic). This is a three-factor design (A, B, and the replicates). In such a trial, the correct procedure is to randomize the assignments of the two two-level factors to four groups of patients, usually with equal numbers in each ($A_1 B_1$, $A_1 B_2$, $A_2 B_1$, and $A_2 B_2$), at each center, independently of the other centers.

9.5.5 Designs without Replication

These designs are discussed only briefly here. Their greatest use is in chemistry, engineering, and some industrial work, in which there may be several factors, perhaps more than three or four. You may never have a need for them, but we include them for completeness. They differ from the cell-replicated designs in having only one patient in each cell. Usually, there is only one full replicate of the design.

Unreplicated designs are randomized in the same way as the cell-replicated designs. You generate a random permutation (or choose one from a table) having the same number of integers as the number of patients who will take part in the trial. For an example of this design, see Figure 9.5. It has 81 cells of one patient each. You will therefore require a permutation of the numbers 1 through 81. Table 9.3 shows random assignments for that design. In this case, I generated the random permutation using a pocket calculator. In such designs, it is clear that the loss of a single cell during execution of the experiment will make one particular set of levels of the factors unavailable for analysis.

9.5.6 Randomizing in Stages

A trial done in complete replicates, for example, in several different centers, should be randomized separately for each center. This should be done even if the centers are close together and drawing upon the same patient pool (as is, of course, not very common for multicenter trials, but may be the rule when the replicates are temporal). As emphasized earlier, be certain that you do

Table 9.3. Randomization of an Unreplicated 3^4 Design

	C_1			C_2			C_3		
	D_1	D_2	D_3	D_1	D_2	D_3	D_1	D_2	D_3
$A_1 B_1$	63	81	33	70	51	13	71	49	19
B_2	64	62	53	24	29	48	55	60	45
B_3	14	11	65	76	52	39	58	69	1
$A_2 B_1$	2	77	68	61	5	59	17	26	28
B_2	57	6	42	66	46	80	18	41	75
B_3	37	56	34	22	50	30	27	36	74
$A_3 B_1$	43	32	10	8	72	31	47	78	3
B_2	38	4	7	44	20	12	40	16	54
B_3	21	25	23	35	67	73	15	9	79

not select patients for any replicate (*or cell*) if they have been used previously in the same trial.

There are some types of multifactor trials for which the randomization *must* be done in two or more stages. One of these is illustrated by the randomized-blocks designs described later (which really illustrate one kind of replication). Note that if you consider that *centers* in a multicenter trial comprise a *random factor*, that trial uses a randomized-blocks design. Another occurs when one of the variables is inherent, for example, when sex is one of the factors in the design.

Suppose that you are planning a trial with two factors, such as drugs and doses. You can and should randomize this in one step, that is, you would assign treatments to patients cell by cell, considering each cell as a patient group within which all patients would receive the same treatment. Table 9.4 illustrates this design, using three replicates per cell (of course, so small a trial usually would be impractical).

But suppose, while you are still planning this trial, that you decide to use a third classification in addition to drugs and doses, namely, that you decide to classify the patients according to sex. Because you have now introduced

Table 9.4. Factorial Design with Two Controlled Factors and Three Patients per Cell

	D_1	D_2
T_1	- -	- -
	- -	- -
	- -	- -
T_2	- -	- -
	- -	- -
	- -	- -

Table 9.5. Factorial Design with Three Controlled Factors and Three Patients per Cell

	D_1		D_2	
	S_1	S_2	S_1	S_2
T_1	- - -	- - -	- - -	- - -
	- - -	- - -	- - -	- - -
	- - -	- - -	- - -	- - -
T_2	- - -	- - -	- - -	- - -
	- - -	- - -	- - -	- - -
	- - -	- - -	- - -	- - -

another two-level factor, sex, into your trial, it becomes a 2^3 design requiring eight patient groups rather than a two-factor design needing only four. Ordinarily, if the third variable was an ordinary factor, this design could be illustrated as shown in Table 9.5, randomizing in one stage by assigning three patients to each of the eight groups (cells) shown. However, in this special case, a better way is to randomize in two stages. The reason is that sex is not a controlled variable in the same sense as drugs, but can be legitimately isolated from the other factors in the design by considering the two levels of sex as two replicates. You therefore should randomly assign the four drug/dose combinations *separately*: the two replicates, women, and men. You can no longer use patient numbers running from 1 to the total number of patients in the entire experiment. Instead, you must begin with two sets of patients, men and women, numbered separately, assigning the two drugs to each individually. You will now have created the following groups: women, drug 1 and dose 1; drug 1 and dose 2; drug 2 and dose 1; and drug 2 and dose 2. The same arrangement will be repeated for the men, making a total of eight groups, four groups repeated in each replicate. This design is shown in Table 9.6. Although the diagram has the same structure as that of Table 9.5, it must be randomized differently, and therefore the analysis will be different.

In cases in which a variable is an inherent characteristic of the patients, the reason that the two stages are needed is clear. You have no choice but to

Table 9.6. Factorial Design with Two Factors in Two Replicates

	Repl. 1 (Female)		Repl. 2 (Male)	
	D_1	D_2	D_1	D_2
T_1	- - -	- - -	- - -	- - -
	- - -	- - -	- - -	- - -
	- - -	- - -	- - -	- - -
T_2	- - -	- - -	- - -	- - -
	- - -	- - -	- - -	- - -
	- - -	- - -	- - -	- - -

sample two separate groups and randomize separately. But even if you are not forced to do that, but you nevertheless want to set up two or more replicates, you should sample and randomize from as many separate groups as there are replicates. First, randomly select the patient groups for each replicate and then make the treatment assignments within each of them.

Contrast these examples with a 2^2 trial in which you have complete control over the assignment of the two levels of both factors, for example, drugs and doses (say, high and low). Here, you can randomly assign each of the four treatment combinations to a group of patients taken from the same pool, so that the randomization is a one-step process.

9.5.7   Summary of Randomization Procedures

As you can now see, the randomization of a multifactor design is often done in about the same way as for a design with a single factor, but it can be a little more complex, as it is when you must or wish to do it in several stages. You can use any of the methods described here and earlier to obtain a permutation of the desired size for each repetition of the design. For a single-replicate design (done in one center, once only), as for single-factor trials, you make your assignments with cells as the basic units. If you are not planning to use full replicates, the only difference in a multifactor design is that the patient(s) in each cell will be assigned to a combination of levels of two or more factors, whereas in the one-factor designs, a cell reflects one level of one factor.

9.6   FACTORIALS WITH UNEQUAL CELL SIZES

In a moderately long and reasonably sized trial, although the cell sizes are usually equal in the beginning, and although the trial may have been managed well, it is probable that some cells will lose patients. In addition, if you plan on too few patients per cell, you run the risk of having some completely empty cells. Therefore, you should be certain that you use adequate cell replication, based upon as good an estimate of the expected attrition as possible.

There are special cases in which it is desirable that one or more of the planned comparisons be done at greater precision than the others, and, to achieve this, trials may be *designed* with unequal cell sizes. Most of the time, however, this arrangement entails no additional benefits over the use of equal sample sizes, and it can be disadvantageous. There are at least three problems associated with factorial data sets having unequal cell sizes; these are, in the order of their importance:

1. As for the single-factor designs, the use of unequal cell sizes will reduce the power of your statistical hypothesis tests. The overall error variance

will not be as small as possible, minimized, even when all the parametric assumptions are satisfied. This means, of course, that your sample size estimates, and thus the cost of the trial, must be increased to compensate.

2. For multifactor designs with unequal cell sizes or missing cells, the analysis methods available are less satisfactory than for so-called "balanced" designs. Your statistician may need to use a so-called *fixed-effects* model in the unequal cell size analysis, although this may not really be what is desired. You may need to do this often enough even when you begin a trial with equal cell sizes, because of noncompleters, but that is unavoidable; see Bancroft (1). There are approximate analyses available, but there is little reason to use them, because the exact procedure is equally convenient on most computers.

3. Any analysis of structures with unequal cell sizes will be more complex than those available for **balanced designs** (designs with equal cell sizes). They are therefore more difficult to explain to nonstatistical management personnel and others.

You may have heard of the "replacement" of missing data values. However, with the present availability of inexpensive computing equipment and sophisticated statistical software, this technique is no longer needed. Formerly, it was used to lighten the labor of analysis in the days before microcomputers (or any computers) were available. Today, almost any microcomputer, with available software, will be capable of rapid completion of the most complex analyses you are likely to encounter in any industrial drug trial. You will find descriptions of many data replacement procedures in Cochran and Cox [11]. Today, these are needed only for analyses done "by hand" (i.e., with a pocket or desktop calculator), procedures that are unlikely to be used except for the purpose of learning statistical techniques.[12]

9.7 ESTIMATING SAMPLE SIZES FOR FACTORIALS

Methods for sample size estimation for factorials will not be discussed in this chapter, but two approaches are described in Part V. One, originated by Bratcher, Moran, and Zimmer (2), involves the use of a special set of tables, also used for one-way studies, and is approximate. The other two are computer programs. One uses a program devised by Borenstein and Cohen [67], and the other (*Design*) was written by Gerard Dallal [66]. It appears that these are approximate only in the sense of the degree of precision with which the programs do the calculations. However, all three approaches will almost always be adequate for the designs for which they are intended. For one

[12]Please do not fail to obtain a copy of this book because of this remark. It is still the best compendium of practical experimental designs available.

thing, the estimates of sigma upon which they are based will always be approximations of those expected in a new experiment, and the values of alpha, beta, and delta, although they are treated as exact quantities, are specified by the user and are thus matters of judgment.

9.8   INTERACTIONS

9.8.1   Introduction

The subject of interactions in factorial designs can be a very complex one. In this book, we will merely wade along the shore, avoiding the deep water. However, you must know something about interactions, because they are common, you will encounter them and sometimes plan to evaluate them, and you will need to interpret them. I believe that the best way to answer questions of the interpretation of interactions that arise after a data analysis is to try to postulate them before the trial begins, considering then what your possible answers may be. The aim of this section is try to help you to do this.

Statistical interactions should not be confused with the idea of *drug interactions*, which are commonly referred to in the medical literature.

9.8.2   Example 9.8: A Simple Two-Factor Interaction

Suppose that you have run a randomized 2^2 trial using osteoarthritis patients, with 10 patients in each cell. Assume that factor A represents two antiinflammatory drugs (let's say a test drug vs. a standard material) and that factor B represents age groups. Age is an important variable in this case, because the severity of the disease would be expected to increase with age. We are therefore using age as a regular variable, but will heed our warnings about the handling and interpretation of such inherent factors. Let's say that you are using joint tenderness index (jti) as a response measurement. Such a design was represented in Figure 9.3. Suppose, now, that the trial is complete and that both **main effects**[13] have been found significant, so that you believe there are important differences both between the drugs and, as would normally be expected, between the age groups (subject to verification in further trials). That is, perhaps you notice that the data for drug A_2 show a lower average joint tenderness value than A_1 that is statistically significant, and, also, you note that there are significantly lower joint tenderness values, on the average, among the patients in the younger group (B_1) than in the older one (B_2). But suppose, in addition to these two significant main effects,

---

[13]A *main effect* is a measure of the response attributed to one of the factors.

that you find a significant **interaction effect** among the levels of A and B. What does this mean?

Any two-factor (AB) interaction can be described as follows: *The differences between levels for one of the factors are not the same as those for the other.* In this case, let's say that you find that the *difference* between the average values of joint tenderness for the two drugs, A_1 and A_2, is not the same, on average, in the over-50 age group (B_2) as it is in the younger group (B_1). This lack of agreement (we sometimes say "lack of linearity") is called an interaction. If the interaction is found to be statistically significant when the data are analyzed, you may state that the differences between drugs varies significantly (in the populations) from one level of age to the other; or you could say, just as correctly, that the difference between age groups varies depending upon which drug was used. Of course, you must be cautious in claiming significance in this case, and should check it carefully in future experiments. Indeed, you should treat any apparently significant result involving an inherent factor such as age with some skepticism. Unless you have designed the trial as discussed earlier, you must recognize that the randomization has not been done in the same way as that for the drugs factor, and the reliability of your conclusions about any factor involving age (including the main effect) must therefore be recognized as questionable.

When such an interaction is detected in your analysis, you can no longer view the main effect differences (the significant differences you found for the drugs and age groups factors, considered separately) as telling the whole (and perhaps not even the correct) story about this system of factors and their levels. To put it another way, you cannot describe the magnitude of the *mean* difference between the drugs without pointing out that it differs depending upon which age group is considered. Similarly, you cannot describe the main effect of age groups without pointing out that although they are different, on the average; the magnitude of that difference depends upon which drug group you look at. In fact, it is not unusual to find that the main effect information per se is no longer relevant at all. In some cases (see the discussion later in this chapter), *neither* main effect is found to be significant, but there is a significant interaction.

Note that if there are interactions, they will not be detectable in a convincing way if you run a one-factor experiment, holding the other factor constant at some level. Even if you were to follow this with a second experiment at another level of the second factor, and find a different outcome, you would not have good evidence of an interaction. It could simply be that the difference you find is due to random variation or some change in conditions between one experiment and the next. The best way to detect an interaction reliably is to run a trial using both factors simultaneously, with appropriate randomization. This was one of Fisher's [16] principal arguments for the use of factorial designs. You may note that this is related to an idea discussed in an earlier chapter, when it was pointed out that a control should be run concurrently in a trial, and that you should not depend for your conclusions upon an historical control or a baseline reading.

In this section, we have just described the simplest kind of interaction. It is simple because there are only two factors, and only two levels of each. Nevertheless, as you will see, there is a wide variety of types of interaction even if you confine consideration to 2^2 designs. Because there are just two factors, regardless of the number of levels each factor possesses, this class of interactions is called **first-order**. There are a number of kinds of first-order interactions, however, and we will exemplify some of them. Following this, we will touch briefly upon higher-order interactions. We will not consider these in much detail, however. Higher-order interactions occur less frequently than first-order interactions, and of course they are impossible to detect unless there are three factors or more in a trial. Furthermore, besides being rarer than two-factor interactions, they are more likely than the latter to merely reflect experimental error. Finally, a detailed treatment is beyond the scope of this book.

In a later chapter, we will mention and briefly discuss the fact that it is possible that one of the assumptions (linearity) is quite wrong in the light of the characteristics of the data, and that the interaction(s) found are evidence of this. There are tests of the data that can be made and remedies that can be applied during analysis to determine whether this may be true. You must also keep in mind, however, that if you are reasonably sure of your **model**[14] and assumptions, and if your tests of the assumptions do not discredit your confidence, the occurrence of an interaction, especially if it is of low order, may be regarded as a credible and realistic event.

9.8.3 Factorial Effects

To help define degrees of freedom in the next section and to help in the following discussions of interactions and other aspects of factorial designs, we need to introduce the idea of factorial *effects*,[15] a term that we have already used without definition.

For a 2^2 factorial, the main effect of a factor is the *mean of all measurements* of that factor at its first level minus that at its second. For instance,

---

[14]The *model* of an experimental design is a formal mathematical expression that describes the sources of variation and their relationships to each other, often supplemented by a statement of certain assumptions that accompany it. Models comprise an advanced topic that is not needed for the purposes of this book, but is important in showing the structure of a design as well as its connection with the eventual data analysis.

This term is not to be confused with the *model* of an analysis of variance (fixed, random, mixed).

[15]This discussion is somewhat simplified, but should assist you in understanding factorial design. For a more thorough discussion, you may wish to refer to Snedecor and Cochran [38], Chapter 16, especially pp. 300–302. If you do so, however, you should read this section first.

suppose that the mean joint tenderness index for drug A_1 in the previous example was 10 (on a joint tenderness index scale of 0 to 34), and that for drug A_2 was 16. The mean value for A_1, 10, is obtained by averaging the data for the 20 patients who received drug A_1 (10 at each level of B). In the same way, the mean value for A_2, 16, was obtained by averaging the data for the remaining 20 patients, those patients who received A_2 (again 10 at each level of B). The **main effect** of factor A, "drugs" would then be $10 - 16$, or -6. The difference may be taken in either direction, so it may be either positive or negative, but you must be consistent. When there are more than two levels of a factor, the definition of a factorial effect is not as simple as this, but that is not of concern at present.

A so-called **double**, or **first-order**, interaction effect in a 2^2 experiment is calculated in an analogous way. The data for the example that we are discussing has four cells, each containing 10 patients' data: A_1B_1, A_1B_2, A_2B_1, and A_2B_2. Suppose that the means of the four individual cells, in the same order (each is a mean of 10 data), were the following: 8, 12, 15, and 17. To calculate the interaction effect, if any, we use these individual cell means. For simplicity, we are assuming here that there were no losses of data so that each of the four cells supplied 10 data.

Remember that the previous interaction was described as a difference between differences (we said that if an interaction exists, the difference between the means for A_1 and A_2 is *not the same* for the B_1 patients as the B_2 patients, on average). This means that the difference between the means for A_1B_1 and A_2B_1 (this is the difference between the means of A_1 and A_2 for those subjects receiving B_1) was not the same as that for A_1B_2 and A_2B_2 (those receiving B_2), or

$$\left(\overline{A_1B_1} - \overline{A_2B_1}\right) \neq \left(\overline{A_1B_2} - \overline{A_2B_2}\right) \tag{9.1}$$

In equation 9.1, the bars over the combinations of A and B representing the four cells signify that they are averages (means). The symbol $\neq$ means "is not equal to."

In this case, Equation 9.1 defines the **interaction effect** for the two factors. Whether its magnitude is great enough to warrant a conclusion that there is a "real" interaction—that is, one among the populations—requires a statistical test.

9.8.4   Degrees of Freedom

Background
The kind of interaction phenomenon introduced in the foregoing paragraphs is a typical example of a first-order single degree of freedom interaction. There is more to say about interactions. But to understand them better on a

practical basis, we must first describe the somewhat elusive concept of **degrees of freedom (df)**. This idea is fundamental in statistics and experimental design, and will be helpful to you in gaining a deeper understanding of interactions, as well as many other quantities in experimental design.

Although the theory is not entirely simple, it is easy to describe the notion of degrees of freedom adequately enough to allow its use and understanding in practical work. Please note that the statistical term does not have the same meaning as it does in other fields of science, such as physical chemistry.

Degrees of Freedom for a Mean

Let's look at the general use and meaning of the idea, and then its application to main effects and interactions. Let's begin with a simple statement: **Degrees of freedom** are equal to the number of data *available* beyond that absolutely necessary when carrying out a statistical procedure.

Suppose that you have a number of data, n, from a trial. To calculate the mean of these data, you need at least one datum. If there were one datum instead of 10, that datum would be equal to the mean of that "set" of data. If there were two data in the set, you would have one more datum than the absolute minimum needed to get a mean, that is, there would be one "extra" datum. If there were 10 data, nine of them would be "extra." The degrees of freedom are the number of "extra" data available. Thus, for the mean of a group of response measurements, it is one less than the total number of data available to calculate it, or, in algebra, $n - 1$, where n is the total number of data.[16]

The concept can be applied more generally. For example, if a factor has two levels, that factor is said to have 1 df. If there are three levels, it has 2 df. And a total of n data also has $n - 1$ df. *But please note carefully that in some calculations other than that for a mean, the df may be $n - 2$, $n - 3$, or still another value.* However, you will not encounter any of these in this book.

9.8.5 First-Order One-df Interactions

First-order interactions are the kind exemplified in Example 9.8. In that example there are two factors, with 10 patients in each cell, so that the design is that shown in Figure 9.3. Let's analyze the degrees of freedom for each part of that design, that is, each source of variation that can affect the response. There are four possible sources: the two main effects, A and B; the AB interaction effect; and the variation or "error" among the subjects within each cell. That error is the **within-cell** variation, and is principally the result of patient-to-patient variation. This variation is exclusive of any varia-

---

[16] If you are calculating a mean, its precision as an estimator of the population mean increases as the number of data used to calculate it increase, and you are almost always concerned with obtaining as precise a statistic as possible. But aside from that, although you *must* have *at least* one datum to calculate a mean, one is enough.

tion in response related to the factors or the interaction, because all 10 subjects *within* each cell are treated identically.[17]

The df for calculating a mean from a group of items was just described. Now, let's tally the degrees of freedom from the sources of variation just mentioned. First, there are 40 patients altogether, so that the total degrees of freedom is $40 - 1$, or 39. Next, each of the two factors has 1 df because each has two levels. Now, what about the interaction? It can be shown that an interaction df is the product of the df's of its individual factors. Algebraically, this means that for the *AB* interaction, you multiply the df for *A* by that for *B*: $(n_a - 1)(n_b - 1)$. Of course, this is equal to 1 in this case, because each of the two factors has only two levels, that is, $n_a = n_b = 2$. If there were more than two levels for one or both factors, however, this would no longer be true.

Finally, we need to find the df "within cells." This is a bit trickier. We have already obtained a value for the total of all of the data, but note carefully that that *includes* those for three parts of the data set: the two factors, their interaction, and that within cells. To get the df **within cells** exclusive of those for the other sources of variation (all of which are **between-cells** properties), you proceed as follows: Note that each cell contains 10 data when the trial is done, so each *individual* cell has 9 df. You now add the df for the four cells, obtaining 36 in this example.

Note that we calculated all four of these df values independently. Now, let's add them:

A	1
B	1
AB	1
Cells	36
Total	39

I have always found that such a group of independently calculated df's adds up to the precalculated total amazing and extremely interesting. In words, the total of the degrees of freedom is the sum of its parts; in this design, the parts are the df's for *A*, *B*, *AB*, and within cells. This characteristic allows you to check your work for errors, which can be useful when the structure of a factorial design is complex. You will find it helpful to remember this idea. It is needed in one way or another in your design planning, and the biostatistician uses it in most statistical data analyses.

A 1-df interaction is the simplest and most common kind, one that you will probably be concerned with frequently in your work. You may even design

---

[17]The within-cells error also includes (i.e., "is confounded with") miscellaneous sources of variation, such as any differences in the way the response was elicited from each subject, and the like. For simplicity, we are considering only the patient-to-patient error here. In addition, in a carefully done trial, it is usually not important to separate out the miscellaneous sources, because they are typically expected to be similar for all subjects and are normally much smaller than the differences between patients.

some trials for the specific purpose of detecting and examining interactions of this kind. Another quite commonplace but more complex kind of first-order interaction occurs, as before, between two factors, but when one of them has more than two levels. For example, suppose you were designing a trial with the two factors, drugs and doses, but that you wish to use three drugs. Factor A would now have three levels. Any interaction between A and B would have 2 df, because the main effect of factor A would have 2 df $(3 - 1)$, and that of B, 1 df $(2 - 1)$, and these two values would be multiplied together to obtain the df for the interaction.

9.8.6   Example 9.9: Interpreting One-df Two-Factor Interactions

Background
Interactions having any number of df's are possible. Two-factor interactions are common and are relatively simple to interpret, especially when they have only 1 degree of freedom. Two-factor interactions with more than 1 df are also common but are a bit more difficult to interpret. These can occur when one or both of the factors have more than two levels. Interactions among more than two factors are less frequently encountered, and can be quite complex.

When you are designing a trial, you must be sure that you understand the meaning of a given interaction if it is found when your data are analyzed. One way to do this is to sketch one or two of the possible configurations it may take and then try to put its meaning into words. This will aid you in creating your design, as well as help prepare you for reporting the trial after the study is complete. If you do find a statistically significant interaction when the data are analyzed, you will need to interpret it in such a way that it can be understood by people with no statistical background. The following figures and examples may be of help to you.

The Case of No Interaction
We will construct a plot of means of the 10 data in each of the four cells calculated from hypothetical data obtained when the design described in Section 9.8.1 and illustrated in Figure 9.3 was run. We are assuming that there was no interaction between the two factors, drugs (A) and age (B). The four means had the following joint tenderness index values. We represent the means of the responses by the symbols for the factors and their levels, with a bar over each:

$$\overline{A_1 B_1} = 5.0$$

$$\overline{A_1 B_2} = 20.0$$

$$\overline{A_2 B_1} = 15.0$$

$$\overline{A_2 B_2} = 30.0$$

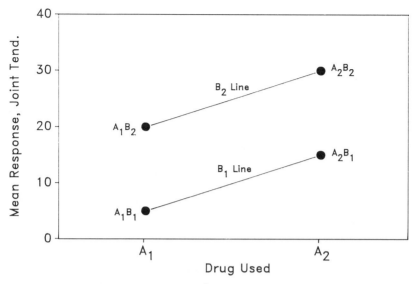

Figure 9.7 Plot of the four cell means from 2^2 factorial design; no AB interaction.

These four means are plotted in Figure 9.7. Note that the four points defining the ends of the two lines represent these means, so that the diagram includes all 40 data that were obtained when the trial was run.

Note that although the ordinate scale is numerical and represents the mean values of the joint tenderness index response, the abscissa is qualitative (because the two different drugs are not described on a numerical scale).[18] Thus, the two points marked A_1 and A_2, representing the two drug levels, are located at arbitrary positions along the drug axis. Of course, the two factors could be interchanged without changing the information conveyed, placing the two factor B levels (ages) on the abscissa of the graph and labeling the two lines with the two levels of A (drugs).

In Figure 9.7, both points representing factor B at its second level lie at equal distances above those showing it at its first level. That is, the difference between the means for A_1B_1 and A_1B_2 (younger vs. older patients taking drug 1) is equal to that between the means for A_2B_1 and A_2B_2 (younger vs. older patients taking drug 2). In other words, the two lines are parallel. Furthermore, the two main effects, A and B, are implicit in the figure. To show this, average all of the data that include A_1 (5.0 and 20.0); the resulting number is 12.5, which is an estimate of the population mean response for that drug. The analogous estimate for A_2 the other drug (the data are 15.0

---

[18]It is sometimes useful to describe the levels of either a quantitative or a qualitative variable with numbers. When there are two levels, this can be done by assigning the quantity -1 to one of them and 1 to the other. When there are three, the numbers -1, 0, and 1 can be used. Similar schemes can be used with greater numbers of levels. There would be no advantage to numbering the levels of the drugs for Figure 9.7, however.

and 30.0), is 22.5. The effect of A is the difference between these two means, which is 10.0. In the same way, the effect of B is the difference between the means for B_1 and B_2 (10.0 and 25.0), and the difference, hence the effect of B, is 15.0. The main effect of drugs, factor A, is $15 - 10$, or 5. (You could have reversed the order of the two means, so that you would then get -5. Either way is correct, as long as you remain consistent.

By looking at Figure 9.7 in a slightly different way, it can be used to investigate the interaction. The two vertical distances (those between the two points at the left and the two at the right) are $20 - 5$, or 15, and $30 - 15$, also 15. Because the difference between these two distances is zero, the slopes of the two lines are equal, which in turn means that there is no evidence of any interaction between A and B. In other words, the difference between ages B_1 and B_2 is the same for drug A_1 as for A_2. Putting it the other way, the difference between drugs A_1 and A_2 is the same for age B_1 as for B_2.

As you can see, the three differences just discussed are estimates of parameters of three theoretical populations. The difference between the two differences (zero, in this case) is an estimate of the mean value of the interaction effect. The difference between the means B_1 and B_2 is an estimate of the main effect of age of the patients, and that between A_1 and A_2 estimates the main effect of drugs. Notice that these estimates are all differences. For the drugs, the estimate is a difference between two means, for the age groups, it is the same. For the interaction, it is a difference between two other mean differences, which, in turn, are each differences between two means. Note also that, as for all factorial designs, you use *all* the data for each of these calculations. This is one of the several advantages of the use of factorial designs.

You can now describe the outcome of this hypothetical experiment in words, including the absence of an *AB* interaction. For example, you might say in your report, "Based upon an examination of the treatment group means, before any statistical hypothesis tests were done, it appeared that there were detectable A and B effects. That is, the two drugs appeared different in their mean responses, as measured by the VAS scale. Similarly, the data for the two age groups indicated that the condition was more severe for older people than for younger, as expected. However, there was no evidence of an interaction, because the difference between drugs remained the same for the two age groups. These tentative conclusions were subsequently substantiated when the statistical tests were done." Note that in a real experiment, it would not be likely that the two vertical distances would be exactly equal, as they were in this case. That is, the omnipresent random variation would make it unlikely that the two lines would be exactly parallel, even in the absence of any interaction. A hypothesis test would then be certainly needed to help decide whether they were *sufficiently* nonparallel to allow you to claim an interaction.

Estimates of effects such as the foregoing, derived from data, are statistics with **expected values** that may equal population parameters. The expected

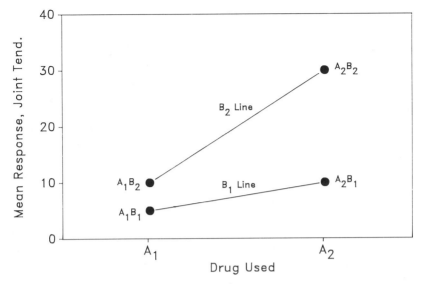

Figure 9.8 Plot of the four cell means from 2^2 factorial design; probable moderate AB interaction.

value of a statistic is the ultimate mean value that would be obtained if samples were taken repeatedly and cumulatively averaged. If the estimates are **unbiased**, their expected values are the parameters of the distributions.

The Case of a Moderate Interaction

If a nonzero interaction is detected when you do your statistical analysis, it might be represented as shown in Figure 9.8. In this case, the interpretation is a bit more elaborate.

In Figure 9.8, there appear to be A and B effects as before, but, in addition, the two lines representing the levels of B are no longer parallel. Therefore, the vertical difference at the left (A_1B_1 minus A_1B_2) and the corresponding difference on the right (A_2B_1 minus A_2B_2) are no longer equal. This suggests that there is an AB interaction, and a test of significance should be run to evaluate this evidence.[19] If you find significance, you might

---

[19]A review: You reason as follows when running **significance (hypothesis)** tests. You postulate four populations of patient data, with the same means as those in your study. You assume that your four treatment groups are samples from these populations. Next, you assume that the treatments had no effect upon the response, so that all four populations have the same means. This is the **null hypothesis**. The **alternate hypothesis**, which you must logically accept if the evidence for the null hypothesis is sufficiently weak, is that there is such a difference, presumably due to the treatments. You then test the data to estimate the probability of obtaining an observed difference by chance as large as that found (i.e., if the null hypothesis is true). If this probability is small (less than alpha), you *reject* the null hypothesis and declare that a population difference, delta, exists. But if the calculated probability is equal to or greater than alpha, you conclude that significance has not been obtained, with a probability beta of being wrong.

explain it as follows: "A significant interaction was found between the two factors, drugs and ages. In this case, the mean difference found between drugs was less for the younger group (B_1) than for the older (B_2)." Alternatively, you can explain the interaction by the observation that the difference between age groups was less for drug A_1 than for A_2. You must then recognize that because of this interaction, any statements about differences between age groups or drugs must be accompanied by a statement as to which level of the other factor it refers. That is, if there is an interaction, the difference between drugs will vary depending upon the age group being considered.

The Case of a Very Strong Interaction

Another, more extreme kind of interaction sometimes occurs. It is noteworthy because it is an example of a configuration in which *neither* main effect shows significance, yet for which there is a strong interaction. In this kind of interaction, the two lines in Figures 9.7 or 9.8 have such different slopes that they cross each other within the range of the values used in the study. The most extreme case of this (to clarify the example) is illustrated in Figure 9.9. In the following, as before, for convenience, we represent the response means by the symbols for the factors and their levels, without the use of bars above them.

In the case illustrated in Figure 9.9, the overall means for A_1 and A_2, $(A_1B_1 + A_1B_2)/2$ and $(A_2B_1 + A_2B_2)/2$, which are the means of the two levels of A, are exactly equal numerically. Therefore, because the estimated

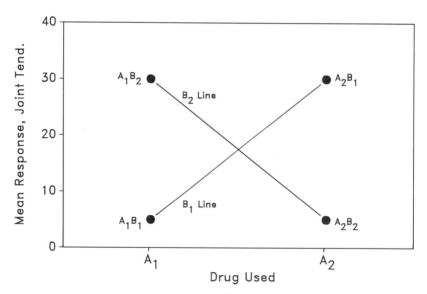

Figure 9.9 Plot of the four cell means from 2^2 factorial design; strong AB interaction.

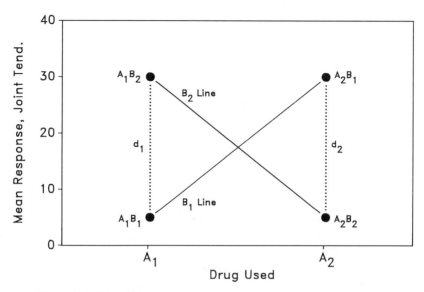

Figure 9.10 Plot of Figure 9.9 showing method of measuring the interaction.

A effect is estimated by taking the difference between these two means, it is seen to be zero, because the signs are opposite. In the same way, the expected value of the *B* effect can also be found to be zero. Nevertheless, although there are no main effects, the interaction *AB* is quite large. Let's illustrate and calculate it.

Figure 9.10 shows the two vertical distances marked off with dotted lines at each side of the same pair of crossed lines shown in Figure 9.9. The difference between the lengths of these two dotted lines is a measure of the interaction, in the same way that we calculated the differences for the less extreme situation in Figure 9.8. Distances d_1 and d_2 represent the lengths of these two lines, or the *differences* between the pairs of points at each side of the diagram. These differences have opposite signs, unlike the two sums we calculated to estimate A_1 and A_2. Remembering that a first-order interaction for a 2^2 factorial is a *difference between two differences*, we see that there is a substantial quantity representing a possible interaction. Although this geometric representation may be clear to you, let's also express the two vertical distances algebraically:

$$d_1 = A_1 B_2 - A_1 B_1 \tag{9.2}$$

$$d_2 = A_2 B_1 - A_2 B_2 \tag{9.3}$$

If you now subtract either one of these distances from the other, you will obtain the "difference between the differences," which we will call *D*, and that is equal to the expression for the interaction. Equation 9.4 illustrates this:

$$D = d_1 - d_2 \tag{9.4}$$

It may appear that the two distances d_1 and d_2 are equal, and the fact is that in this extreme example, they are *numerically* equal. But their signs are different. The interaction effect can be defined as the difference between the high and low levels of B (i.e., $B_2 - B_1$) at the first level of A (this is d_1) minus the same difference at the other level of A (this is d_2). When you subtract one from the other to get D, using Equation 9.4, if you correctly manage the signs, you will get a large difference, actually equal to the sum of d_1 and d_2. This sum will be positive or negative depending upon the direction of your subtraction, but the sign does not matter as long as you are consistent. There is thus a large apparent interaction. Using the values of the four means of the $A_i B_j$ as given before, $D = 15 - (-15) = 30$.

You might explain this interaction in your report in words similar to these: "The two drugs did not differ from each other in any simple way, nor did the age groups. However, an interaction was found between the two factors.[20] In terms of the drug factor, this interaction consisted of a difference between the two drugs that was equal in value but opposite in sign for the younger compared to the older patients. In other words, there was a strong drug difference in the mean values of joint tenderness obtained, but its direction depended upon the drug used." Therefore, the drug effect cannot be discussed without taking the age of the patients into account.

Thus, you see that it is quite possible to carry out a trial in which both main effects are zero, but in which there is nevertheless a nonzero interaction. Such extreme interactions, or situations approaching them in which the two lines in a diagram like those we have been discussing, are less uncommon than might be supposed. What is to be learned from this was mentioned earlier, but now takes on more emphasis: If a statistical analysis of data indicates that there is an interaction, the meanings of the corresponding main effects must be interpreted with caution, considering carefully the meaning of the interaction. Sometimes, as in this extreme example and in similar cases, if the interaction is accepted as real and does not appear to be the result of an error in reading or recording data, then the interaction, not the main effect(s), is relevant in interpreting what is happening.

9.8.7   Interpreting Interactions with Two or More df's

The understanding of interactions, even of first order, becomes more difficult as their dfs increase. Perhaps, fortunately, there are few clinical trials with more than three factors, and many are run using two, each of which may have

---

[20] If significance is found when a hypothesis test is done. We reemphasize that you do not have any statistical support for such a statement until then.

no more than two or three levels. For your practical work, therefore, you only really need to understand systems with first-order interactions between two or possibly three factors, having one or a few df's.

The class of first-order interactions of least complexity beyond the 1-df cases that we have just discussed are those occurring when there are still only two factors, but for which one factor has two levels and the other three or more. Because few factors with more than three or four levels are used in industrial clinical trials, and because a consideration of a 2×3 experiment will exemplify any trial of this type quite well, we will consider one of these as representative of the class of $2 \times m$ experiments (m greater than 2).

9.8.8   Example 9.10: Interaction in 2×3 Factorial Study

Suppose we plan a study, then, in which factor A will have two levels, represented by two drugs as before. But now let's assume that factor B, representing patient's ages, has three rather than two levels (let's say, 18 to 30, 31 to 43, and 44 to 56). Also, let's assume that we have the same kind of variables as before (drugs and age groups, using two drugs but three instead of two age groups).[21] Finally, let's again use 10 data per cell, and the same response measurement (joint tenderness index). This experiment will have two factors at two and three levels, so there will be 2×3, or 6, means of 10 patients' data each when the trial is done and the means calculated.

The six means of the jti data are the following, each comprising 10 patients:

	A_1	A_2
B_1	5	7
B_2	10	15
B_3	12	30

Figures 9.11 and 9.12 illustrate two ways of plotting these six means, and show one possible and common configuration of the cell means when there is an interaction between the two factors.

In Figure 9.11, the two drugs are plotted along the X-axis (A_1 and A_2), and the three levels of age are shown as three straight lines, each plotted against the two drugs. As before, the ordinate is a quantitative axis showing values of the joint tenderness scale. You may find this arrangement easier to explain in your reports than the alternative that follows, because of the simplicity of the three straight lines. Of course, this is possible only when one

---

[21] Note that the age groups are equally spaced. It can be helpful in the data analysis and presentation of results if the spacing between levels of a quantitative factor is either equal, as here, or follows some other regular rule, such as the use of logarithmic spacing. The latter includes logs to any base, for example, the series, $2, 4, 8, 16, \ldots$ is logarithmically spaced, using logarithms to the base 2.

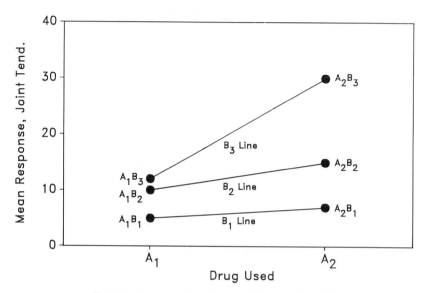

Figure 9.11   Illustration of a two *DF* interaction *AB*.

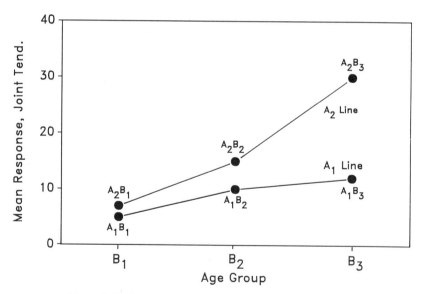

Figure 9.12   Interaction of Figure 9.11 with *A* and *B* reversed.

of the factors has only two levels. The pattern of the results is typical of multiple df interactions; the interaction seems to exist principally, if at all, between the two levels of factor A (1 df) and the second and third level of B (2 df). There seems to be little or no interaction between A and levels 1 and 2 of B.

In Figure 9.12, the age groups (B) instead of the drugs (A) are plotted on the X-axis and the two "lines" represent the two drugs.

If the analysis shows this interaction to be significant, two ways to describe it are the following (the two are equivalent). The first corresponds to Figure 9.11 and the second to Figure 9.12:

1. (See Figure 9.11): "For the two lower age groups, there is only quite a small difference, if any, between the two drugs, in favor of drug A_1, which showed smaller jti's. Among the older patients, there appears to be a substantial difference, although still in favor of A_1. This increase in the two drug differences, which depends upon the age group used, was found to be significant in the statistical analysis ($p = 0.01$). Thus, age should perhaps be taken into account when comparing or recommending one of the drugs. However, there is little evidence that drug A_2 was poorer than A_1 for the younger patients. Drug A_2 appeared superior for the older patients (remembering that *lower*, not *higher*, values of the response represent improvement)."

2. (See Figure 9.12): "For drug A_1, results for all three age groups were similar, with possible slightly better scores for the younger groups. With A_2, however, the older group of patients fared substantially more poorly than the other two groups, showing joint tenderness scores that were considerably higher. Thus, age should be considered, at least when recommending drug A_2."

Again, remember, as in all preceding cases, that these examples and those given earlier are intended as suggested ways to explain your results when writing your reports. Because the data in the examples have not been subjected to statistical tests, the conclusions are tentative at best. In an actual study, after significance tests have been done correctly, the statements given would incorporate the statistical information. In addition, it is important to bear in mind that every interaction requires a separate explanation—each will be different. There is no "boiler plate" or standardized explanation.

9.8.9 Higher-Order Interactions

When there is cell replication, finding interactions of first order (i.e., two-factor interactions) such as those just considered is not unusual, and the results are relatively simple to interpret. Clinical trials having three or more factors (so that higher-order interactions are possible) are less common than simpler trials. But even when such studies are used, it is quite unusual to find significant higher-order interactions. Nevertheless, in a trial having three factors and cell replication, three-factor (triple) interactions as well as two-factor interactions are possible and can be detected when they are present. For example, in a study having three factors involving factors A, B, and C, with cell replication, the following interactions, as well as the three main effects A, B, and C, may exist and can be tested statistically:

First-order (two-factor) interactions:
  AB
  AC
  BC

Second-order (three-factor interaction):
  ABC

Studies having four factors, as indicated, are quite rare in industrial practice, and interactions among the four factors are even rarer.

A second-order (triple) interaction, like ABC, can be viewed as an interaction between interactions. For instance, suppose that the two-factor drugs/age groups trial was run as a multicenter trial, with 10 cell replicates in each of the four cells used at each of, say, five widely separated centers. Now suppose that the three-factor interaction (drugs × ages × centers) was found to be significant, and the drugs × age groups interaction illustrated in Figure 9.9 was found to occur in two of the centers, but was not detectable or was less severe in the other three. Under some circumstances, this phenomenon could be regarded as a meaningful triple (second-order) interaction.

9.9 SUMMARY OF THE CHAPTER

This chapter introduced the use of full-factorial (multifactor) experimental designs in clinical drug trials, and to their randomization and interpretation. Although this book emphasizes experimental design, some discussion of interpretation of results was necessary because planning cannot be done properly without considering the outcome of an experiment.

A factor is a controlled, independent variable used in an experimental design. All factors possess two or more levels. For example, a two-factor clinical trial might use "drugs" as one factor (e.g., drug A vs. drug B) and "doses" (e.g., high vs. low) for the other. Factorial designs and their randomization were introduced by Sir Ronald A. Fisher in the 1920s. They eventually replaced the traditional "one factor at a time" methods of experimentation, and true randomization replaced the bias-prone systematic assignment of treatments to experimentation units. These innovations not only made more efficient experimentation possible, but for the first time allowed the effective evaluation of interactions between factors.

By using a number of brief examples, the concepts underlying crossed parallel factorial designs were explained, and their advantages over older methods of experimentation were shown. Various experimental structures were then discussed, beginning with the simplest multifactor arrangement, the 2^2 design, and eventually discussing two-factor designs in which the factors do not necessarily have the same numbers of levels. Finally, three-factor designs were described.

Two kinds of replication were discussed; cell replication, in which each factor combination is present for more than one experimental unit, and what we call full replicates, or the repetition of an entire design through space or time. Designs having no replication were also discussed briefly.

The randomization of various factorial designs was described, with examples. The estimation of sample size for multifactor designs was not covered, but will be discussed in Part V.

The concept of degrees of freedom (df) was explained from a practical point of view, in preparation for its use in discussing interactions and other concepts of statistics and experimental design. The distinctions between simple 1 df interactions among two-level factors and more complex structures having more than 1 df were shown. Finally, there was an introduction and explanation of two-factor interactions and their interpretation. Three-factor interactions were mentioned briefly. Several examples and diagrams were given to help clarify these. It was emphasized that the reliable discovery and evaluation of interactions can only be accomplished with factorial experimentation.

The next chapter will present a group of examples of parallel single-factor and multifactor clinical drug trials for your study and reference.

9.10 LITERATURE REFERENCES

(1) Bancroft, T. A., *Topics in Intermediate Statistical Methods, Volume I*, Iowa State University Press, Ames, Iowa, 1968.
(2) Bratcher, T. L., M. A. Moran, and W. J. Zimmer, "Tables of Sample Sizes in the Analysis of Variance," *Journal of Quality Technology*, 2, 156–164 (1970).

CHAPTER 10

Parallel Factorial Designs: Examples

10.1 BACKGROUND

10.1.1 Visual Comparisons of Means

This chapter presents five examples of practical factorial designs for your information and future reference. We give no broad attention to the statistical analysis of these examples or other trial data in this book, leaving that for your statistics department. However, in Part IV, we describe a few simple procedures with which you should be familiar. In this chapter, we will continue to substitute the calculation and visual examination of means of the data for complete statistical analyses, as we did when discussing interactions, although we report the results of more formal procedures in one case.

Such a simple visual comparison of means of data is *not* a statistical analysis. When a statistician speaks of the "comparison of means," the reference is not to the calculation of means and their visual comparison. Rather, what is meant is the following: He or she uses one or more of many kinds of hypothesis tests or confidence intervals to manipulate the data from the **sample** of patients representing the effects, if any, of the several factors and their interactions. Then, by utilizing the results, conclusions about differences among treatments or groups of treatments in hypothetical **populations**, such as the population of patents sampled (see Section 10.1.2, which follows), are drawn. The substitution of visual inspection for the more formal mathematical comparison of treatment groups is merely a very crude substitute for a mathematical analysis, lacking the verification afforded by hypothesis testing. However, it will serve the purpose of an analysis in these examples. At times, we will state the outcome of a correct statistical analysis done on the data. It should be understood that in any actual trial, appropriate statistical procedures must be used in lieu of or in addition to the simple examination of means.

When we calculate treatment means from a sample (i.e., means of the groups or combinations of groups of data representing the levels of a factor), we say that we are estimating certain population means (μ values). The following equation is not intended to instruct you in the calculation of an arithmetic mean, which you already know. Rather, it illustrates the notation we use here for individual data, sums, and means. Equation (10.1) shows the calculation of the mean of a set of data, the individual members of which are represented by y_i:

$$\bar{y} = \frac{\Sigma_i y_i}{n} \tag{10.1}$$

This equation states that to get the mean, $\bar{y}$, of a set of data, y_i, you must add all values of the data ($i = 1, 2, \ldots, n$) and divide the result by n, the number of data that was summed. This is not exactly an arbitrary rule, as it can be justified by the application of the **least-squares** principle.

10.1.2 Patient Populations

We spoke of hypothetical patient populations before. Although this matter has been mentioned earlier (see Chapter 2), it is so important that the earlier discussion is worth supplementing here.

Complete guidance for the use of a new treatment based upon the results of a clinical study *cannot* be obtained using *statistical* inference. It is impossible to obtain a random sample of patients for a clinical study who will represent those who will later use the drug(s) or treatments of interest if they become available generally. If for no other reason, the population of interest is composed of patients who may use your new drug *in the future*. Furthermore, a random or stratified random sample from an existing population is virtually never taken. Instead, practically always, patients are selected as representatives of those who *it is believed* may later benefit from the new treatment. Thus, any *statistical inferences* based upon the trial can refer only to these patients. *Inferences to any patient population, including one comprising future patients, must be drawn by the use of your professional experience and knowledge.* The statistical analysis of the trial supplies a basis for such nonstatistical inferences, and thus is eminently necessary despite its limitations. And such inferences are clearly needed before taking further action. For example, if you were to conclude that a treatment was *not* effective, based upon a clinical trial and its analysis, you surely would not draw the opposite inference respecting a future population. Of course, the entire process is customarily reinforced by the use of repeated trials. See Chapter 2, Section 2.2.3, the section entitled "The Population Sampled." See also Deming (1) and Nelson (2), both of whom discuss this problem very clearly and pragmatically.

10.1.3 Experiments with Two or More Factors

When two or more factors must be studied, factorial experiments are much more practical than groups or series of single-factor studies, as were formerly used (and still are, at times). There are two major reasons for this. First, during the analysis of a factorial, *all* the data can be used to calculate *each* effect mean. Second, and even more important, only with the use of a multiple-factor design can interactions be *reliably* detected. Furthermore, because two or more factors are tested at the same time, a multifactor factorial experiment is more efficient than a series of single-factor designs (i.e., requires fewer patients).

These benefits have a cost, although it is usually trivial. For the same total sample size, all other things being equal, the power of a two-factor factorial design for detecting either of the two main effects is slightly lower than that for detecting the single main effect in a one-factor trial of the same size. This occurs because of the loss of 2 df from the error estimate, which will be used in the comparison of treatment means. However, this small disadvantage is reduced as the total sample sizes of the two types of design are increased, and for most practical trials, it can be ignored. Thus, the two-factor design is well worth this small cost, because, using almost the same number of patients, you obtain the ability to evaluate two main effects rather than one, and you will be able to test for a possible interaction effect between them. When there are two or more factors to evaluate, the only practical way to do so is with a factorial design.[1]

10.2   DESCRIPTIONS OF EXAMPLES

There will be five examples in this chapter. Like most of the others in this book, they are not descriptions of trials that were actually run in industry, because such information is proprietary and is rarely available. However, in all cases, except for their size, they closely resemble actual trials in which I have been involved. For clarity, most are smaller than similar studies that would actually be run in practice.

The first three are reviews of one-factor trials, each using a different kind of response. Each of these is described in some detail. The first illustrates the planning and the calculation of means for a one-factor experiment with two levels of the factor, using a multiple-point judgment scale as a response (more than two possible scores). By way of a crude analysis, we summarize the two levels and compare their means visually. We also report the results of both *t* and rank tests, although we leave the details of those procedures for Part IV.

The second example illustrates the use of a binomial (two-valued) response and is another one-factor trial. For the third example, we describe a

---

[1]There are some multiple-factor designs that are not factorial. For example, a common type is used widely in engineering work, the Box-Wilson response surface designs. Some of these are factorials, but others, called *central composite* designs, for example, are not. To my knowledge, none of these has been used in clinical studies.

similar one-factor design, this one with three levels. However, in this case, we use an objective variable (number of days), considered to be continuous, as a response. The fourth example uses a two-factor arrangement in which each factor has two levels (i.e., a 2^2 design), and for which the responses are scores (SPID). Using the resulting data, we calculate the two means for each factor. We then calculate the interaction means to see if their difference appears large. The fifth and final example in this chapter is a three-factor experiment in which the factors have 2, 2, and 5 levels. This is a fairly common design; for example, it is widely used in multicenter trials. Because there are five centers, this is merely a 2^2 design done at each of five locations. The response is a continuous variable (FEV_1).

10.3   ARRANGEMENT OF EXAMPLES

To make these five examples convenient to compare and understand, the same outline will be used in describing each one. The outline will consist of nine steps. Other steps that could have been included are either not the concern of this book (such as the execution of the trial) or have not yet been covered (e.g., hypothesis testing, Chapter 13). The two primary purposes of these examples are to provide prototypes for your use as references and to further clarify the design of full factorial designs. Any discussion of further activities such as hypothesis testing is included only to the extent necessary to elucidate your planning. Some procedures previously described, such as randomization and sample size estimation, will not be explained again at the same length. Finally, all these designs will be of the sort commonly called **completely randomized**, and will be **double blind**. The term *completely randomized* means that there are no major restrictions upon the randomization (such as the blocking described in the next chapter). A *double blind* trial is one in which both the patients and those working with them during the trial are unaware of which patient is receiving which treatment, although both groups should be aware of what treatments are being tested.

Here is the outline:

1. Objectives
2. Factors and levels
3. Selecting responses
4. Planning analyses of data
5. Selecting patients
6. Estimating sample size
7. Randomization
8. Examining data
9. Conclusions

10.4 EXAMPLE 10.1: ONE FACTOR, TWO LEVELS (SCORES)

10.4.1 Objectives

This experiment was a small, double blind, parallel, one-factor trial, and was run for the purpose of comparing two antiinflammatory drugs for their relative efficacies in the treatment of rheumatoid arthritis.

10.4.2 Factors and Levels

There was one factor, drugs, at two levels.

10.4.3 Selecting Responses

Although most clinical trials use more than one response measurement to assure completeness of information, we used just one in this and each of the following examples, because any additional kinds of measurements are pedagogically unnecessary and would require adjustments of the sample sizes and irrelevant complexity in presenting results.[2] Let's assume that the experimenter used a manipulated joint tenderness index. In this procedure, the investigator, a rheumatologist, manipulates each of a number of joints, scoring each according to whether the patient states that there is no pain (score = 0), some pain (score = 1), or severe pain (score = 2) (other scoring schemes may be used instead). The final test value for each patient is obtained by adding all these scores. If there are 17 joints, for example, the possible scores for a given examination of a given patient could range from 0 to 34. Sometimes other scoring procedures are used, such as the use of different numbers for the scores (e.g., 1, 2, and 3 instead of 0, 1, and 2), more or less than 17 joints, or longer judgment scales. The use of several joints and the addition of the scores to give a single final total score make the data behave more like samples from continuous distributions. This is an advantage when certain kinds of statistical tests are to be used.

10.4.4 Planning Analyses of Data

In this example, the two drugs were compared by computing the mean values of the responses and comparing them visually. On the other hand, if you were to run a similar design for your sponsor, you would anticipate that the biostatistician would plan and describe the expected final statistical analysis. In this case, for this response, that analysis could consist of a single t test or a rank test, with the latter slightly preferable. Although the purposes of this book do not include descriptions of many statistical procedures, these two

---

[2]A reminder: When more than one kind of response is used in a trial, appropriate sample size adjustments must be made during the planning stage. If multiple-comparisons tests are used properly, the significance test probabilities will be correct, but without an a priori sample size increase, the power of the tests will suffer. See Chapters 5 and 15.

simple procedures are described in Part IV. We include them not because we expect you to make frequent use of them, but rather because they incorporate several fundamental concepts underlying statistical analysis. It is important that you, as a trial designer, learn these procedures in order to gain a fuller understanding of the relationship between design and analysis.

10.4.5 Selecting Patients

A limited patient population was used; the sample was taken from among the outpatients at a certain rheumatology clinic. As patients appeared at the clinic, each was asked whether he or she would be willing to take part in the trial. Each who agreed was interviewed, and, if there were no negative considerations, was entered into the trial until the number needed was secured.

10.4.6 Estimating Sample Size

A pilot trial gave an estimate of sigma of 4.00 in joint tenderness index (jti) units for a response using 17 joints, scored as described before. The experimenter wished to use 0.20 for beta, 0.05 for alpha, and to be able to detect differences between drugs of one sigma, or 4.00 jtu's (delta = 4.00). Delta divided by sigma is thus equal to 1.00. Entering Table A.3c in the Appendix with these specifications and this value of delta/sigma gave a sample size of 17 patients for each drug in a parallel study.

10.4.7 Randomization

The design was randomized using one of the methods described in Chapter 6. The result is shown in Table 10.1.

10.4.8 Examining Data

We will calculate the two group means and compare them visually, as indicated earlier. However, a parametric statistical test such as a t test would probably be used if the data of this example were analyzed conventionally. We estimated the sample size under that presumption, because Table A.3 is designed for that purpose. However, the use of a t test requires the assumption, among others, that the errors of your data have been sampled from normal distributions. This cannot be true for this example, although perhaps the departure is not severe. For one thing, the joint tenderness index data do not use a continuous scale as is assumed for weights or temperatures; rather, they are integers.[3] Another assumption, that of homogeneity of variance between the two treatment groups, must be tested, because it is

---

[3]On the other hand, because the data are sums of 17 individual data, they are not likely to be greatly different from normally distributed values.

Table 10.1. Randomization of a Single-Factor Design for the Comparison of Two Antiinflammatory Drugs in Patients with Rheumatoid Arthritis (Example 10.1)

Patient Numbers	
A_1 (Drug 1)	A_2 (Drug 2)
22	33
27	26
3	18
13	29
6	24
5	1
14	17
8	32
20	2
19	28
7	21
11	30
31	16
15	23
4	10
34	9
12	25

required when applying an ordinary t test. Further assumptions, in the present study, are either likely to be true (independence) or to be unnecessary in this case (additivity).

Although the t test or an equivalent such as an analysis of variance are probably robust enough to be appropriate in this case, it is correct to recognize that the data are not really normal and it is preferable to provide for that fact. To be conservative, therefore, a rank test, the Wilcoxon Rank Sum test, was used in the actual analysis.[4] In this case, we also ran a t test so that you might compare results. The Wilcoxon test is designed for comparing two independent groups, actually comparing their medians. When the data are known to be normal, its asymptotic (long-run) efficiency is 96.5% relative to the t test. That is, 100 patients tested with a Rank Sum test would be expected to have the same efficiency as about 97 using the t test. If the data are not normally distributed, the t test, strictly speaking, is not appropriate (although, in the present case, its "robustness" would very likely make it adequate). Both tests require that the two samples come from populations whose variances are the same or reasonably so. This example was created in

---

[4]This test is equivalent to the Mann-Whitney U Test, although it was published two years earlier. It is described in Chapter 14.

Table 10.2. Joint Tenderness Index Values (jti's)
(Comparison of Two Antiinflammatory Drugs in Patients with Rheumatoid Arthritis)
(Example 10.1)

A_1 (Drug 1)		A_2 (Drug 2)	
Patient No.	jti	Patient No.	jti
22	12	33	15
27	8	26	16
3	16	18	20
13	18	29	14
6	8	24	21
5	14	1	10
14	12	17	19
8	10	32	18
20	14	2	26
19	11	28	20
7	6	21	13
11	14	30	14
31	17	16	14
15	8	23	22
4	17	10	12
34	16	9	17
12	11	26	16

a way that guaranteed equal variances in the populations, so this assumption was satisfied. In your work, the statistician should test the data for conformance to this assumption.

After the trial was completed, the data shown in Table 10.2 were obtained. Because it happened that the jti responses, as described earlier, can range from 0 to 34, which happens to be exactly the range of the patient numbers, care must be taken not to confuse the two. The responses could have been rescaled, for example, by scoring each joint on a scale of 1, 2, and 3, but this was not judged necessary.

All patients completed the trial. To estimate the effect of the drugs, we averaged all the data in the two jti columns separately, as follows.

The values of n_i and Σ_j for each drug were needed. Both n_1 and n_2 are 17, and the sums of the data are 212 for drug A_1 and 287 for drug A_2. Using Equation (10.1), we get the two means:

$$\bar{A}_1 = \frac{212}{17} = 12.5$$

$$\bar{A}_2 = \frac{287}{17} = 16.9$$

10.4.9 Conclusions and Remarks

The mean jti for drug A_2 was larger than that for A_1, so the data suggest that if the difference was not entirely due to error (random variation among the data), drug A_1 had a lower mean jti than drug A_2, and hence may have been superior by the criterion set up by the experimenter. Later, it was found that drug A_1 was indeed superior, because, according to a Wilcoxon Rank Sum test, the difference between the two treatment means was indicated to equal or exceed delta at a low probability level (p was less than 0.006, using the normal approximation method described in Chapter 14). This means that if the null hypothesis of a difference less than delta were true, the probability of a difference as large as that observed (17.4 − 12.6 = 4.8) was less than 0.006. This is a much smaller value than 0.05, the value specified for alpha, and the null hypothesis was therefore rejected. As a matter of interest, a t test was also done, and gave a probability less than 0.005, thus agreeing well with the Wilcoxon test despite the discontinuity of the jti data.[5] It was concluded that a difference of delta or greater existed between the population means of the two drugs, in favor of A_1.

The data of this example were created by using a computer to produce two samples of random normal numbers. Equal standard deviations but different means were specified. To simulate jti data, each datum in the resulting samples was rounded to produce an integer. This violated the continuous-scale property of a normal distribution. In spite of this, as you have seen, there was little disagreement between the t test, which assumes that the samples are from normal distributions, and the rank test, which does not. In cases in which there are greater differences between the probability values obtained with a parametric and a "nonparametric" test, the latter should be considered the more reliable. In any event, it is strongly recommended that you be sure that normality and, especially, homogeneity of variance tests are run on your data before you or the biostatistician decide how to test them. These procedures are discussed and described in the appendix to Chapter 14. However, you willoften find, as in this example, that when there are equal numbers of data in a trial with two or more treatments, the t test is quite **robust** to nonnormality.

One more point should be made. In running the trial of Equation 10.1, we assumed that the object was to compare two treatments, and that no other important variables were expected to affect the system. If this assumption were valid, there should be no important criticism of the trial except that perhaps it ought to be repeated for verification, and eventually run in one or two multicenter trials, especially if it were planned to market drug A_1 and recommend it for treating seriously ill patients. On the other hand, if there were a possible interaction between the two drugs and the magnitudes of the

---

[5]Good agreement in the face of some nonnormality is not unusual when the sample sizes are equal and are not extremely small.

doses of each, the design would have been inappropriate.[6] In other words, if there were a possibility that the difference between drugs was not the same at dose levels other than those used in this trial, a two-factor study should have been planned, using the same two drugs, but with a "doses" factor consisting of at least two levels of doses for each drug. Of course, the two doses would have been likely to be different for the two drugs unless they were closely related pharmacologically, so that the "high" and "low" doses should be decided upon by a knowledgeable rheumatologist. If an interaction were found, the conclusion that drug A_1 is superior to drug A_2, based upon a one-factor trial, could be strongly misleading.

10.5   EXAMPLE 10.2: ONE FACTOR, TWO LEVELS, PARALLEL (BINOMIAL)

10.5.1   Objectives

Two antacid drugs are to be compared. The first of the two, D_1, is a currently marketed drug and will be used as a standard. The second, D_2, is the test drug. Volunteers experiencing occasional stomach upsets will take part in the trial. The sponsor believes the test drug is more effective than the marketed drug. This will be a small study, with the object of trying to determine whether the test material is sufficiently more efficacious than D_1 to warrant mounting a major trial. There will be no interest in the test product unless the trial indicates a superiority of at least 20 percentage units, that is, a value of delta (δ) of 20 percentage units. It is planned to use a "one-tailed" statistical test, reflecting the desire on the part of the sponsor that the delta value must favor the new drug. To explain this a bit further, a two-tailed test would be used if there were interest in finding a difference in either direction between the two drugs, if one exists. There is not expected to be any safety question; the standard has been marketed for several years without serious problems, and, on the basis of hundreds of trials of similar materials, the test drug is not expected to produce any disagreeable or toxic effects. This is an example of the rare case in which a *one-tailed* test is appropriate. The response will be binomial (*success or failure*) and the two groups to be compared will be *independent*.[7]

---

[6]The use of doses as a second factor was merely an example. You may often decide to choose other variables in your two-factor or multifactor trials.

[7]The independence is exactly analogous to that in an experiment in which continuous-response data are analyzed with the use of an *independent t* test. Separate groups of patients receive each drug (each patient receives only one of the drugs). A *dependent* test would require that each patient receive both drugs, and, of course, in accordance with correct experimental design, in random order.

10.5.2   Factors and Levels

The two drugs to be compared constitute one factor at two levels.

10.5.3   Selecting Responses

Equal numbers of patients will receive each drug. This is a preliminary test and must be completed as soon as possible, so each patient will be asked to use the drug for **one** upset stomach attack and to rate the results at the time of use on a form supplied by the clinic. Since the response will be binomial, the ratings will be either "no relief" or "at least some relief." The patients will be asked to use either of these responses, but no other (i.e., they should not respond with "don't know" or with any phrase other than one of the previous two).

10.5.4   Planning Analyses of Data

For each drug, the proportion of patients reporting relief will be calculated (this is the number reporting relief divided by the total number of patients receiving the drug). These proportions will be compared visually. No analysis of the data beyond this comparison will be discussed in this chapter. We will discuss one kind of statistical analysis for such data in Part IV. An excellent reference for tests using this kind of response is Fleiss [41], although other texts among those recommended in the Bibliography, notably Snedecor and Cochran [38], also discuss it.

10.5.5   Selecting Patients

The study will be double blind. Patients will be selected from those attending a local clinic who have complained of occasional digestive problems. The patients must have been judged by the clinician(s) to be suffering from simple GI problems and are not presenting symptoms of any more serious condition. Each will be asked to take part in the trial, and, upon agreement, will be given three separately packaged doses, an instruction sheet, and a report form. All three doses will be used during one attack, if needed; any unused drugs are to be returned to the clinic and the amount recorded. To ensure that the instructions are understood, each patient will be asked to read them and request clarification, if necessary, before leaving the clinic. They will be told that the report sheet should be mailed to the clinic after one attack has been treated and recorded. If a response is not received from any patient within a reasonable time, a telephone follow up will be done.

   This system for obtaining responses from the patients is obviously less satisfactory than one that requires them to report to the clinic at the first sign of an attack, receive the dosage there, and then remain at the clinic for an hour or two so that the effect of the treatment can be observed and the patient interviewed. Such an arrangement can greatly increase the reliability of the data. This scheme is often difficult to implement, however. It requires substantial effort from the patients, especially if they live at a distance from the clinic. Because neither the patients nor the investigators will know beforehand when a visit may occur, this additional effort will be considerable and will also add to the difficulty and expense required of the clinic personnel. Furthermore, there will be more difficulty recruiting patients (and perhaps also investigators) for the study, and the noncompleter rate will be higher. And these disadvantages will be multiplied if, unlike this example, the protocol requires more than one occurrence of the symptom(s). For these reasons, many industrial studies are run using the self-dosing procedure just described, as long as there is no safety problem and the procedure for dosing and recording the results is simple.

Thus, for the purpose of drawing conclusions, the population will have been defined by these procedures to be one consisting of patients from one clinic who experience occasional simple stomach upsets. The patients taking part in the trial will be considered to be a representative sample taken from such a population, although not a random one.

10.5.6 Estimating Sample Size

Based upon the literature, the monitor believes that the standard drug, D_1, will produce about 40% positive responses. She plans to consider the new material as a candidate for further trials if at least 60% of the patients using it respond favorably, thus specifying the delta value of 20 percentage units. She chooses a value of alpha of 0.05 and a beta value of 0.10. For this kind of trial, in which the response is binomial (good/bad, yes/no, plus/minus, etc.), a value of sigma need not be specified explicitly, because in a binomial distribution, the value of sigma is implicitly related to the proportions of successes and failures. You can also view the proportion of successes as estimating the mean probability of success in future trials. In the proposed comparison, we are considering two different binomial distributions—one with a positive response frequency of 60% or more and another with one of 40%. This is analogous to a parametric test in which we postulate two normal distributions, each with a different mean.

Table A.7h in the Appendix, which is designed for estimating sample size when comparing two independent proportions, gives 115 patients per treatment for the above values of alpha, beta, one tail, and the proportions specified. The use of this table will be explained further in Part V. Because the patients are to mail in their results, however, which may result in some nonresponders, the planner decides to add about 20% to this value; therefore, she will use 138 patients per treatment, or 276 altogether. To preserve her specified values of alpha, beta, and delta, however, she plans to use the data from only the first 115 patients who complete the test for each treatment.

The sample size of 276 may impress you as unexpectedly large when a difference as great as 20 percentage units is the smallest of interest. This is typical of trials with binomial responses, however, You may pay dearly, in terms of the numbers of patients required, for the simplicity of the design, execution and analysis and its relative lack of restrictive assumptions. In fact, it is not uncommon for some trials to be too small to detect a clinically important difference because they have been designed without giving thought to the kind of analysis to be used and without using sample size estimates. The experimenters in such a case may then conclude that there is no difference large enough to be of interest. Yet when a trial is too small to demonstrate a specified difference (delta), the experimenter has no way of knowing whether such a difference really does exist between the hypothesized populations.

10.5.7 Randomization

The randomization of this trial is simple, because all that is needed is to decide, at random for each patient, whether he or she will receive D_1 or D_2. This can be done with the random-number function of a scientific calculator, such as the Hewlett-Packard 42S, being sure to select a unique seed value to provide a unique series of numbers. Of course, you may wish to use a table of random numbers from one of the references in the Bibliography, or a computer, either of which will be equally satisfactory. In this case, however, one of the "manual" methods will probably require less time than the computer, when you consider waiting time, loading a program, executing it, and printing the output. By using the random numbers from the calculator for this example, if the first two digits form an odd number, drug D_1 is assigned to the current patient; if the number is even, the patient gets D_2 (remember that "00" is even). Of course, this procedure is not likely to result in exactly equal numbers assigned to the two treatments. Therefore, when 138 patients are assigned to one drug, the remaining patient numbers of the 276 can then be "used up" by assigning them to the other. Another method is to continue in the original manner until all 276 patients are assigned, which will usually result in moderately unequal numbers receiving the two drugs. A moderate inequality in sample sizes between groups is not likely to create any difficulty, particularly when the sample sizes are fairly large, as in the present case.

The results of this randomization are shown in Table 10.3. Of course, they were generated before the trial started.

10.5.8 Examining Data

For a trial of this size, there are often data losses due to noncompleters, but to everyone's surprise, in this case, it happened that all patients reported their results, so there were no missing data. Of the first 115 patients who

Table 10.3. Random Assignment of Two Antacids to 138 Patients Each (Example 10.2)

Patient Numbers							
Drug 1 (D_1)				Drug 2 (D_2)			
3	70	145	209	1	73	135	216
4	71	146	210	2	74	136	218
5	77	148	212	6	75	137	219
10	79	153	214	7	76	143	220
11	80	158	215	8	78	147	222
12	83	160	217	9	81	149	224
13	84	161	221	15	82	150	226
14	87	164	223	18	85	151	228
16	92	166	225	20	86	152	230
17	94	168	227	22	88	154	231
19	96	171	229	23	89	155	233
21	101	172	232	25	90	156	236
24	102	173	234	26	91	157	239
27	103	174	235	31	93	159	240
28	104	175	237	33	95	162	242
29	106	176	238	36	97	163	244
30	107	177	241	38	98	165	245
32	108	178	243	39	99	167	248
34	110	179	246	40	100	169	249
35	111	180	247	42	105	170	252
37	113	183	250	44	109	181	253
41	122	184	251	46	112	182	254
43	124	185	255	48	114	186	256
45	125	190	257	50	115	187	258
47	127	191	259	51	116	188	261
49	128	192	260	53	117	189	262
52	129	193	263	56	118	195	265
54	132	194	264	59	119	198	266
55	133	196	267	60	120	200	268
57	138	197	271	62	121	202	269
58	139	199	272	64	123	203	270
61	140	201	273	65	126	205	275
63	141	204	274	68	130	206	276
66	142	207		69	131	211	
67	144	208		72	134	213	

used D_1, the standard, 49 patients, or 42.6%, reported it to be effective, and 66 found it ineffective. For D_2, the test drug, there were 61 (53.0%) effectives and 54 ineffectives. The difference in the sample proportions was therefore only 10.4 percentage units. A one-tailed statistical hypothesis test did not show significance ($p > 0.050$), which means that the population proportion in the test drug group did not appear to exceed that in the standard by as much as delta.

10.5.9 Conclusions

The outcome of this trial indicated that it was unlikely that a difference as great as 20 percentage points existed between the proportions in the two populations. The experimenter noted that a difference of that magnitude had not been shown to exist. The subsequent larger trial was cancelled.

10.6 EXAMPLE 10.3: ONE FACTOR, THREE LEVELS (RESPONSE = TIME)

10.6.1 Objectives

Two drugs were to be compared with each other and with placebo for their ability, if any, to promote wound healing. There was interest if even a small degree of efficacy was found for either of the test drugs. There was no safety problem, because both drugs had been in use for some years for other indications. The patients were volunteers who were to undergo a common minor surgical operation.

10.6.2 Factors and Levels

The two test drugs were represented by D_1 and D_2, and the placebo by D_3. All three were prepared in the form of tablets identical in appearance, and were to be taken orally, b.i.d., beginning on the day of the operation and continuing until the sutures were removed.

10.6.3 Selecting Responses

The elapsed time in days between the completion of a patient's operation and the removal of sutures was to be recorded as the only response. Of course, if there were differences among the treatments, the shorter the average time before the sutures were removed, the better the treatment.

10.6.4 Planning Analyses of Data

In this example, as in the others in this chapter, the only analysis to be demonstrated will be the calculation of mean times to removal of sutures for each drug, followed by a visual comparison of the means. For a statistical analysis, residuals calculated from the data would first be examined to determine their suitability for a parametric analysis, and then an appropriate transformation would be found, if necessary. An alternative would be to use a kind of analysis not sensitive to lack of normality, if the variances among the treatment groups were reasonably close to equal, and the observations were independent. These points are discussed in Part IV.

10.6.5 Selecting Patients

The patients who were to take part in the trial were selected from among these scheduled to undergo a minor operation in a large hospital. All patients underwent the same procedure. They were interviewed before the operation, and the study was described to them at that time. Each one who agreed to take part was enrolled in the study as soon as it was certain that the operation would be performed, and one of the drugs was then randomly assigned. The trial was double blind.

10.6.6 Estimating Sample Size

Because of the nature of the operation, it was judged unlikely that more than about 30 patients could be enrolled within the time available for planning, execution, and analysis of the data. Accordingly, 30 (10 per treatment) were chosen. No sample size estimation procedure was used, as it was believed, based upon earlier work, that the sample size chosen was near the minimum necessary. However, it was planned to calculate the sigma and delta values obtained in the trial during the statistical analysis.

10.6.7 Randomization

The random assignment of drugs to patients was done in this case by selecting a permutation of the numbers 1 to 30 from Moses and Oakford [49]. The second permutation, $12, 29, \ldots, 18$, in the fourth row on page 63, was selected. Each patient was given a sequential number, beginning with 1, as he or she was enrolled in the trial. By taking the numbers in the permutation as representing patient numbers, the first 10, reading by rows, became the patient numbers to whom the first drug (D_1) was assigned. The next 10 received the second drug (D_2), and the final 10, the third (D_3). The final arrangement is shown in Table 10.4.

10.6.8 Examining Data

A Wilcoxon Rank Sum test was used for the three treatment comparisons. Had a parametric test been planned, it would have been necessary to precede it with a test of normality and of homogeneity of variance among the three

**Table 10.4. Randomization of Three Drugs
to Patients in a Wound-Healing Trial (Example 10.3)**

	Patient Numbers	
Drug 1 (D_1) (Test)	Drug 2 (D_2) (Test)	Drug 3 (D_3) (Placebo)
12	27	23
29	16	6
28	1	20
11	10	14
24	13	5
26	8	17
25	7	21
22	19	4
9	3	15
2	30	18

groups and to take steps to remedy any important departures from these assumptions that were found. For the rank test, only a test of the equality of the variances of the three treatment groups was necessary. Both parametric and rank tests assume independence and homogeneity of variance of the errors of the data, although with equal sample sizes, they are both somewhat robust to violations of homogeneity, so that moderate departures are permissible. The independence assumption is important, but lack of independence is often obvious from a knowledge of the way the randomization and other procedures were done.

The data of this trial are given in Table 10.5 and represent the surgeon's record of the numbers of days, to the nearest day, between the completion of

**Table 10.5. Data for Wound-Healing Trial
(Times Sutures Remained in Place, Days) (Example 10.3)**

Drug 1 (D_1)	Drug 2 (D_2)	Drug 3 (D_3)
12	27	23
29	16	6
28	1	20
11	10	14
24	13	5
26	8	17
25	7	21
22	19	4
9	3	15
2	30	18

each patient's operation and the removal of sutures. Note: The data are in the order of patient numbers given in Table 10.4.

The means of the three treatment groups, in days, were

Treatment	Mean
D_1 (test drug)	18.8
D_2 (test drug)	13.4
D_3 (placebo)	14.3

Their absolute differences were

Treatment Pair	Absolute Difference
D_1 vs. D_2	5.4
D_1 vs. D_3	4.5
D_2 vs. D_3	0.9

The three treatment comparisons were made, using the Wilcoxon test. As we will discuss in Part IV, there is a new difficulty to overcome when more than one comparison is made with a hypothesis test, as was planned in this trial (each drug vs. the other and vs. the placebo). In such a case, multiplicity is introduced, and one of the multiple-comparisons procedures must be used to preserve the specified alpha risk value. In this case, a Bonferroni procedure was used. Because there were three comparisons to be done and the specified alpha value was 0.050, this gave 0.050/3, or a "working" alpha value of 0.017. This was changed in a conservative direction to 0.010 for easy reference to the tables for the significance test (because the Bonferroni test is somewhat conservative, of course, this made the results still more so). The results showed no statistical significance for any of the three comparisons.

Although the data were probably quite nonnormal, the value of delta, assuming a parametric test, was calculated as planned.[8] For your later reference, the calculation was done with one of the equations given in Part V, using a value of 0.010 for alpha, 0.100 for beta, and a pooled value of sigma of 16.927. A two-tailed test was assumed. These values yielded an estimate of 16.9 days for delta. The reason for using a somewhat more rigorous value for alpha (0.01 instead of 0.05) was to make a conservative correction for the multiplicity.

The treatment differences shown before are much smaller than the calculated value of delta. Using this value and the estimate of sigma just given,

---

[8]The sample size procedure used was in reality appropriate only for data suitable for the use of a *t* test, but only an approximation of delta was needed. The multiplicity problem was handled as shown in what follows.

Table A.3b in the Appendix indicates that for delta/sigma of 16.9/16.927, or approximately 1.0, about 32 patients per treatment would have been needed. Obviously, the sample size was much too small, despite the original judgment that it was perhaps appropriate, and, if these values of delta and sigma are good estimates, one could not have hoped to obtain significance with 10 patients per treatment. Whether significance could have been obtained had 31 patients per treatment been used is unknown, because the value of sigma is an estimate based upon this experiment, and had a smaller value of delta than 16.9 been used to enter Table A.3b, a still larger sample would have been needed.

10.6.9 Conclusions

The sponsor concluded that, because none of the test drugs was shown in this trial to possess efficacy, and, further, that it was unlikely that differences, if any, could be discovered without the expenditure of considerable additional time and money, the project would be abandoned.

10.7 EXAMPLE 10.4: A 2 × 3 DESIGN (SCORES)

10.7.1 Objectives

This experiment was an example of the comparison of three analgesics for the control of pain in moderate osteoarthritis. One of the drugs (buffered aspirin, used as a standard) is also an antiinflammatory and was expected to reduce joint inflammation and edema as well as pain. The sponsor hoped that at least one of the other two treatments (the test drugs) would also have antiinflammatory properties. Therefore, responses to measure those effects were included in the trial. In this example, however, because our purpose is primarily to illustrate the application of an experimental design, we will be concerned only with the control of pain. Furthermore, as usual, to illustrate the principles involved more clearly, the example will use fewer patients than would be used in actual trials of this kind.

The object of this experiment, then, was the comparison of two new analgesic drugs with each other and with buffered aspirin for the control of subjective pain in osteoarthritis patients. There was to be no placebo, because, although their pain was relatively mild, most placebo patients would have experienced unnecessary discomfort. In fact, if the treatment given any patient in the study appeared to be ineffective, the investigator agreed that such patients would be dropped from the study and the experimental treatment replaced with his or her regular medication.

10.7.2 Factors and Levels

As indicated, one of the two factors was the drugs, at three levels (three drugs). To help preserve blinding, all were prepared as powders in opaque capsules. Because some patients experience some stomach upset with aspirin, and others may have a fear of such effects even if they have not experienced them, all patients were told at the initial interview that one of the drugs would be *buffered* aspirin, and asked whether they objected to taking it. Those who did object were not entered into the trial. All patients were also told that there would be no placebo among the three drugs, and that it was believed that all three would be effective, although perhaps to different degrees. They were informed that any patient, however, if he or she requested, could be dropped from the trial and returned to his or her regular medication. Finally, each was told that the two test drugs were neither ibuprofen nor acetaminophen, the two which, with aspirin, are the only ones currently approved as OTC analgesics by the FDA. They were told that these two were new materials that, however, had given no evidence of any serious adverse effects during safety testing.

The second factor was doses, at two levels, high and low. The three drugs differed chemically and pharmacologically, so the definitions of "low" and "high" were set up by an experienced rheumatologist familiar with earlier trials of similar drugs. Each patient was to take one capsule per dosage period, but the capsules were to be large enough to contain either the low or the high dose of any of the three drugs. The low-dose capsules contained a mixture of the drug and an inert, harmless material, to make their total weight and volume approximately equal to that in those containing the high doses.

Patients were asked to take their medication t.i.d., at each meal during the day. They were also allowed to take a dose at retiring and once again during the night, if they felt it necessary.

10.7.3 Selecting Responses

As indicated before, only one of the responses originally planned is used in this example; it is a pain "measurement" based upon judgment scores. As in an earlier example, however, the procedure was such that the scores (SPIDs) were analyzable by parametric methods robust enough to be little affected by the inherently nonnormal distribution. The use of a pain response in this way is now common in clinical work. For more information about the so-called SPID response, see Buncher and Tsay [19], Chapter 9, by Jack W. Green, pages 189–204. Further information may be found in Beaver and Feise (3) and Beaver et al. (4), among others.

The responses are obtained as follows: At the beginning of the trial, a so-called baseline response is obtained from each patient. Because arthritis is a disease that varies in intensity (and in the area affected) from time to time, each patient was asked to report to the clinic on three mornings a week apart, and a baseline reading was taken each time. These three readings were then averaged for each patient to help ensure more reliable data. These means were later utilized as described in what follows.

The scoring system and the derived responses will remind you of the joint tenderness indices described in Example 10.1. In this example, we call the responses recorded by the clinician "pain intensity responses," or "pain intensity scores." These are subsequently modified (see what follows) to produce "derived responses," called "sums of pain intensity differences." The latter are then used in the calculation and examination of the treatment and interaction means.

The pain intensity (PI) scores were to be elicited by interviews with each patient. All interviews in this trial were conducted at about $1\frac{1}{2}$ hours after the first dose of medication had been taken at breakfast. The scoring scale had five points, as follows:

1. No pain
2. Slight pain
3. Moderate pain
4. Substantial pain
5. Severe pain

The scores were to be assigned by the investigator, who was a rheumatologist experienced with the disease. Separate scores were to be assigned to each of several joints during each of several patient visits (see what follows), and the results averaged. As a check and for the record, certain other tests were also to be conducted at each visit.

After the last of the baseline readings was taken, each patient was given a week's supply of medication and asked to return in a week, in time for a reading to be taken approximately $1\frac{1}{2}$ hours after breakfast. There were four such weekly interviews, on four successive weeks, and a pain intensity (PI) score was obtained for each joint each time, after which the several scores were averaged. At each visit except the last, a fresh supply of medication was given to each patient and each returned any unused portion of the previous week's supply. Every effort was made to encourage patients not to drop out of the trial prematurely. A single missing visit, if not made up within 48 hours, was deemed sufficient to disqualify the patient's data from use in the data analysis. As it happened, there were no such events.

10.7.4 Planning Analyses of Data

The derived responses were computed as follows: The original data were the average PI (pain intensity) and BL (mean baseline) scores. When the former were received, the statistician subtracted each from the mean BL for that patient; this operation and the formation of the SPID scores that follow were built into the database program for this trial, but the original data were also preserved. Each weekly difference from a patient's mean baseline score was called a PID, or pain intensity difference. If a PID is zero, it reflects no change relative to the baseline; if it is positive, it shows improvement, because the mean BL must then be greater than the PI; if it is negative, it shows degradation in a patient's condition. After the PID values for each patient were calculated, all four PID scores were added together to create a SPID value, or sum of pain intensity difference. This procedure and the earlier averaging tends to normalize the distribution of the resulting SPID values and eliminates any autocorrelation[9] among successive weekly pain intensity measurements. Thus, a single composite response was obtained for each patient, covering the entire period of the trial. The SPID values were then analyzed statistically.

Despite the expected normalizing effect of combining the weekly PID averages to form a SPID response for each patient, a Michael normality test of the residuals of the data and, of course, a test of the homogeneity of the cell variances (Levene test) would normally have been done.[10] There was no expectation of violation of the independence assumption once the SPIDS were calculated, because (a) the successive measurements through time had been eliminated by the addition of the weekly averages, and (b) each patient was examined individually, often on different days. It is true that the same investigator examined each, but he was asked not to refer to the results for other patients when interviewing a particular one, and it was assumed that results between patients were therefore unlikely to be correlated.

In this case, however, neither a normality test nor a test of the variances was done. There were fewer data than would usually be needed for these procedures, so that significance was very unlikely even if the errors were nonnormal or the variances nonhomogeneous.[11] However, the statistical procedures to be used were quite robust to nonnormality and heteroscedasticity, especially in the case of equal sample sizes, and the SPID values were more precise than ordinary single measurements, because they were based upon several observations for each patient.

---

[9]Analyzing a set of measurements or scores taken on the same patients at intervals throughout a trial is likely to seriously violate the parametric assumption of independence among the errors of the data. This might be avoided by analyzing the data separately for each time interval, but the multiplicity resulting from the analysis of more than one measurement per patient in the same trial would then need to be taken into account. The Bonferroni method might be used to do this, employing a larger sample size to compensate for the use of the smaller working value of alpha that Bonferroni requires. But often a simpler and better procedure is to average or add the weekly responses as is done for the SPID, producing a single response for analysis and avoiding any multiplicity.

[10]Both of these procedures are described in the appendix to Chapter 14.

[11]Statistical tests concerned with the assumptions of normality and homogeneity of variance commonly use the terms *tests of normality* or *tests of homogeneity of variance*. We mention these in this volume. They are really tests of *non*normality, or *heterogeneity* of variances. Findings of significance mean that there is nonnormality or lack of homogeneity of variances. The reason is that these tests are usually performed without prior specifications of beta or delta. If significance is *not* found, it cannot be concluded that the data tested have errors that are *not* normal or *not* homogeneous, but only that non normality or heterogeneity of variance have not been shown, either because they are absent or because the sample size is too small.

Normally, in most trials you will do, except early Phase I, you will probably require substantially more than the 18 patients used in this example. Because this sample was too small for an adequate test of the variances, and probably also for a normality test, we will assume that the data are reasonably normal and homoscedastic and that the statistician will use parametric methods for the analyses. This is not unreasonable in the case of SPID values; see Jack W. Green, Chapter 9 in Buncher and Tsay [19]. Incidentally, that chapter is a useful source of information about SPID and related scales in analgesic testing.

As before, we do not show statistical analyses of these data but only the calculations of means and the results of their visual examination. In a real situation, however, you should outline your expected analyses at this point in the planning. This outline should include provision for checking the parametric assumptions, as mentioned before. Furthermore, any rank tests that might be used also assume independence and homoscedasticity, so you should plan tests for these even if you do not expect to do parametric analyses.

10.7.5 Selecting Patients

The patients will be taken from those seeing the rheumatologist who serves as investigator. The criteria will be mild to moderate osteoarthritis, a willingness to take part, and the usual medical and health requirements.

10.7.6 Estimating Sample Size

The sample size actually calculated will be substantially larger than that used in this example, as just discussed. The sample size estimation method used would be that described by Bratcher et al.; cf. reference 2, Chapter 9. This will be discussed in Part V. In this example, there were three patients per treatment group.

10.7.7 Randomization

There are six cells in this example, represented by drug 1 at the low dosage (A_1B_1), drug 2 at the low dosage (A_2B_1), through drug 3 at the high dosage (A_3B_2). This trial used the same general method of randomization as that for the three preceding examples. For maximum power and, less importantly, for simplicity of analysis (not as critical as a few years ago because of the availability of computer programs), each of the six cells should be designed to have the same number of experimental units (patients). In this example, this number is 3. You simply randomly assign 18 patients to the design, three to each of the six cells. Any method of obtaining six different combinations of three of the numbers 1 through 18 will do, but, as before, perhaps the use of the excellent Moses and Oakford [49] book of permutations is most convenient.

Table 10.6. Random Assignment of Treatments to Patients for Example 10.4

Doses	Drugs		
	A_1	A_2	A_3
B_1	6	9	11
	7	3	10
	4	12	5
B_2	18	16	2
	15	17	14
	8	13	1

We now set up Table 10.6, having three columns and two major rows, with each of the latter consisting of three subsidiary rows to accommodate the three entries in each cell. Turning to the Moses and Oakford table of permutations of the numbers 1 through 20 (Table 3, pages 24 to 51), we arbitrarily select one page, row, and column. I chose page 40, column 2, and row 8; this is the one beginning with the integers 6, 7, and 19. The resulting randomization is shown in the table.

10.7.8 Examining Data

Tables of Data and Means

Table 10.7 shows the data obtained. The subject numbers are those shown in the same positions in Table 10.6. To examine the mean responses for the three drugs and two doses, and to examine the interaction means, we first get two sums, one from each of the two sets of nine data for the two doses (the first and last sets of three rows). Then we add each for the three columns of six data each for the sums for the data for the three drugs. Finally, we obtain the six cell sums of three to be used to get the interaction means. We then divide each of these sums by the appropriate divisor (the number of items summed in each case) to get the means we need. Looking at Table 10.7, you

Table 10.7. Data for Example 10.4 (SPID Values)

Doses	Drugs		
	A_1	A_2	A_3
B_1	8	3	6
	4	3	5
	2	5	7
B_2	11	7	8
	7	8	9
	12	5	9

**Table 10.8. Cell, Row, and Column Means for Example 10.4
(Original Data in Table 10.7)**

	A_1	A_2	A_3	Means
B_1	4.7	3.7	6.0	4.8
B_2	10.0	6.7	8.7	8.4
Means	7.3	5.2	7.3	6.6

can see that the three drug means must be averages of six data each, the dose means, averages of nine, and the interaction (cell) means, averages of three each. These means are shown in Table 10.8. If you wish, you may calculate these yourself and compare them with the means in the table. The body of the table contains the six means of three data each for the cells; the cells are identified by the row (dose) and column (drug) headings of the table. The two marginal row means in the table are the means of nine data each for the doses. The three column means are the means of six data each for the three columns, representing the drug means. The figure at the lower right (6.6) is the grand mean of all 18 data.

A logical rule of thumb for suggesting the fact that means have greater precision than individual data (smaller variances or standard deviations) is to use one more decimal place than that which appears in the individual data for means of 3 to 10 data, then 2 up to 100, etc. This rule is a little more liberal than the one commonly taught, which starts with means of 10 rather than 3 or 4, but I find it reasonable.[12] This rule was used in constructing Table 10.8.

The means in Table 10.8 were calculated from the original data of Table 10.7. The marginal means shown there will not necessarily agree exactly with averages calculated from the cell means in the body of the table, because of rounding errors.

Main Effect Means

The pain intensity (PI) scores assigned during each interview are in ascending order, that is, the higher the score, the greater the discomfort. However, the

---

[12]As a review, we point out that the precision of a mean in terms of the units of the original response can be represented by its standard error, SEM (the standard error of the mean, or the standard deviation of the mean). The SEM is the standard deviation of an individual item divided by the square root of the number of items, n, used to calculate the mean. Thus, as n increases, SEM decreases. A mean of two items has a SEM that is 0.7 times that of the single items; its precision is about 1.4 times better (i.e., the square root of 2) in the units of the test. The SEM for a mean of 3 is about 1.7 times better; its precision is about 0.6 times that of a single item. For a mean of 4, this figure is 0.5, so the precision of the mean is now just twice that of a single measurement. The improvement in precision becomes smaller as n increases; see Table A.3 in the Appendix. It seems reasonable to reflect this substantially greater precision by the use of an additional decimal place for means of 3 or 4, rather than insisting that no improvement be implied until a mean is derived from 10 or more items.

results (SPID values) in Table 10.7 were obtained by first subtracting the PI values obtained subsequent to the first drug dosage from the mean of the three obtained at the baseline. If these differences are positive, as they all were in the example, the *larger* SPID values represent greater efficacy than the smaller ones, because they signify *improvements* over the baseline scores.

As you can see by examining the column means (drug A_i) in Table 10.8, drug A_2 appears less effective than the other two. Of course, this observation needs the support of a statistical hypothesis test, as do the rest of the comparisons to be made at this time. For purposes of discussion, however, let us say that A_1 and A_3 seem superior to A_2, based upon the main effect means.

In the case of the dose factor, the higher dose, B_2, has a mean SPID value almost twice as large as the low dose. This is reasonable, of course, if one or more of the three drugs are effective at all and the dosage range was chosen correctly. We here discuss the dose means averaged over all three drugs, but in the case of a dose factor, this estimation of the dose effect may be of little interest. However, the same calculations and reasoning apply to any single factor, as it was for the drugs in this case. In the absence of a statistical hypothesis test comparing the dose means with each other, this observation should carry a little more weight than the comparison of the drug means, because the two dose means are averages of nine individual differences from the baseline, whereas the drug means used only six. In terms of their SEMs, assuming that the sigma values for all of the data are the same, the dose means are 1.22 times (about 20%) more precise than the drug means (this is the ratio of the square roots of the numbers of items in the two kinds of means). If you use statistical hypothesis tests to compare the means for drugs

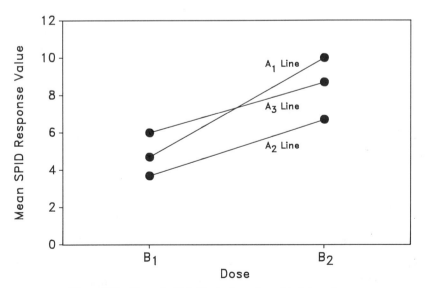

Figure 10.1   Example 10.4: Illustration of possible interaction.

and for doses, and if both factors show significance, you may conclude that the indicated differences are significant, because the tests take the SEMs into account. Note that, unlike a design in which both factors have the same number of levels and the cell sizes are equal, in this trial, there are small differences in precision among the main effect means. This will result in slightly more power for the comparisons using the larger means.

It remains to examine the data of Table 10.8 for a possible interaction. To do this, each of the means of three patients' data in the body of Table 10.8 were plotted, and the plot is shown in Figure 10.1. It appears that there is a moderately strong interaction between drugs and doses for drugs A_1 and A_3 and a similar but slightly smaller one between A_1 and A_2. The differences between the third pair of drugs, A_2 and A_3, are almost equal; thus, their two lines are almost parallel and therefore show little or no evidence of interaction.

In Figure 10.1, the extremities of the lines are not labeled as they were on the earlier plots. The labeling was omitted to keep the graph from appearing too crowded. These six points can be identified, however. For example, the ends of the lowest line are A_2B_1 and A_2B_2, because this is the A_2 line.

10.7.9   Conclusions

The conclusions were partially outlined before. The higher dose appeared more effective than the lower, as might be expected. Drug A_2 may be less effective than the other two. The apparently strong A_1/A_3 interaction suggests that although there is only a small difference between the two drugs at either dose level, when taken together, this difference is reversed from one dose to the other. That is, A_3 is numerically superior to A_1 at the low dose, whereas at the high dose, the reverse is true. On the other hand, the apparent interaction between A_1 and A_2, although showing differences in slopes almost as great as that for A_1 and A_3, and therefore suggesting almost as strong an effect, does not show the same kind of reversal. However, this is simply because the difference between the average values of the two treatments is greater within the dose range used. These two possible interactions illustrate the difficulty of describing an interaction in words, although a diagram is quite clear. We conclude tentatively that the two main effects should be ignored and attention centered on their interaction. Of course, significance tests must be run first, to test these visual impressions.

10.8   EXAMPLE 10.5: THREE-FACTOR MULTICENTER TRIAL (FEV$_1$)

10.8.1   Objectives

Our final example of simple factorial designs is a multicenter trial. The design was the $2^2 \times 5$ structure (i.e., $2 \times 2 \times 5$, of Example 9.5, which was described briefly in Chapter 9, Section 9.4.2, and illustrated in Figure 9.6). The object of the trial, which was a middle Phase II study, was to compare two drugs, each in two different forms, in each of five centers. The treatment groups were chosen from patients at each center who suffered from a restrictive lung condition. The effects of the four drug and drug form combinations upon the patients' conditions were to be compared. The patients were informed that if the assigned treatment did not appear to be effective and there was substantial discomfort, they could of course revert to their usual treatment. Although such incidents were to be reported, the patients concerned would be treated as noncompleters during the analysis, and marked *failure* in the data records.

10.8.2 Factors and Levels

The factors and their levels were the following:

A_1 = test drug

A_2 = standard drug

B_1 = salt form of drug

B_2 = free base form of drug

$C_1, C_2, \ldots, C_5$ = centers

Thus, there were four patient groups to be set up *at each center*, with a group assigned to A_1B_1, the test drug in the salt form; one to A_1B_2, the test drug as the free base; a third to A_2B_1, the standard drug in the salt form; and the last to A_2B_2, the standard drug as the free base.

Fixed and Random Factors

Although the drugs and drug forms used were four of many that might have been sampled from four defined populations, as usual in the case of variables of interest for comparison in a clinical trial, they were *not* randomly selected samples. Instead, the four comprised the only ones in which there was interest for this study. In this sense, therefore, the two drugs comprised **complete populations** of drugs defined in this way. The same reasoning applied to the two drug forms. Such factors are referred to as **fixed-effect**, or **model I**, variables. On the other hand, the five centers could have been considered as a representative **sample** of all appropriate centers, although not a random one. If it were not for the lack of random sampling, such a sample of k levels of a factor would be a **random-effect**, or **model II**, variable or factor. However, although random sampling of the centers for a trial is almost never done, it is often assumed. The alternative, that is, to consider centers to be fixed, is also common. This assumption is also not completely accurate, however, because it implies that the particular centers chosen are the only ones of interest or relevant to the objectives of the trial.

It may not always be difficult to select centers in a truly random fashion for a multicenter trial, although this is not often done. To do so, one would list all the centers in the relevant geographic area *that are expected to be available for the trial*, and *that are acceptable by reason of having properly-qualified specialists and other features required*. All the centers having these attributes comprise a defined population, although not an infinite one. The required number of centers could then be selected by any of the random procedures we have used to select patients for drug assignment.

This will be the only discussion of the ideas of fixed-effect and random-effect variables, Eisenhart's so-called analysis of variance models (5), in this book. It is a somewhat advanced topic, but one with which your biostatistician is undoubtedly familiar and about which he or she may have strong opinions. It is discussed briefly here because it must be considered during the design of a trial. In single-factor designs in clinical studies, the concepts of fixed and random effects should never arise, because the single factor, usually treatments, will always be fixed. However, this will often not be the case in multifactor studies. One example, as you will see in the next chapter, is the blocking variable in a randomized blocks design, which is usually considered to be a random-effect variable (Model II). The question of whether *clinics* in a multiclinic trial should be fixed or random is discussed by Fleiss (6), and he concludes that they should probably be considered to be fixed. Whether to use a fixed-effect or random-effect model in a design is one of the factors that determine the manner in which the data analysis is done. The decision affects the kind of analysis appropriate, and therefore must be addressed during the planning of a trial.

10.8.3   Selecting Responses

To simplify this example and eliminate further discussion of multiplicity (which, however, must be taken into account in any actual trial by adjusting the sample size accordingly and by using the appropriate statistical procedures during analysis), we will consider only one response variable here, the FEV_1. This measurement, forced expiratory volume, measures the number of liters of air that a patient is able to discharge in 1 second after inhaling fully. The FEV_1 for a normal patient averages about 4.0 liters. In practice, in a trial of this kind, several other pulmonary function tests would probably be used in addition to this one.

10.8.4   Planning Analyses of Data

As was done for the other examples, the data analyses at this stage were simply examinations of means. Again, we emphasize that when the formal data analyses are begun, tests of the parametric assumptions should be done first. If the errors of the data are not found to be approximately normally distributed, with treatment group populations having fairly equal variances and independent errors, suitable transformations of the responses can be done before any analyses using these assumptions are performed; see Part IV.

The analysis of the data from this trial is more complex than the use of a t test, ranking procedure, or multiple-comparisons method (all of which are described in Part IV), and is not covered in this book. It is called the analysis of variance, or ANOVA, and is appropriate when there are more than two levels of the variable in a single-factor design, or when there are two or more variables, whatever their levels. In the first of these two cases, there are alternate methods of analysis, but, for any normal purposes, the ANOVA is by far the more suitable method of analysis for the latter case. Thus, although you will be unlikely to find yourself performing a data analysis using an ANOVA, you should know when such an analysis is needed when you plan a trial.

10.8.5 Selecting Patients

The patients were selected from those being treated at each of the five centers. All apparently suitable patients reporting to each center and having the condition of interest were asked if he or she would be willing to take part. Numbers were assigned patients entering the study in the order of their acceptance, beginning with the number 1. It is important in this and any trial that the patient numbers be assigned only after each patient has agreed to enter the trial, has been found qualified, and has actually been enrolled.

Each patient was given a battery of tests, including the FEV$_1$, the latter to be used as baselines. Each was then given a 1-week supply of his or her assigned drug, asked to take it daily (see what follows), and to report to the clinic in 1 week to return the container and obtain a second week's supply. This was done to allow a check of patients' condition and to help ensure that they were using the medication as instructed. In addition, the FDA has been known to ask for counts of unused medication when the data are submitted. On the third visit (after 2 weeks of dosage), each patient was tested again and the results of the tests recorded on CRFs. This concluded the trial for each patient.

10.8.6 Estimating Sample Size

As before, we shall assume that an appropriate sample size was chosen for the trial, in this case, five patients per treatment combination. The sample size would have been arrived at by taking data from all five centers into consideration, of course. Suitable references are Dallal (see Wilkinson [66]), Cohen [27], and Borenstein and Cohen [67], as mentioned in Part V. Our specifications were

$$\alpha = 0.050$$
$$\beta = 0.200$$
$$\delta = 0.5 \ liters$$

A value of sigma was available, because, as you would expect, several smaller trials of the same drugs and dosage forms had been done before this trial was mounted. Of course, the sigma value found when the data were analyzed was not expected to be identical with that obtained earlier, both because of random variation and because the present trial encompassed a wider variety of sites and investigators.

Note that this trial uses both cell replication and full replication. We are using cell replication (10 replicates per cell), but are also doing the entire experiment in five replicates (five centers). In the language of experimental design, the centers would be called **blocks**. This kind of structure is discussed at more length in Chapter 11.

10.8.7 Randomization

The kind of randomization procedure used for this design has been described previously, but will be recapped here. Because this was a multicenter trial, with five different and independent clinics taking part, a separate randomization was needed for each clinic. The randomization is not shown here, but could be done by computer, or by the use of the Moses and Oakford [49] tables, independently for each center (separate table for Moses and Oakford in each case, as if it were a completely independent study). Thus, in each center, five patients were assigned to each of the four cells $A_i B_j$.

10.8.8 Examining Data

The data are given in Table 10.9. There were no missing data.

The means for factors A and B and their combinations, calculated from the data in Table 10.9, are given in Table 10.10. The four means of the AB combinations $(A_1 B_1, A_1 B_2, \ldots, A_2 B_2)$ in the body of the table are means of 25 items each. Note that each mean includes the same number of data from each of the five centers. The means of each row and column shown at the right and bottom are, of course, means of 50. The grand mean of all 100 data is shown at the lower right-hand corner.

There are three factors in this study, so additional tables could be constructed, and if the statistician were doing the analyses "by hand" or with a desk calculator, they would be necessary. When the analysis is done using a statistical analysis package, the tables are not usually printed out, although most software can supply them if needed. Table 10.10 is a "two-way" AB

Table 10.9. Data from Trial of Example 10.5 (FEV_1)

	A_1		A_2	
	B_1	B_2	B_1	B_2
C_1	2.9	5.2	3.9	3.5
	4.0	3.9	3.9	2.7
	3.4	3.9	3.3	2.4
	3.2	3.5	4.3	3.6
	3.8	5.4	3.2	2.1
C_2	3.4	5.7	4.9	4.6
	4.4	4.6	4.6	3.5
	3.8	4.3	4.0	3.7
	3.9	3.9	5.3	4.7
	4.3	5.7	4.2	2.9
C_3	2.6	5.1	4.0	3.8
	3.9	3.9	4.0	3.0
	3.4	4.1	3.4	2.6
	2.9	3.5	4.4	3.5
	3.3	4.9	3.3	2.4
C_4	2.5	4.7	3.9	3.6
	3.4	3.6	3.7	2.5
	3.0	3.4	3.1	2.5
	2.6	2.9	4.3	3.8
	3.2	4.8	3.0	2.2
C_5	3.1	5.5	4.5	4.3
	4.1	4.5	4.2	3.2
	3.4	4.5	3.9	3.0
	3.4	3.7	4.9	4.4
	4.0	5.1	3.8	2.9

Table 10.10. Example 10.5: Means of Factors A (Drugs), B (Chemical Forms), and Their Combinations

	Level of B		
Level of A	B_1	B_2	Row Mean
A_1	3.44	4.41	3.92
A_2	4.00	3.26	3.63
Column Mean	3.72	3.83	3.776

table of means. There are two other two-way tables possible, an AC and a BC table. Because C had five levels, each of these tables would have two rows (A or B) and five columns (C) or five rows and two columns. Although there are four cells in the AB table (Table 10.10), the AC and BC tables would each have 10 cells (five columns times two rows or five rows times two columns). Finally, there is one possible three-way table, the ABC table. This would have five rows or five columns labeled with the five levels of C, and four rows or columns for the four A_iB_j combinations, so that the table would have 20 cells. It should be mentioned here, however, that the blocks (clinics) in a multiclinic trial usually may be of little interest, but merely serve to segregate any effect of differences among centers from expanding the error estimate in the analysis. On the other hand, centers' data should be examined, and any unusually different center or centers investigated.

The means of the five centers, averaged over both A and B, were the following (each is a mean of 20 measurements of FEV_1, liters):

$$\overline{C}_1 = 3.61$$

$$\overline{C}_2 = 4.32$$

$$\overline{C}_3 = 3.60$$

$$\overline{C}_4 = 3.34$$

$$\overline{C}_5 = 4.02$$

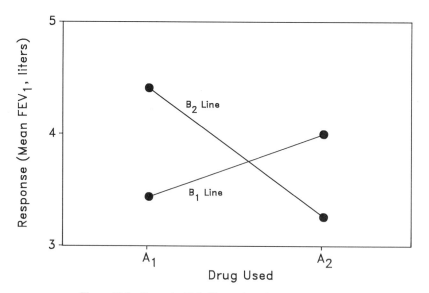

Figure 10.2 Example 10.5: Illustration of AB interaction.

The reasonable uniformity of these five averages suggests that the results from no center differed greatly from the others.

Neither main effect was significant, suggesting that the population differences were smaller than delta. However, the interaction was very strong and was significant in the analysis. Figure 10.2 is a plot of this interaction. The slopes of the two lines were very different. As you can see, in the sample, there were indeed sizable differences between main effect levels for the drugs, so much so that the signs of the slopes were reversed in going from the low to the high dose.

Note that because there were three factors in this experiment, there were four possible interactions and three main effects. A statistical analysis showed AB only to be significant. Neither A nor B was significant. C was not tested because there was no interest in comparing centers per se in the absence of any unusually large difference in means or in variance for one or more of them.

10.8.9 Conclusions

Because of the strong interaction, the report of the statistician centered upon that. Discussing the mean levels of the two main effects, drugs and drug composition, without considering the interaction, even had they been significant, would have led to distorted conclusions.

For the B_1 form of the two drugs, drug 2 gave a higher mean FEV_1 value than drug 1. For the B_2 form, however, drug 1 gave a higher mean. This interaction appeared strong, and this impression was verified when the statistical analyses were done. Obviously, any future choice between the two forms might depend upon the difference between the properties of the two, such as the seriousness or prevalence of adverse effects, for example. On the other hand, Figure 10.2 does show that the combination of these two factors that is numerically best is A_1B_2 and this might influence the choice. Of course, this trial was not the last in the investigation, and, as it happened, both drugs and both forms were used in further trials.

Finally, the data were carefully checked for errors of transcription, because such "crossed" interactions are frequently the result of a mistake in reading an instrument or recording results. In this case, however, no such error was found.

10.9 SUMMARY OF THE CHAPTER

This chapter presents five examples of parallel factorial designs to illustrate the principles given earlier, and for use as reference material. In general, a standard outline was followed: (a) objectives of the study, (b) factors and levels, (c) responses, (d) planning analyses, (e) selecting patients, (f) estimating sample size, (g) randomization, (h) examining data, and (i) conclusions. Because no descriptions of statistical methods for data analyses have yet been represented, and because the emphasis in this volume is on experimental design and planning rather than statistical methods, analyses of the data from these examples were not given, although some procedures were mentioned, which are discussed later in Part IV. Instead, in each case, means of the relevant variables were shown and discussed. The five examples were the following.

Example Number	Description
10.1	One factor at two levels (two drugs), with 25 patients assigned to each level. The form of the responses was joint tenderness index (jti) scores.
10.2	One factor (drugs) at two levels, with 138 patients assigned to each, and a binomial response.
10.3	One factor at three levels (two drugs and a placebo). The response was time in days, and 10 patients were assigned to each of the three groups.
10.4	Two factors at three and two levels (three analgesics at two doses each). The response exemplified was the sum of pain intensity differences, or SPID scores. In the example, six patients were assigned to each cell, but it was noted that for any serious trial, the sample sizes would have had to be larger.
10.5	A multicenter trial, using three factors (including centers). The trial was a $2^2 \times 5$ design. There were two drugs (one factor at two levels), two chemical forms of each (a second factor at two levels), and five centers (the third factor). The patients suffered from a restrictive lung condition. Although the actual trial used several pulmonary function responses, the example was confined to FEV_1 data. Ten patients were used in each cell; therefore, each center treated and measured 40 patients (two drugs and two forms of each, with five patients assigned to each of these four groups at each center—100 patients altogether.

10.10 LITERATURE REFERENCES

(1) Deming, W. Edwards, *The American Statistician*, 29, 148–152 (1975).

(2) Nelson, Lloyd S., *Journal of Quality Technology*, 22, 328–330 (1990).

(3) Beaver, W. T., and G. A. Feise, *Journal of Clinical Pharmacology*, 21, 461–479 (1977).

(4) Beaver, W. T., S. Wallenstein, R. Houde, and A. Rogers, *Journal of Clinical Pharmacology*, 7, 741–751 (1966).

(5) Eisenhart, Churchill, *Biometrics*, 3, 1–21 (1947).

(6) Fleiss, Joseph L., *Controlled Clinical Trials*, 7, 267–275 (1986).

CHAPTER 11

Parallel Factorial Designs: Blocking

11.1 RESTRICTION OF RANDOMIZATION: INTRODUCTION

11.1.1 Confounding

One of the purposes of the random assignment of treatments to subjects when planning a study is to eliminate any possible systematic effects due to patient characteristics, as these might distort the treatment comparisons. When patient characteristics affect the responses, a kind of **confounding** exists and can change the conclusions drawn from the data.

Confounding means the "mixing" of sources of variation in data so that they cannot be distinguished from each other. The sources of variation can be factors introduced by the experimenter or unknown variables introduced by the patients or the environment. An exaggerated example might be a diet study in which random assignment is not used. Because of the lack of randomization, an excess of overweight patients might be assigned to an effective weight-reducing regimen, and less heavy patients to a less effective treatment, or vice versa. The treatment effects would then be confounded with the patients' weights.

Confounding can be employed for constructive purposes in **fractional factorial** and **split-plot** designs. Fractional factorials, including latin squares, are widely used in chemistry and engineering, but only rarely in clinical trials. They are not discussed in this book because of their infrequent use, and also because an adequate discussion of the subject is beyond the scope of this book. For anyone interested, excellent discussions of fractional factorials per se and in the form of latin squares can be found in Davies [14], Cochran and Cox [11], and Snedecor and Cochran [38]. Split-plot designs are rarely, if ever, used in clinical trials, although they are widely employed in agriculture, chemistry, and engineering. Descriptions and explanations can be found in several of the items in the Bibliography. For example, see Cochran and Cox [11], Chapter 7; Snedecor and Cochran [38], Chapter 16, pages 325–29; and Wooding (1).

Confounding can also exist between main effects and interactions among the factors of interest in an experiment.

11.1.2   Restriction of Randomization

The difference between **completely randomized** designs and those in which **blocking** is used lies in the fact that the latter **restrict** the randomization in some important way. Even a completely randomized design uses restriction of the randomization in the sense that the levels of each factor are segregated, so that it later becomes possible to evaluate their effects in the analysis of the data. That is, we separate the subjects into groups, each associated with a different level of each variable, and, in effect, randomize them separately, thereby making it possible to compare data later among groups. However, there may be possible identifiable **nuisance variables** that, if ignored, could be confounded with the effects of the factors of interest, thereby weakening the ability of an analysis to detect the latter. These nuisance variables can be isolated in **blocks**. Their presence then does not affect the evaluation of the factors of interest. Because randomization is done to eliminate the effects of any unidentified and unwanted variables upon the response(s), but these particular variables have been identified and accounted for in the design by the blocking, their randomization becomes unnecessary.

Random assignment would be unnecessary if we knew that there would be no confounding of unknown effects with treatment effects. One purpose of an experimental design is to make it possible to isolate the effects of those sources of variation that are known and obvious. If we could identify every unwanted source of variation, leaving only the factors of interest, randomization would become unnecessary. But such knowledge is impossible. A good researcher knows from experience that regardless of how certain it is that there are no confounding variables, he or she could be wrong. The use of randomization makes it possible to separate any confounding by variables originating with patient characteristics or the environment from the treatment effects of interest. Randomization is usually easy to do, and its benefits far outweigh its cost.

In a sense, the principal function of randomization is to spread out the effects of any unknown variables more or less evenly throughout an experiment, rendering the analysis less powerful, but helping to ensure that the response measurements are as unbiased as possible. But randomization is an imperfect tool; we use it because there is no substitute. And although we can never expect that our treatment factors will be the only differences in responses among patients, we can sometimes make a reasonable guess as to the identity of one or a few of the undesirable "lurking variables." If this can be done, it is then often possible, in turn, to use a design that will allow the elimination of these effects from the treatment or error calculations. Even in such cases, however, randomization must still be used to handle other, unknown variables. But if one or a few of the bothersome sources of variation can be eliminated in the analysis by using such a special design, randomization can then be applied in a more limited way than in the "completely randomized" designs we have discussed so far. Such designs are said to employ **restriction of randomization**.

In medicine and elsewhere, all experimental designs except those that we call **completely randomized designs** use some form of restriction of randomization. In this book, we discuss only **randomized blocks**, and some common types of **changeover** designs, some of which include blocking. However, there are many kinds of designs, using several different methods of restriction of the randomization. All of these are widely used in applied statistics, but many of them have never been used in clinical trial designs.

The most commonly used designs in medical trials are completely randomized parallel arrangements, such as those already discussed and illustrated in Chapters 8, 9, and 10. With the exception of multicenter trials (which can be viewed as randomized blocks designs with centers as the blocks), parallel designs in which there is restricted randomization are less common in clinical work than in other fields (an exception is the category of changeover designs, discussed later). This may be because the use of statistics and experimental design is quite new in medical clinical work, having become widespread only in the 1960s. Another reason is that because they are more complex structurally, they are more difficult to manage when trials are run. Relatively small departures from their structures as laid out during planning can more easily result in the production of unusable or less usable data, or the reversion of a design to a simpler, less efficacious arrangement. However, you will often find blocking well worth the extra effort. They are usually more efficient and powerful than the simpler designs, so that they will generally require fewer patients. If you can be sure of close supervision of your trial and careful adherence to the design and the protocol, you will often be rewarded with worthwhile savings in sample size and completion time if you use such designs.

11.2 NUISANCE VARIABLES

11.2.1 Blocking and Restricted Randomization

An example of blocking and the use of restricted randomization with which you are already familiar is the employment of similar techniques in fully replicated designs and multicenter trials. In any fully replicated design, as we have used the term, the replicates are blocks, each of which embodies a complete set of the design variables and their levels. In a multicenter design, where a complete replicate is run at each location, the centers (replicates) are the blocks. In this example, there were five levels of the variable centers, labeled C_1 through C_5. The repeated portion of the structure consisted of two drugs (A_1 and A_2), each used in two chemical forms (B_1 and B_2). This design also used cell replication; at each center, five patients received each of the four combinations of the factors A and B.

In any design that is repeated several times, whether spatially, as in a multicenter trial, or temporally, in which a design is repeated at successive intervals, the replicates, the part of the design that is repeated, are often called blocks. As an example, see Figure 9.4 in Chapter 9. In this figure, a three-factor design is shown. Two of the factors, A and B, represent two variables of interest, such as drugs and doses. The third factor, C, represents weeks, which are the blocks (temporal in this case). Factors A and B form a 2^2 design that is repeated in each of 14 weeks (C).

11.2.2 Nuisance Variables and Blocking

Both of the examples mentioned earlier used restricted randomization and both involved what we called **nuisance variables**. The restriction was accomplished by randomizing the assignments separately in each block (week or center), instead of employing the method used in completely randomized designs, in which the randomization would have been applied in a single step to the entire design. The centers or replicates, the nuisance factors, were used to broaden the applicability of any inferences from the trials or to increase the sample size to an amount required. They were so-called because any differences among them were of no particular interest, and could have reduced the power of the statistical tests. With proper randomization, ignoring the weeks factor in the design and analysis would not have biased the results. But if that had been done, the experimental error estimate, needed to do the significance tests, would have been inflated, reducing the power of any analysis. The isolation of the centers or temporal replicates accomplished by the use of the blocks prevented this from occurring.

A nuisance variable is one that you wish wasn't there. For examples, in the "weeks" design of Figure 9.4, if you could have been certain that there would be no important difference in results among the several different weeks (aside from chance variation or experimental error[1]), you would not have needed to provide for the weeks factor in the design. You could have merely ignored that factor, safe in the knowledge that you had minimized the influence of any lurking variables having different levels at different times. But, of course, you could not have made this assumption. You could not have predicted beforehand that there would *not* have been influences acting from week to week that might have affected the patients' responses to factors A and B. The technique of isolating the weeks in blocks to make it possible to

---

[1]Even "chance" variation is really the total effect of all of the unknown variables that influence the responses.

separate any such effects, if they are present, from those of A and B, solves the problem.

In the case of a multicenter trial, the problem is analogous, because centers are the blocks and comprise the nuisance variable. In running such a trial, if you can be sure that the responses from each center will not vary because of unknown differences among the centers (different patient characteristics, differences in investigator use and reading of the FEV_1 instrumentation, etc.), you might run the trial without dividing the design into blocks. In such a case, you would then have randomized the patient numbers to form a continuous series. However, experience suggests that this would have been poor science. There would almost certainly have been differences among centers that could distort your results.

11.2.3 Reducing Experimental Error

To summarize, the use of blocking reduces experimental error. Properly done, blocking of a nuisance variable reduces error if there are differences among the levels of that variable. This occurs because it then becomes possible, during the data analysis, to separate the effects of the nuisance variable from the remaining error. If you ignore that variable in the randomization and analysis of a design, any differences among responses due to changes in conditions from week to week would become part of the error estimate. The statistical tests are essentially comparisons of the magnitudes of effects due to treatments with those due to error, so the data analyses would then lose power.

11.3 RANDOMIZED BLOCKS

11.3.1 Discussion and Description

A brief mention of the two principal kinds of randomized blocks used in clinical studies is necessary at this point to avoid confusion. One kind is discussed here and the other later.

In clinical trial work, unlike fields of experimentation that do not involve human beings, it is important to distinguish between the two kinds of randomized blocks designs. In the first kind, discussed in this chapter, the **blocking variable** may represent any source of variation *except* patients. Frequently, in the second kind, the only blocking variable is *patients*. In a clinical trial using the second kind, we no longer use the term "parallel" design. When patients comprise blocks, each patient receives two or more treatments. The error estimate necessary to carry out the hypothesis (significance) tests is then derived from an estimate of the aggregate **within-patients** or **within-blocks** difference. This overall **within**-patients difference is usually smaller than that **between** patients, although that is not always true. If the within-patients difference, and therefore the experimental error, is made smaller, the hypothesis test becomes more powerful in the detection of treatment effects.

In addition to randomized blocks designs in which the patients are the blocks, there are a number of other designs that use two or more treatments, given successively to each patient, with separate responses measured for each. In this book, we call all these arrangements, including the randomized blocks designs in which the patients comprise the blocks, **changeover**[2] designs. In such designs, patients are still blocks, but that characteristic may not be obvious. Such structures will be discussed in detail in the next chapter. In changeover designs, the experimental units are no longer "patients," as in parallel designs. Instead, they are called **plots**, or "treatments within patients." Each patient "contains" more than one experimental unit, because he or she receives more than one treatment.

Thus, to summarize, you can see that **parallel** randomized blocks designs are included among the arrangements with which you are already familiar, typified by multicenter trials or studies with full replicates repeated at successive intervals. They include *any* design in which each patient gets one treatment level or combination of factor levels (i.e., in which patients are the experimental units), and that includes repetitions in space or time, with any variability created by spatial and temporal differences controlled by blocking. In contrast to these, designs in which patients are blocks (where each patient receives more than one of the treatments) are so different from the parallel designs we have studied so far that they are treated by most biostatisticians and monitors in clinical work as a separate category, which we call **changeover** designs in this book. This chapter is concerned with blocked designs that have parallel structures. The next chapter is devoted to changeover designs.

When centers are the blocks in a trial, we have an example of a randomized blocks design in which the blocks are spatial.

11.3.2 Randomization Procedure for Parallel Randomized Blocks

In Chapter 9, Section 9.2.4 and Figure 9.4, and again in Section 9.3.2 and Figure 9.5, we discussed two designs in which one of the variables represented successive weeks (Figure 9.4) or months (Figure 9.5 and Section 9.3.3). When we use the blocks (time or space) to represent nuisance variables, these two examples can be considered to be randomized-blocks designs. The randomization of such a temporal randomized blocks experiment has not yet been exemplified. However, it is done in exactly the same way as that for a

---

[2]The term "crossover" has been used as a general term to characterize this kind of design. However, to avoid ambiguity, we use the terms "two-period crossover" to describe a particular kind of changeover design, and "changeover" otherwise.

spatial arrangement. The randomization of a trial in which the blocks are spatial was outlined briefly, in a previous example. We give another illustration here, this time in more detail; the blocks can represent either temporal or spatial variables. If you have read up to this point, you already know how to design both types, but the information has been scattered. Having the descriptions here will make the reference easier for you in the future.

11.3.3   Example 11.1: Randomized Blocks

The following illustration is suitable for a randomized-blocks trial in which the blocks are either time periods or locations. We plan to use five blocks. In the first case, we could postulate that the five blocks represent five full replicates done on each of five successive weeks. In the second, we could make the blocks represent clinics. The essence of the randomization procedure, as you will see, is to assign each treatment or treatment combination to a randomly selected "position," where the "positions" are time periods from a prescribed group, such as successive days, weeks, or months, or locations in a group; for example, several different clinics.[3] To make this example concrete, let's say that we adopt the latter identification—the blocks will be spatial and will represent clinics. We plan to compare three antibiotics, and patients in each of five clinics will take part. We designate the five blocks as factor C. Thus, we now have factor C at five levels: $C_1, C_2, \ldots, C_5$.

The Other Factors

In addition to factor C, this example will have two other factors, both qualitative—the first, the antibiotics at three levels (three different drugs), and the second, methods of administration at two levels, oral and parenteral (the latter, in this case, intravenously). We will symbolize the three drugs as A_1, A_2, and A_3, and the two modes of administration as B_1 and B_2. Multiplying the levels together, we see that we need 3×2, or six, groups in each center (block). We have estimated that we need six patients per cell, or 36 per block. Because there will be five blocks, 180 patients will be needed for the trial.

Recall the discussion of fixed and random effects in Chapter 10, Section 10.8.2. In this trial, after consultation with the biostatistician, you decided that the clinics would be regarded as fixed. The other two factors (see what follows) are obviously fixed, so the trial as a whole employs a **fixed model** (Model I), with three fixed factors.

---

[3]If blocks are clinics, the number of clinics to select from is usually limited to one of the several that have been initially selected for various reasons and that agree to take part. Obviously, this is not a "random" factor, but a "fixed" one. Nevertheless, the patients within each block are assigned randomly to the treatments or treatment combinations. If the blocking variable is time periods, it is likely that the extent of these will also be limited, so that this factor also could be called "fixed," because it must be selected from a finite and usually small range of periods.

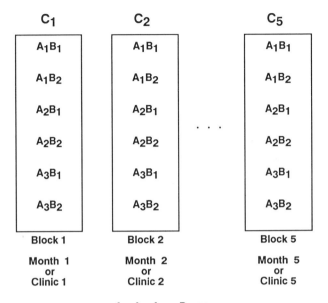

Figure 11.1 Example 11.1: A randomized-blocks design with embedded factorial (randomization not shown).

When you are planning your trial, whether centers are random or fixed will have a critical effect upon the method of data analysis. The reason is that this choice will determine what is used as the error term in the statistical analysis. *Therefore, it is important that you consult your statistician before a decision is made regarding the degree of cell replication or the number of centers to use.* We will assume, as is nearly always the case, that the factors in your trial, other than centers, are fixed (drugs and methods of administration in this example). If the statistician agrees that centers (which comprise the blocking variable) are also to be regarded as fixed, cell replication furnishes the error estimate when the data are analyzed, and the amount of cell replication you use becomes important. On the other hand, in a trial like this example, if centers are not fixed but all other factors are, an interaction term between one of those factors and centers must be used as the error estimate. In that case, the number of centers used and the number of levels of the treatment factor(s) become critical, and must not be too small. Of course, you should nevertheless use some cell replication to ensure against empty cells.

Figure 11.1 shows the three factors and their identifications. Each $A_i B_j$ factor combination within a block stands for six patients. The blocks have been labeled with both months and clinics to remind you that either is a valid

	C_1		C_2		$\cdots$	C_5	
	B_1	B_2	B_1	B_2	$\cdots$	B_1	B_2
A_1	--	--	--	--	$\cdots$	--	--
	--	--	--	--		--	--
	--	--	--	--		--	--
	--	--	--	--		--	--
	--	--	--	--		--	--
	--	--	--	--		--	--
A_2	--	--	--	--	$\cdots$	--	--
	--	--	--	--		--	--
	--	--	--	--		--	--
	--	--	--	--		--	--
	--	--	--	--		--	--
	--	--	--	--		--	--
A_3	--	--	--	--	$\cdots$	--	--
	--	--	--	--		--	--
	--	--	--	--		--	--
	--	--	--	--		--	--
	--	--	--	--		--	--
	--	--	--	--		--	--

Figure 11.2   Detailed structure of the randomized-blocks design of Figure 11.1 (randomization not shown).

blocking variable. Hereafter, in this example, we assume the blocks are clinics.[4]

11.3.4   Structure of the Trial

Figure 11.2 is a more detailed diagram of the design when the complete structure of the five full replicates—the clinics or centers—is indicated. The double hyphens in the figure represent the data in each cell, so that the

[4]The analysis of this design will not use an error term derived from the six cell replicates in each block, but the interaction of blocks and treatments. The cell replicates are used to obtain a better representation of the patient population. See Snedecor and Cochran [38] or Davies [4].

diagram is an abbreviated picture of the data (three of the five centers) as it will appear, with response values substituted for the hyphens, after the study is completed.

11.3.5 Random Assignment of Patients

Numbers of Patients
We will go through the assignment procedure in some detail, using the Moses and Oakford Tables [49], so that you will have a detailed example available for reference. Remember that any valid method of obtaining the necessary permutations would be satisfactory. We use the tables here because they clearly illustrate the process. Alternatives are (a) to use a statistical package that will do the assignments for you or, (b) if you are a programmer, to write a routine to supply a specified number of random permutations of any range of numbers.

A cell in this design consists of all of the patients identified by one combination of the levels of the three factors, such as the six patients receiving the combination $A_1B_1C_1$. Thirty cells altogether are represented in Figure 11.2, although, because all the replicates are alike, only the first, second, and fifth are shown. For this design, five separate random assignments are needed, one for each replicate (center). Each of these will contain six cells, and each of the cells with contain six patients. For example, for center C_1, we need to assign treatments to 36 patients, six to each of the six cells in that center, that is, $A_1B_1, A_1B_2, \ldots, A_3B_2$. This procedure will be identical for each of the five replicates, but you must use a different permutation table of the numbers 1 to 36 for each. If you use Moses and Oakford, [49], you will need to use the permutations of the numbers 1 to 50, omitting any numbers over 36, because those tables are the nearest having 36 or more numbers.

Again, you should remember that it is also *very* important that you use an entirely different set of 36 patients for each replicate—no patients should be entered into the trial more than once. Because centers are usually separated spatially, this is unlikely to happen in a multicenter trial, of course, but someone may suggest it to save expense if the replicates are time periods, such as weeks or months. The 36 patients at each center can be numbered from 1 to 36, each of these sets representing a different group of patients. Alternatively, if you wish, you can number the five sets sequentially (1–36 in center 1, 37–72 in center 2, etc). If you use the latter scheme to avoid confusion in the data records, you will need to "translate" the numbers 1–36 in Moses and Oakford's tables to 37–72, 73–108, etc. We recommend that you do not do this, however, as it could lead to confusion if the patients are arbitrarily numbered at each center in the order of their acceptance into the trial. You could distinguish among centers if you use patient numbers 1–36 in each by adding the center number as a suffix, for example, 17.1, 36.3, etc. For use in recording the entire set of patient numbers, you should prepare a table similar to Figure 11.2 without the hyphens, providing space to record the patient numbers for each of the five replicates. You will need five groups of 36 patients, therefore five permutations of the numbers 1 through 36 from Moses and Oakford. The permutation sets nearest to this in size are those composed of the integers 1 through 50 on pages 68 through 92; we will use five of these.

Assigning Patients to Factor Combinations

I chose the following permutations at random, numbering those on each page by columns, beginning with the left-hand column, and by permutations within each column: page 73, column 2, permutation 4 (5, 20, 19, . . . , 24); page 76, column 2, permutation 2 (43, 26, 30, . . . , 42); page 80, column 1, permutation 7 (41, 45, 26, . . . , 31); page 83, column 1, permutation 1 (39, 49, 44, . . . , 31); and page 89, column 2, permutation 5 (20, 25, 33, . . . , 42).

The first permutation was used to obtain the patient numbers in replicate 1 (C_1), starting with cell $C_1A_1B_1$, then $C_1A_1B_2$, ending with $C_1A_3B_2$. Six of the numbers in that permutation were placed into each cell, starting with the first number that was 36 or less. The numbers selected were assigned to the first group, $A_1B_1C_1$, in the order in which they appeared in the permutation. This procedure was repeated for each of the remaining five groups in that center, using the remaining numbers that were 36 or below in the same permutation. This procedure ensured that there would be 36 patient numbers altogether for the portion of the trial to be run in clinic C_1, numbered from 1 to 36 in a random manner, with six of them assigned to each treatment combination.[5] Any numbers encountered in the permutations that were greater than 36 were ignored. An analogous procedure was used for each of the remaining four clinics. Table 11.1 shows the completed set of random assignments.

Remaining Steps

We need go no further with Example 11.1. The next steps would be to complete the planning, run the trial, and analyze the data. As mentioned earlier, the analysis of multifactor designs is not covered in this book, but you should be familiar with their structure. The appropriate statistical procedures should be very familiar to the biostatistician who analyzes your data.

This design was made a bit more complex than might have been used to illustrate a simple randomized-blocks design, because it is an example of a practical structure that you may well use quite often. Like many multicenter clinical trials designs, the "treatments" within each block are the combina-

---

[5]It is not correct to randomly choose a group of 12 numbers for each of the three levels of A and then assign one of each of the 12 to one of the two-factor B groups within that level of A, as is sometimes done. This procedure makes it impossible for any of the remaining 24 patients to be assigned to that A group.

Table 11.1. Patient Numbers Assigned to Treatments in a $2^2 \times 5$ Clinical Trial (Example 11.1)

	C_1		C_2		C_3		C_4		C_5	
	B_1	B_2	B_1	B_2	B_1	B_2	B_1	B_2	B_1	B_2
A_1	5	20	26	30	26	8	11	2	20	25
	19	32	22	7	12	35	12	24	33	1
	1	30	5	31	20	10	18	22	16	23
	36	15	34	35	36	17	13	1	8	22
	6	10	18	20	11	23	35	21	13	9
	28	33	33	11	29	28	33	10	18	29
A_2	7	31	27	29	27	19	5	28	12	3
	17	27	9	2	30	33	17	4	10	21
	16	18	21	25	18	3	14	25	14	15
	26	21	15	19	13	21	29	27	6	28
	34	25	36	16	2	7	15	8	32	2
	35	2	14	4	25	32	26	3	30	11
A_3	22	3	24	3	22	4	9	36	32	34
	29	12	17	13	16	14	7	19	31	36
	4	23	12	6	24	34	23	6	4	17
	9	13	1	28	15	9	32	30	19	7
	8	14	23	32	5	6	16	34	5	26
	11	24	10	8	1	31	20	31	27	24

tions of the levels of a full factorial, so that each center actually runs a small two-factor study.

A simpler and similarly common design would use just one factor of interest in addition to centers, say, drugs: a test drug, a standard drug, and a placebo. In this case, the three levels of the drug factor would be assigned in replicate to three cells in each center. For example, there might be five centers, each running four subjects assigned to each of the three levels of drugs, so that there would be 12 patients run at each center. If both centers and drugs were fixed factors, the study would be exactly analogous to Example 11.1, but simpler in structure. Of course, the choice of three cell replicates, making 12 patients per center, was used here as an example, and might well be greater in your trial.

Finally, a still simpler randomized-blocks design might be formed as follows: A single-factor design at, say, four levels (of course, any number of levels might be used), comprising four drugs to be compared with each other, might be needed. As is frequently the case, it might be that patients could only be assembled gradually, so that the trial would need to extend over a period of time. One way to handle this problem and reduce the likelihood of important nuisance variation would be to run one small block every month, planning on enough such blocks to supply the needed amount of replication. For example, you could run four patients in each block, *one* assigned to each level of the drugs factor. Then there would be *no* replication of the levels of the drug factor within each block. This is a very common randomized-blocks design, although it is probably used much less often in clinical studies than more complex designs like that of Example 11.1.

11.4   COMMENTS AND SUMMARY OF THE CHAPTER

11.4.1   Restricted Randomization: Parallel Randomized Blocks

If there is a source of variation that may become confounded with the responses intended to supply treatment information in a study, an experimenter can introduce a **blocking variable** into a design to allow isolation of such a confounding effect from the treatments and error effects during analysis. Such blocking variables are often called **nuisance variables**. It is rarely possible to assign patients at random to the several levels of the blocks, whether the latter are temporal or spatial. However, if the blocking variable is a nuisance variable such as weeks or centers, as is usually true, there will be no interest in evaluating blocks or comparing them statistically with each other per se, because purpose of blocking will merely have been to avoid the influence of the blocking variable on the other comparisons in the trial. And if hypothesis testing is not to be done, randomization is not necessary. This is an argument for classifying blocks as Model I, because in that case, any investigation of the blocks in the analyses can be avoided.

Despite these considerations, blocking in this way is a better method of dealing with a nuisance variable than the use of a completely randomized design, in which all replications of all treatments are assigned to patients in random order. Although such a completely randomized design will yield unbiased results if done properly, the power of the statistical tests will be less than it would be for a randomized-blocks design if the suspected nuisance variable exists.

11.4.2   Other Blocking Designs

The blocking discussed in this chapter is only one of many kinds, most of which are beyond the purview of this book. Incomplete blocks designs, latin squares, incomplete latin squares, chain blocks, and response surface designs comprise a few of these. One kind of latin square, the Williams square (see Cochran and Cox [11], pp. 133–141) is widely used in bioavailability studies when there are more than two treatments. The others are not widely used in clinical work, with the exception of an incomplete latin square design

(Youden square), which is a very common design in proprietary antiperspirant testing. We discuss none of these in this book at any length, because of their rarity and complexity. You can obtain information about any of these in Cochran and Cox [11], Davies [14], Box et al. [32], Fleiss [8], and Armitage [18].

11.5 LITERATURE REFERENCE

(1) Wooding, W. M., "The Split-Plot Design," *Journal of Quality Technology*, 5, No. 1, 16–33 (January 1973).

CHAPTER 12

Changeover Designs

12.1 INTRODUCTION

12.1.1 Nature and Origin of Changeover Designs

Changeover designs are mentioned briefly in earlier chapters, and they were defined in Chapter 11, to distinguish them from parallel designs.

To review, in clinical studies, the fundamental concept of a changeover design is to use the ideas of **blocks** and **plots** as described for the parallel designs in Chapter 11, *but to identify the blocks with patients or subjects*. The plots can be **temporal** or **spatial**, as before, but the most common case is temporal. In such a design, each patient (block) is assigned two or more treatments, which are given in succession. Thus, in that design, the plots represent successive time periods.

In a spatial changeover design, each patient may have a group of treatments applied simultaneously to several different locations upon the body (1). Thus, the "changeover" from one treatment to the next is a change of *location* rather than of *time periods*. Under our definition, nevertheless, the design is a changeover, because the patients are the blocks, and the plots are within patients, just as for the temporal designs. If a design possesses a temporal or spatial factor that is not identified with locations on patients' bodies or with successive treatment times, we do not call it a changeover. For example, a multicenter trial is not a changeover design, nor is a trial with several full replicates done in a series of time periods. These are designs using blocks, but the blocks are not the patients.

As mentioned earlier, modern experimental design began in the early years of this century with the work of Sir Ronald A. Fisher at the Rothamstead (pronounced "Romsted") Agricultural Experiment Station in England. One of his books, *The Design of Experiments*, was the first monograph ever published on that topic, and appeared in seven editions from 1935 to 1960 [16]. But before that book was published, he had published a number of papers on the subject. Fisher appears to have introduced into the literature some of the terms we use in experimental design and statistics, such as **blocks** and **plots**.

In agricultural experimentation, the total space in an experimental farm is divided into a number of **fields**, and each field is called a **block**. So that more than one treatment can be used in a given large field, the blocks are often further divided into **plots**, with one of several levels of factors such as crop varieties, soil, or plant treatments randomly assigned to each plot. The assignments are spatial, that is, each level of a factor in its plot has a randomly determined location. The response is usually the yield of the crop(s), such as bushels per acre or a similar measure. When there is no such subdivision, but, instead, a single large area such as a farm is divided into fields with a single treatment per field, larger areas are necessary for an experiment. The experimental error then reflects the substantial differences in location and fertility among the group of fields. When plots instead of fields are used as the experimental units, each with its own treatment, this error is likely to be smaller, because the within-field plots are less widely separated than the fields. Of course, as you may imagine, variations in yield, independent of treatments and due solely to fertility differences among locations, can be very large, so that the use of plots quickly became an important tool, increasing the power of the experimenters' data analyses.

As you have seen, the terms *block* and *plot* used in Fisher's day continue to be used today, not only in agricultural research all over the world, but also in the many other applications of statistics and experimental design, including clinical trials. But in modern experimental design, the idea of a plot within a block is extended to temporal as well as spatial structures, as you will see in a moment.

Like the analogous situation in agriculture, when a changeover design is used, the differences due to random variation among successive responses measured for the same patient, by their nature, must be equal to or smaller than the differences between patients. In fact, in the real world, they will always be smaller, because the *between-patients* variation includes any variation *within* patients. Therefore, a changeover would be expected to have more statistical power than a parallel study, all other things being equal (such as the number of patients being used). Conversely, a changeover design of the same power as a parallel design would be expected to have fewer patients. Of course, this means not only a less expensive trial, but often one that can be completed in significantly less time.[1]

12.1.2 Difficulties with Temporal Designs

Despite all their advantages, temporal changeover designs, especially, introduce their own set of problems that must be resolved for a study to be

---

[1]The likelihood that random within-blocks variation will be less than that between blocks is the reason for using blocking designs even when blocks are not identified with patients or subjects, as in Chapter 11. In clinical trials, however, using patients as blocks is a particularly important design, because the random variation found between plots (*within* patients) is almost always smaller than that between blocks (*between* patients).

successful. In spite of this, changeovers are quite often desirable if for no other reason than economy of patient group sizes. As we discuss each individual type, we will expand upon the kinds of difficulties that may arise, and suggest methods for overcoming them.

12.2 BIOAVAILABILITY STUDIES

12.2.1 General

Perhaps the most common use of changeover designs today is in bioavailability studies, so the discussion and examples in this chapter are limited to such cases. Of course, changeovers can be used for other purposes, but such uses are much less frequent in industrial clinical work.

Bioavailability studies necessarily use temporal changeover designs, because variation in the concentration of a drug or metabolite in the blood or urine must be recorded and followed over a period of time for each individual subject. One such design, in particular, is the two-period two-treatment crossover, which is very commonly used for this purpose. This subject is broad and complex, and our treatment will be necessarily abbreviated. The limited coverage in this chapter is necessary, however, because bioavailability studies are needed in most organizations concerned with clinical studies.

Bioavailability studies are most often used in early Phase I trials when new drugs are being evaluated for safety, but they are also needed when a new dosage form is to be compared with the old, or a change in formulation is made. For example, the FDA requires their use by organizations contemplating the marketing of an established drug as a generic, to ensure that the bioavailability of the generic product does not depart significantly from the original. Two-period crossover designs are most often used for these purposes, but these designs have inherent problems that require careful and frequently complex analyses to manage. We are accordingly suggesting a procedure whereby, if serious problems are encountered with a two-period crossover during its analysis, a randomized blocks analysis, with patients as the blocks, can be used instead. This is possible in this unusual case because the kind of randomization used for the two-treatment randomized-blocks design is also suitable for the crossover, although the reverse is not true.

Both the design and the analyses of data from a two-period crossover trial are not infrequently done incorrectly. You should be certain that the biostatistician is quite familiar with the structure of changeover designs and their use (and their special pitfalls, if a two-period crossover is used), as well as the complexities of their analyses. At the end of this chapter, we provide a selected set of references both for the designs and the analyses. These are mentioned in more detail later in the chapter.

The problems just referred to apply particularly to two designs: the two-period crossover and the multiple-period changeover design, properly called the Williams latin square (2). The former is very widely used, and often incorrectly, because its apparent simplicity is deceptive. The Williams design is more straightforward, but it is inherently more complex and more difficult to manage during a trial. However, that design is used only in special situations.

12.2.2   The Nature of Bioavailability Studies

Bioavailability or "bioequivalence" studies can consist of single-dose or multiple-dose studies, and the designs can be two-treatment two-period designs or multiple-treatment multiple-period arrangements. When there are only two test drugs or dosage forms to be compared, a study can be designed and analyzed either as **randomized blocks** or as a **two-period crossover** arrangement. Trials using more than two drugs or drug variations are much less common, but when they must be run, randomized blocks may still be used, and is the simplest method. The Williams squares mentioned before may also be used in these cases. Its analysis is more powerful than randomized blocks, and its special properties allow the isolation of any *first-order carryover effects* (the influence of some treatments upon the next ones), without dependence upon washout periods. However, the procedures necessary for this design, including planning, administration, and analysis, are more complex. Therefore, you may prefer to use a multiple-treatment randomized-blocks design, which is simpler. If so, the problem of possible carryover effects can usually be handled by using an adequate washout period between drug dosages. As for the two-period designs, there can be some loss of power if this is done.

Multiple-dose studies are trials in which each drug is given repeatedly in order to create an approximate equilibrium condition; see Ritschel [76], pages 249–271. As Ritschel points out, multiple-dose studies are often used to estimate doses and intervals needed to maintain a given level of drug or metabolite concentration in the body. Such studies are beyond the scope of this book, however; the material here is limited to the single-dose procedure. Except for a brief description of multiple-treatment studies (Williams squares) later in this chapter, we also limit our discussion to trials using only two drug products. However, the statistician at your organization should be familiar with both multiple-dose and multiple-treatment designs, and the FDA guidelines that are available for some of them.

The term **bioavailability** refers to the response for any single material. A "bioequivalence" study is one in which two or more materials or drug forms are compared. We prefer the term **comparative bioavailability** rather than "bioequivalence"; that term is an inexact description of the trial process, because two treatments cannot be shown to be the same by the use of a statistical test with a finite sample size.

For a single-dose comparison of two drugs, using either randomized blocks or the two-period crossover design, one of the two materials to be compared is given orally or parenterally to healthy volunteers, and a series of blood and (sometimes) urine samples are then taken over a period of time. Following this, preferably after a washout period, the same procedure is carried out with the other drug. After chemical analyses of these samples of blood or urine have been completed, the responses described in the next paragraph are derived and analyzed statistically.

For the blood tests in comparative bioavailability trials, all the following responses are usually obtained: (a) the time required after dosage for the concentration of each drug or its metabolite(s) to reach a peak in the bloodstream (time to peak, T_{max}); (b) the total quantities of such materials detected in the blood over the entire session (area under the curve, AUC); (c) their maximum concentrations in the blood (peak concentration, C_{max}); and (d) their half-lives in the body ($t_{0.5}$). The urine responses, if used, are analogous. Typically, concentration versus time plots of the responses for each drug are reported, and statistical comparisons of the drugs using each of the previous four kinds of derived responses based upon these plots are made. Of course, the multiplicity resulting from the repetition of the significance tests on each response should be provided for. Note that the time to peak and the peak concentration are usually highly correlated, but both are nevertheless measured and used in most cases. A representative single-dose study will require 24 to 48 hours or more for each of the two periods, and will usually involve the collection of approximately 12 to 18 blood samples from each subject. A washout period between the two drugs should be used, and should be several estimated half-lives long.

For clarity, we will use the same bioavailability study for both of the examples in this chapter (the randomized-blocks and the two-period crossover designs). Both are changeover designs, and they are very similar in structure. However, the method of randomization can be different, and the analyses are always very different. The two-period crossover is the most common design used for two-treatment single-dose studies. However, there are difficulties in planning, using, and analyzing it (e.g., the incorrect use of baseline data, incorrect preparation for evaluating the so-called carryover effects, and the use of incorrect methods of analysis). These usually are the results of inexperienced use of the design and its analysis, because the pitfalls are not widely known or understood except by the few who have studied them carefully. There is no other design for which it is more important to ensure that a statistician is part of the team from the first moment of planning. In this chapter, therefore, we suggest a special planning procedure that will allow the design to be analyzed as randomized blocks if the two-period crossover analysis is found to be inappropriate.

12.2.3 The Need for Bioavailability Studies

Most workers in clinical trials will need to run bioavailability tests at one time or another. If your organization applies for an IND or NDA, or changes the dosage form of a marketed drug, the new form must be compared with the old before it can be approved. If you plan to market a generic drug, the FDA requires you to carry out some evaluation work, regardless of the fact that such products, if on the market, will have been tested and approved earlier by the original manufacturer. There can be important differences in the absorption and metabolic rates between the original manufacturer's drug and the dosage form your company wishes to market. Even if the dosage form is the same, there can be differences in bioavailability related to different manufacturing methods and equipment. Often, the only tests required are one or more two-drug single-dose comparative bioavailability tests, in which the generic product is compared with the original manufacturer's material using the four responses mentioned before.

12.2.4   Example 12.1: Single-Dose Two-Period Bioavailability Trials

Randomization

This example describes the planning of single-dose trials, using either the randomized-blocks or the two-period crossover design. Provided that the randomization is done in a manner that makes a randomized-blocks analysis possible, as described in what follows, the design may be analyzed either as a two-period crossover or as randomized blocks. On the other hand, as will be shown, a different randomization, actually the one more commonly used, will necessitate analysis of the data as a two-period crossover. Then, if a so-called sequence effect is found, the study must be analyzed by a method resulting in a catastrophic loss of power, which will be likely to show no significance even if the specified difference between drugs exists. You would then find it necessary to repeat the trial.

Healthy volunteers (subjects) are normally used in these studies. The sample size is usually relatively small, in the neighborhood of 20 to 40. Every subject receives both drugs, each in a separate test period. *For either the randomized-blocks or the two-period crossover design*, the randomization can be done by independently choosing, for each subject, which of the two products, T_1 or T_2, is to be given first. This can be done by computer, by drawing random numbers from a table, or by the use of a scientific calculator, assigning "T_1 in the first period" to a subject if, for example, the random number is odd, and "T_2 in the first period" if it is even. You should use four- or five-digit random numbers to avoid duplication or ambiguity. *It is not necessary that equal numbers of subjects be assigned to each of the two orders of administration, although that arrangement is acceptable.* If the group sizes are unequal, the analysis of the data as a two-period crossover design is very slightly more complex. For randomized blocks, however, the analysis is the same whether or not there are equal numbers in each order. It is important that no restriction in the direction of maintaining equality or near equality of the groups be used. However, it is unlikely that there will be serious differences.

A second commonly used procedure that ensures equal group sizes may be used. That is, to restrict the randomization by determining for each individual subject which treatment he or she will receive first, as just described, but when half of the required number of subjects has been so chosen and assigned to one sequence of doses (one "order"), assigning the other sequence to the remaining subjects.

The first procedure is recommended. *If randomization is done by that method, the data can be analyzed as either a randomized blocks design or a two-period crossover. The second method produces data suitable only for analysis as a two-period crossover.* If you use that method, the difficulties to be discussed in connection with the crossover design may then force the use of an analysis with insufficient power, and, at times, may make any useful analysis impossible. If that happens, a completely new study will then be necessary. On the other hand, if you use the first kind of randomization, the statistician can try analyzing the data as a two-period crossover. If that cannot be done because of a problem discussed in what follows, a randomized-blocks analysis can be used instead. When there are no difficulties with it, analysis using the two-period crossover will usually be the more powerful procedure.

12.2.5 Execution of the Trial

Usually, the two parts of a comparative bioavailability trial should be separated by at least seven or eight estimated drug half-lives or more. This separation is called a **washout** period. Thus, if the longest half-life is estimated to be 1 day, at least a week should be allowed to elapse between the first and second drug administrations. Sometimes your estimates of half-life may be a bit shaky; in such cases, longer periods, within reason, do no harm and will provide greater assurance of valid data.

Many workers use baseline data taken before drug administration at the beginning of each of the two periods, later analyzing the data as differences from the appropriate baseline value. However, if your statistician is planning to analyze the data as a crossover design, this *must not* be done. Fleiss, Wallenstein, and Rosenfeld {6} have found that the use of baseline data taken before each of the two periods can severely distort the results of an analysis of a two-period crossover design.

Each subject is given a single dose of his or her assigned drug, carefully recording the time of dosage. On a predetermined schedule based upon the expected shape of the resulting curves of concentration vs. time, and your estimates of the absorption and elimination rates, the blood and (perhaps) urine samples are then taken periodically. Generally, the rise in concentration of the drug or a metabolite in the blood or urine following dosage will be more rapid than its eventual reduction after passing a peak, and this is usually assumed in planning the frequency of sampling. These procedures are repeated for the second drug, following the washout period.

The blood and urine samples are protected from deterioration and analyzed as soon as possible for the quantity of drug or metabolite. The method used must have been carefully developed and tested for accuracy and precision prior to the bioavailability test.

12.2.6 Results

Figure 12.1, taken from an actual study, is a plot of the concentration vs. time for one subject. It was selected to show a close approach to the theoretical shape; many depart much further from the ideal shape than this one. As you might expect, curves based upon averages of data from several individuals will display a still closer approach to that paradigm. This drug was an analgesic. The data were concentrations of a metabolite of the drug in the blood, in micrograms per milliliter, vs. time. Note the rapid increase in concentration during the first few minutes, and the much slower decrease after passing the peak; this general shape is typical for many drugs. A theoretical or a power curve is *not* fitted to the data points; such a curve is not needed for the empirical procedures commonly used to obtain the responses detailed earlier. Instead, each adjacent pair of points is simply joined by a straight line.

Because interest lies in the concentration of material found in the blood or urine vs. time, the measurements can be interpreted as rates, for example, the numbers of micrograms/milliliter in a given time interval. At the beginning of a session, the absorption rate of a drug predominates, and the concentration rises. After the concentration reaches a peak, the elimination rate predominates. In a two-period single-dose study, there are two or more drugs, and the object is to compare them in terms of the four responses derived from the concentration measurements.

12.2.7 About the Examples of This Chapter

Because bioavailability is important to almost everyone concerned with drug trials in industry, the two examples given here are bioavailability studies. Although it is generally very difficult to obtain suitable proprietary data for use as real-data examples, in this case, these data originated in a series of trials designed and analyzed by the author for a client, and are used here with permission. The bioavailability test data used in both Examples 12.2 and 12.3 were part of a single study. In no case have any of the data been altered, although not all of the available data have been used, and a simplification of the structure of the design was made. Subjects (healthy volunteers) were used.

Because of this emphasis upon bioavailability testing, it must be made clear that the two designs in which its application is illustrated—randomized complete blocks using patients as blocks, and the so-called two-period crossover—may be used for other purposes as well. These designs are both

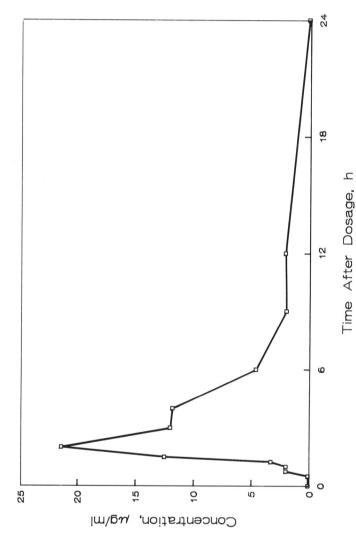

Figure 12.1 A typical bioavailability plot for one patient (concentration of drug or metabolite vs. time).

classified as changeovers as long as the randomized blocks are identified with patients or subjects in the first case, and the columns of the crossover are so identified in the second. The plots in the randomized blocks may be spatial rather than temporal, as mentioned earlier; this arrangement is often used in certain kinds of skin testing. Similarly, the rows in the "two-period" crossover may not be used to represent periods of time at all, but can represent locations. When the crossover is used in this way, many of the problems encountered with the design disappear and/or change their nature.

12.2.8 Literature

Details of the calculations of the derived responses and the analyses of these two designs are not within the scope of the goals of this book. However, an excellent reference is available in the Bibliography (Buncher and Tsay [19]), which contains a chapter devoted to the design and analysis of bioavailability trials; see Chapter 10 by Daniel L. Weiner, a recognized authority in the field. Some newer works are in preparation. Another reference that should be available to anyone planning to run bioavailability trials is Ritschel [76]. A third is Tallarida and Murray [78]. You can read Weiner to gain a practical knowledge of bioavailability studies. Ritschel's handbook will help you to gain a basic understanding of the kinetics of the process that is hypothesized to take place within an organism during such trials. Tallarida and Murray supply a collection of the mathematical concepts and equations underlying this and many other pharmacological procedures. There are also some examples in Bolton [7], on pages 160, 195, and 205.

At the end of this chapter, in addition to the usual chapter references, as a matter of interest, we present a fairly large group of references to the design and analysis of the two-period crossover. That literature is included because of the frequent misuses of the design, to refer you to methods that have been found reliable, and to show you the extent of the problems that may be encountered if a crossover is used without knowledge of its idiosyncracies. The regular chapter references appear in parentheses and the special references are in braces. Most of the information contained in the references is not repeated here.

12.3 RANDOMIZED BLOCKS (RBs)

12.3.1 Description

Randomized blocks have not been widely employed in industry for two-treatment comparative bioavailability studies. If, after reading the following material on both the crossover and randomized blocks, you plan to use RBs in a submission to the FDA, it might be well to seek FDA comments. However, in the past, many biostatisticians have gone on record in pointing out some of the problems that can be encountered with the use of the two-period crossover; and at least one paper suggests randomized blocks as a safe substitute; see Hills and Armitage {10} among the special references at the end of this chapter.

We will show in the following that under some circumstances, in bioavailability tests and other applications, the randomized-blocks design possesses a major advantage over the conventionally used two-period crossover and overcomes a serious problem that may arise.

When the randomized-blocks design is used as a changeover, the patients themselves become the blocks. The experimental units are the plots. There will be at least two plots, imaginary divisions, "within" each block. Each plot receives one treatment. The plots are usually temporal, that is, each represents a separate treatment period. At the beginning of each period, a new treatment is given to each patient and the measurement of a new set of responses begins. The assigned sequence of the treatments thus defines an order of treatments as well as the separate treatment intervals.

In some studies, plots within patients are spatial instead of temporal. One common example is the use of changeover designs in dermatological studies; see Kligman and Wooding (1). In such studies, there is interest in a comparison of the effects of several topical treatments upon the skin, so that different sites upon the body of each patient, each comprising a different plot, are used for each treatment. These treatments are often applied during a single session rather than over a period of time.

In a temporal study, the lengths of the periods are usually equal for a given trial but may vary from trial to trial. In a spatial study, in which the plots represent locations upon the body, corresponding areas are usually used for each patient or subject. The terms "changeover" and "crossover" have sometimes been used to refer exclusively to temporal studies, but in this book we use them in connection with either temporal or spatial designs. The three examples in this chapter, including previous Example 12.1 and the two (Examples 12.2 and 12.3) in this section, use temporal designs, but you will be able to design spatial studies by analogy, if needed. Except in dermatological work, ethical drug evaluation is usually temporal.

The preparations for running a changeover randomized-blocks design have much in common with the randomized-blocks designs described in Chapter 11 (the parallel designs), but there are some important differences. These will become apparent as we describe the procedures.

12.3.2 Sample Size

Methods for estimating sample size have not yet been described for any designs other than completely randomized structures. A convenient tabular method for this design will be described in Part V. The information and specifications needed, however, are the same for all designs. As described in Chapter 5, to estimate sample size in the most effective manner, four quantities are needed regardless of the kind of design that you are planning. These quantities are delta (δ), alpha (α), beta (β), and sigma (σ). If you are estimating the sample size during planning, delta, alpha, and beta are specifications; you set them to any values you feel suitable when planning your trial. Sigma must be estimated, however, either from experience or by running a pilot trial.

To review, delta is the smallest difference between two treatments, in terms of a response variable, that is of practical (i.e., clinical) importance. Alpha is the probability of being wrong that will obtain if, after a test, it is claimed that statistical significance (a difference of delta) exists in the population for some such contrast. Beta is the probability of being wrong if you do *not* find significance and, as a result, claim that any difference that exists is smaller than delta. You should specify the desired values of alpha, beta, and delta when you plan a trial. Sigma is your estimated experimental error.

Once you have specified alpha, beta, and delta and estimated sigma, the estimation of the necessary sample size follows almost mechanically, often merely by the use of a table. In applied statistics, sample size estimates are always approximations, because sigma is never known; it is always *predicted* from past data. In addition, in most cases, the tables or equations used to estimate the sample size are based upon approximate relationships. All the estimation procedures given in this book are approximations. However, all of them are entirely adequate for the usual clinical study.

In Part V, an approximate method for the sample size in a randomized-blocks design, using tables, is given; the reference is to Bratcher et al. at the end of Chapter 15 and to the abridged Bratcher et al. table in the Appendix, Table A.6. You will note that that the Appendix table is labeled as providing sample size estimates for one-factor studies. However, as the authors point out, it is possible to use it for randomized-blocks designs as well.

12.3.3 Randomization

In a **parallel** design using randomized blocks, each plot in a block represents a different patient, and the blocks themselves usually represent some "nuisance" variable. You randomize the assignments by allocating treatments at random to each of the several patients, repeating the procedure with an independent randomization for each block.

If, in a **changeover** design using randomized blocks, for example, the treatments are several drugs, they are also assigned at random to the plots within each block. However, the blocks are now patients, and the plots represent a sequence of time periods. Thus, the arrangement is temporal; you are determining the *order* in which *each patient* (block) receives the treatments.

The randomization procedures for both temporal and spatial RBs changeover designs is the same—you randomly assign treatments to the plots, independently in each block. The only difference between the two is the nature of the plots.

12.3.4   Example 12.2: A Two-Treatment RBs Changeover Trial

Outline of Study Procedure

This example illustrates a typical application for a single-dose two-period changeover design. The two treatments consisted of a single common analgesic drug made by each of two different manufacturers. The formulations and manufacturing processes used for the two may have been different, but the dosage forms and the active ingredients were the same. The trial was to be a small pilot study. The purpose was to estimate an approximate value for sigma and to accomplish other goals of the study, but it was expected to be too small to yield the necessary sensitivity to treatment differences (power). It was one of several trials intended to evaluate a new set of facilities for bioavailability testing. Blood tests only were used. The two periods comprised two dosing and blood-sampling sessions a week apart. For the first session, the drug to be given to each subject originated from one of the two manufacturers, and was assigned randomly to one of the two periods for each patient. In the second session, each received the remaining drug.

At the beginning of each period, a "zero-time" blood sample was taken from each subject, and a single dose of the assigned drug was then immediately given. The responses derived from the zero-time measurement were *not* used as baseline data, but merely to record initial conditions. Thereafter, a series of blood samples was taken over a period of 24 hours, as described in the next paragraph. The procedure in the two periods differed only in the drug assigned to each subject. It was planned to separate the serum from each blood sample, preserve it by freezing, and then analyze it several days after the trial to determine the concentration of drug or metabolite.

Blood Sampling

Based upon knowledge of the drugs being tested, it was decided that blood samples would be taken from each subject 13 times in each of the two sessions. Figure 12.1, shown earlier, displays the results of the serum analyses for one of the subjects. The intervals between blood samplings were the same for all subjects: 0.00, 0.50, 0.75, 1.00, 1.25, 1.50, 2.00, 3.00, 4.00, 6.00, 9.00, 12.00, and 24.00 hours following the single dose. The 0.00-hour point represents the sample taken just prior to dosage. A maximum variation of ± 5 minutes was allowed in these intervals during the trial, but, as it happened, the work was carefully done, and all the intervals varied by less than 2 minutes from the specified times. The increases in the intervals reflected the expected rate of change of the drug concentration in the blood of an average individual, and the expected shape of the curve. The half-lives of both brands were expected to be close enough to allow the same intervals to be used for each.[2] The units of concentration used by the analytical laboratory were micrograms per milliliter (μg/ml), as shown in Figure 12.1.

Some simplifications have been made in the remaining descriptions of the design and procedures that follow to allow the essential points to be displayed as clearly as possible.

Blood-Serum Analysis

Before the trial began, an acceptable and reliable quantitative laboratory method for the measurement of the drug or a metabolite in the blood was needed. In this case, a method already existed, but some modifications were necessary. It was essential that it be both specific and sensitive, that is, interferences from other common materials found in human blood had to be prevented; and it was necessary that quite low concentrations of the drug or metabolite be detectable. The work required some preliminary blood samples from subjects who had been dosed with the test products, and these were arranged for and supplied by the sponsor. These samples had to represent a wide range of concentrations of the active material to ensure that there were no problems related to the level present in the blood. The analytical laboratory that developed the methods also did the analyses of the blood samples after the trial.

Sample Size

In the usual bioavailability study, unlike most hypothesis tests, the tests used to analyze the data look for *lack* of significance between drugs, rather than for a significant difference. Normally, following the spirit of several FDA Guidelines on bioavailability tests, the sample size of a test comparing a new dosage form or the product of a new manufacturing procedure to a previously satisfactory product should be that giving a beta of, at most, about 0.20, and preferably 0.15 or 0.10, with an alpha value of 0.05 or less.[3] In many cases, these specifications result in a sample size of 20 to 40 subjects. This often is sufficient to conclude that there is adequate similarity in the bioavailability of the two drugs if, when the hypothesis tests are done, significance is not found. For the present pilot study, however, only 12

---

[2]Although the two products contained the same active ingredient, and were supplied in the same dosage form (tablets), it is not unusual for the responses to vary somewhat as a result of different manufacturing conditions and perhaps different "inert" ingredients. For example, differences in pressure used in forming the tablets may affect their bioavailability because of differences in rate of solution of the tablets in the stomach.

[3]The FDA issues periodic Guidelines for this and other drug-testing and related procedures. This description is based upon Guidelines available from the FDA, which may not be current when this book appears. You should secure the latest Guidelines before planning any bioavailability trial, however, as they are subject to change. It should also be pointed out that although you are not required to follow the Guidelines in this or any other procedure, you may find it helpful to do so.

Week 1	D_2	D_1	D_2	D_1	D_1	D_2
Week 2	D_1	D_2	D_1	D_2	D_2	D_1
Subject:	S_1	S_2	S_3	S_4	S_5	S_6

Week 1	D_2	D_2	D_2	D_1	D_1	D_2
Week 2	D_1	D_1	D_1	D_2	D_2	D_1
Subject:	S_7	S_8	S_9	S_{10}	S_{11}	S_{12}

Randomization Data

Block	Random Digit	First Drug	Block	Random Digit	First Drug
S_1	even (4)	D_2	S_7	even (2)	D_2
S_2	odd (1)	D_1	S_8	even (0)	D_2
S_3	even (6)	D_2	S_9	even (2)	D_2
S_4	odd (3)	D_1	S_{10}	odd (1)	D_1
S_5	odd (7)	D_1	S_{11}	odd (3)	D_1
S_6	even (4)	D_2	S_{12}	even (0)	D_2

Figure 12.2 Example 12.1: Randomized-blocks design showing randomization of orders of dosing.

healthy volunteers were selected for the trial. No sample size estimate was used, and it was expected that the study would be too small to compare drugs. However, as indicated, comparing the bioavailabilities was not the purpose of the trial.

Randomization
For each subject (block), the order of giving the two drugs (i.e., which of the two plots was assigned to each drug) was determined randomly. For this small trial, this was done by the use of odd and even five-digit pseudo-random numbers, using a random-number function on a pocket calculator. A random "seed" value was used to ensure that the sequence obtained was unique. Drug 1 (D_1) was given in the first session if the number ended with an odd digit, and drug 2 (D_2) was given first if the last digit was even. Figure 12.2 is a diagram of the complete design with the randomization shown. In the lower portion, the 12 blocks are listed, showing the last digit of each random number and the drug given first as a result.

Running the Trial

There was an interval of a week (washout period) between doses.[4] The interval was established upon the basis of prior estimates of the half-lives of the two drugs. As will be seen from the data, the greatest half-life calculated a posteriori for either drug and any individual subject was 3.46 hours. The separation of 7 days, therefore, constituted over 48 half-lives, making the washout more than adequate.

It was arranged for all 12 subjects to assemble at the clinic on the same day for each of the two sessions. Each one remained for 12 hours, returning the next day for the 24-hour sampling. It was not possible to blind either the subjects or the investigators, because the drugs were used in their commercial forms. However, the randomization schedules were not made available to the investigators, and the subjects were informed only that each dosage would consist of one of two commercial analgesics. The subjects were numbered from 1 to 12 in the order in which they arrived at the clinic on the first day of the trial.

Results

The results of the chemical analyses of the serum samples are given here, as are the derived responses, but only brief explanations of the calculation of the latter are given in this book. If the statistician associated with your organization is experienced in clinical trials generally, he or she will be familiar with them. For further information for anyone in your organization, a special group of literature references with item numbers in braces, { }, appears at the end of this chapter. In addition, there are several books available on the subject, including those appearing in the Bibliography and referred to in this chapter (Cochran and Cox [11] and Buncher and Tsay [19]).

We will not reproduce the complete set of raw data for this study, but Table 12.1 shows the original data for subjects 1 through 4. The units of measurement used in the table are micrograms per milliliter, referring to the concentration of the metabolite of the test products found in the chemical analyses of the blood samples. You will note that none of the readings at time zero is zero, although the subjects had not yet taken any drug. Such results are common for chemical analysis data. To compensate, sometimes the initial "blank" reading is subtracted from each of the readings obtained. In Table 12.1, if that were done, row 1 in the table would become zero and each of the other values would be reduced by 0.1 μg/ml. However, this is not necessary, and no alterations were made to the original data.

---

[4]In some studies, each subject is asked to undergo a "break-in" period of a week or two, during which he or she is not to take any drugs resembling the test products. This serves as a washout period *preceding* the trial.

Table 12.1. Original Data for First Four Subjects (Example 12.2) (Micrograms per milliliter)

Hours after Dosage	Block 1 (B₁) (Subject 1)		Block 2 (B₂) (Subject 2)		Block 3 (B₃) (Subject 3)		Block 4 (B₄) (Subject 4)	
	Drug 1 (D_1)	Drug 2 (D_2)	Drug 1 (D_1)	Drug 2 (D_2)	Drug 1 (D_1)	Drug 2 (D_2)	Drug 1 (D_1)	Drug 2 (D_2)
0.00	0.1	0.1	0.1	0.1	0.1	0.1	0.1	0.1
0.50	0.1	0.1	0.1	0.5	4.8	13.1	10.4	1.3
0.75	2.0	2.4	1.7	1.0	4.9	16.8	16.3	3.5
1.00	2.0	10.5	0.1	2.4	7.0	23.0	23.8	7.1
1.25	3.3	14.9	0.1	5.2	6.2	20.0	23.9	8.7
1.50	12.5	14.4	0.1	13.7	13.3	27.3	20.1	18.3
2.00	21.4	37.8	0.1	12.1	14.7	42.3	45.8	13.2
3.00	12.0	21.4	15.8	11.5	14.6	36.5	14.0	11.6
4.00	11.8	3.4	2.5	13.1	14.3	23.2	10.9	14.8
6.00	4.6	4.8	7.6	6.2	8.3	3.3	5.0	9.3
9.00	2.0	0.1	1.0	2.5	2.3	0.1	0.1	2.8
12.00	2.1	0.1	4.8	2.3	2.5	1.7	0.1	1.1
24.00	0.1	0.1	0.1	0.1	0.1	0.1	0.1	0.1

Derived Responses

The methods of calculating the four responses shown in Table 12.2 are described briefly in this section. They are based upon the data in Table 12.1, and no further information is needed, but a plot of the data for each subject is helpful, and can also serve to present the results when the data analysis is

Table 12.2. Derived Responses for Four Individual Subjects (Example 12.2)

Subject	Drug	Derived Responses			
		AUC (μg-h/ml)	C_{max} (μg/ml)	T_{max} (h)	$t_{0.5}$ (h)
1	D_1	86.18	21.4	2.00	2.98
	D_2	80.91	37.8	2.00	0.87
2	D_1	78.80	15.8	3.00	3.46
	D_2	88.58	13.7	1.50	2.95
3	D_1	105.41	14.7	2.00	2.87
	D_2	155.05	42.3	2.00	3.27
4	D_1	106.31	45.8	2.00	0.85
	D_2	96.40	18.3	1.50	2.79

AUC: Area under the curve between 0 and 24 hours.
C_{max}: Maximum concentration reached.
T_{max}: Time to reach maximum concentration.
$t_{0.5}$: Half-life.

complete. The plots are empirical estimates in the sense that they use actual data points, rather than functions fitted to the points. The straight lines joining the points in the plots shown in this chapter (Figures 12.1 and 12.3) were drawn merely to assist in visualization. The calculations of the four derived responses reflect that empiricism. This procedure is the usual one employed in industrial bioavailability testing, and ensures that the actual data obtained in the trial are the basis for the derived responses, with no assumptions made about the mathematical function that may give rise to the curves. In any event, for individual subjects, the shapes of the curves vary widely, and, in many cases might depart substantially from any such model.

Reference to Figure 12.1 will help in understanding the following brief descriptions:

C_{max}

This is the y coordinate of the highest point found on each subject's curve. It is the estimated highest concentration of drug or metabolite found in the patient's blood; its units are micrograms/milliliter.

T_{max}

This is the estimate of the time required to reach C_{max}, in hours.

AUC

The AUC (area under the curve) is an estimate of the total quantity of drug or metabolite found in the blood samples during the entire period of measurement; its units are microgram-hours/milliliter. It is calculated by the use of a numerical integration; a method called the **trapezoidal rule** is widely used by clinical trial biostatisticians, but any method of estimating the area under each curve between the limits of zero hours and the time of the last blood sample will be appropriate. This function and other methods of numerical integration are given in Beyer [47].

$t_{0.5}$

Finally, $t_{0.5}$ is the estimated elimination half-life of the drug, based upon the rate information given by the declining portion of the curve, expressed in hours. That quantity is the time required for half of the original quantity of drug to be eliminated from the body. One source of the function needed for this calculation is given in Tallarida and Murray [78].

Comments

You will often find that analyses of C_{max} and T_{max} lead to the same conclusions, although there will probably be differences in the precision with which they are measured, because T_{max} is likely to be a cruder measurement than C_{max}. That they are closely related is to be expected, because the position of T_{max} is *defined* by C_{max}. However, most monitors prefer to report both. The value of the AUC, on the other hand, depends upon all of the points. The value of $t_{0.5}$ is also dependent upon all the points, in a sense, because it is derived from the slope of the tail portion of the curve, which, in turn, is related to C_{max} and therefore to the earlier points as well.

These four derived responses, calculated from the data of Table 12.1 for the first four subjects, are given in Table 12.2, with their units.

Data Processing

The four responses, C_{max}, T_{max}, AUC, and $t_{0.5}$, were each subjected to a separate statistical analysis. You may have heard of a technique called multivariate analysis, whereby a group of *dependent* variables (responses) may be analyzed together (in a single statistical procedure). Superficially, that might seem to be ideal for data that invariably consist of several responses, but multivariate analyses are almost never used for clinical data. The reason is that the results are often extremely difficult to interpret. Therefore, in cases like this example, you are advised to use separate univariate analyses. If you do so, you should allow for the multiplicity introduced by the use of four responses in calculating the sample size during planning.

Some of the literature occasionally refers to the analysis of multifactor data (multiple *independent* variables) as multivariate, but this is not the statistical meaning, and can cause confusion. Univariate analyses can be done with data representing any number of factors, as long as only one response is used in each analysis.

In this example, as in the previous chapters, we will content ourselves with calculating the average values of each response for each drug. Table 12.3 shows the means of each of the four responses for the two drugs and the first four subjects, calculated from the individual results shown in Table 12.2. Because of the small sample size, the differences between the pairs of drug means (means of T_1 and T_2) shown there could quite easily be due to random fluctuation, however (of course, we are considering only four subjects). Even though these differences between treatments may be influenced only by within-subject error (and not to any population difference in location between drugs), such variation can be substantial, especially for small sample sizes. In addition, another characteristic of a small sample is that it may not

Table 12.3. Means of Derived Responses for Each Drug for Four Subjects (Example 12.2)

Name of Response	Response Means	
	Drug 1	Drug 2
AUC (μg-h/ml)	94.18	105.24
C_{max} (μg/ml)	24.4	28.0
T_{max} (h)	2.25	1.75
$t_{0.5}$ (h)	2.54	2.47

Table 12.4. Means of Original Concentration Data for Four Subjects and Each Drug (Example 12.2)

Hours after Dosage	Mean Concentration, $(\mu g/ml)$ (4 Subjects)	
	Drug 1	Drug 2
0.00	0.10	0.10
0.50	3.85	3.75
0.75	6.23	5.93
1.00	8.23	10.75
1.25	8.38	12.20
1.50	11.50	18.43
2.00	20.50	26.35
3.00	14.10	20.25
4.00	9.88	13.63
6.00	6.38	5.90
9.00	1.35	1.38
12.00	2.38	1.30
24.00	0.10	0.10

be an accurate (i.e., unbiased) representation of the population, because the samples of subjects were undoubtedly not selected randomly.

Table 12.4 gives the averages of the original concentration vs. time data shown in Table 12.1 for the same four subjects, using drugs 1 and 2. Note that these figures are the means at each sampling time, whereas those in Table 12.3 are averages of the *maximum* concentrations, at whatever time they occurred. Only four subjects were used to simplify the presentation of the derived responses. The data of Table 12.4 are plotted in Figure 12.3. The plot using the small hollow squares is that for drug 1; that using the small solid circles represents drug 2.

We now briefly describe the analysis of data from all 12 subjects, but we will use only the C_{max} responses.

Results of C_{max} Analysis (12 Subjects)
Complete univariate analyses for all 12 subjects were done separately for each of the four responses, although we discuss the C_{max} analysis only. Remember that this trial was a pilot study and was not run to compare drugs. However, we discuss the comparison procedures here so that they will serve as a reference for you. The details of the randomized-blocks analysis, which is best done using an analysis of variance, are not described, because this book does not cover the use of that technique. However, your biostatistician will be very familiar with the procedure; if you are interested and have time, you can find it described in any of several of the books listed in the Bibliography: for example, Neter et al. [37], Dixon and Massey [33], Snedecor and Cochran [38], and Davies [14].

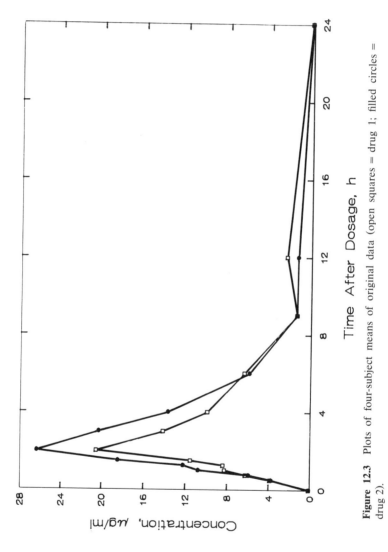

Figure 12.3 Plots of four-subject means of original data (open squares = drug 1; filled circles = drug 2).

Table 12.5. C_{max} Data for Randomized-Blocks Changeover Analysis for 12 Subjects (Example 12.2)

Subject	Drug T_1	Drug T_2
1	21.4	37.8
2	15.8	13.7
3	14.7	42.3
4	45.8	18.3
5	32.5	28.5
6	30.0	25.2
7	34.5	46.1
8	19.9	28.1
9	31.6	69.1
10	39.5	85.2
11	50.5	49.5
12	34.5	26.2
Sum	370.7	470.0
N	12	12
Mean	30.89	39.17
Difference	8.28	

The two drugs compared in a bioavailability study almost invariably have the same or very similar active ingredients. But despite this identity or close similarity, they will represent two different dosage forms or two different formulations, will have been made by two different manufacturing procedures, or will otherwise have been treated in two different ways, so that their bioavailabilities may be different. The purpose of the statistical analysis is to look for any such differences that appear greater than delta.

Table 12.5 shows the C_{max} data for all 12 subjects. The sums and mean values for the 12 data for each of the two treatments, and the difference between the means, are also given. In this example, there were 12 blocks of two data each. The blocks were the 12 subjects, and the two data occupied the two plots (experimental units) within each of the subjects. In Table 12.5, each row thus represents one block. These data were analyzed statistically as a randomized blocks model to assess whether the sample difference was large enough to justify the conclusion that the population values of the two C_{max} means were different, using preset values of alpha (0.05) and beta (0.10). Because the trial was not originally designed to compare treatments, no preset delta value had been specified. Delta was nevertheless calculated a posteriori and found to be approximately 21 $\mu g/ml$.

In the analysis, the treatments were not significantly different (the probability found was between 0.10 and 0.25). The difference between the sample means is given in Table 12.5; it was 8.28 $\mu g/ml$, substantially smaller than the delta value found. Sigma was estimated from the data to be 14.7327.[5] By using the Bratcher et al. tables in the appendix, it was estimated that about 70 subjects would be required to detect a difference between the population means if delta were 8 (the approximate difference found here) and such a difference continued to exist.

It is recommended that the statistician analyzing any data of this kind for your firm follow the usual careful practice of plotting residuals from the RBs model and examining them carefully to ensure that the data form a reasonable fit. This suggestion sounds obvious, but it is often not followed.

Final Remarks

This concludes Example 12.1 and the section on randomized blocks as a changeover design. Again, although the example was presented in terms of a bioavailability study, similar procedures would be used for any changeover study with k treatments, using patients or subjects as randomized blocks.

Both the randomized-blocks changeover design and the two-period crossover described next can be extended to more than two treatments. The extension of the two-period crossover is called a Williams latin square design in this book, and is described briefly in this chapter. The extension of the randomized complete blocks design is still called randomized blocks; it merely uses larger blocks (i.e., more plots per block).

12.4 THE TWO-PERIOD CROSSOVER DESIGN

12.4.1 Description

This design, like the previous one, can be used for other purposes in addition to bioavailability studies. The difficulties mentioned here may not exist in such cases.

The two-period crossover superficially resembles the two-treatment randomized-blocks design with patients as blocks. The differences are in the randomization procedures (sometimes) and in the statistical procedures used in the analysis (always). For the randomized-blocks design, the sequence of the two treatments is determined randomly *and independently* for each block (i.e., disregarding the order of the treatments in any other blocks). For the crossover design, there are two possible randomization procedures, both of which can be analyzed correctly. In the first, the same procedure as that just described for randomized blocks is used. In the second, a constraint is imposed; viz., *equal* numbers of patients or subjects are randomly assigned to receive drug 1 and drug 2 first. When the first procedure is used, more patients may be assigned, by chance, to one sequence than to the other. But

[5]This is S_{xi}, the sample standard deviation for individual measurements, obtained by taking the square root of the error mean square in the randomized blocks analysis of variance.

unless the trial is very small, the proportions of patients assigned to the two sequences will nearly always be reasonably similar. That procedure is the one we recommend in this book,[6] although it is not yet widely used.

12.4.2 Problems and Advantages of the Design

Today, the clinical use of the two-period crossover design is restricted almost entirely to bioavailability tests. It was formerly broadly employed in a variety of small clinical trials, but its widespread misuse, especially the employment of incorrect analyses,[7] has gradually reduced its popularity. The design (in some cases) and the analysis (always) of the two-period crossover design are different from those appropriate for randomized blocks. As well as the risk of misuse, the design can have a possible inherent problem, which can be severe. If the restricted randomization method (equal sample sizes) is used, and a sequence effect test is used before the planned crossover analysis, the statistician may find that the second period data are not analyzable. The remaining alternative is then to analyze the first period data only, as a simple parallel design. However, it will be likely that the sample size is too small to permit an informative analysis, both because that single period comprises a parallel design, and also because it now provides only half of the observations originally done. There is then no recourse but to begin over with a new trial.

The major advantage of the two-period crossover is that its analysis isolates the effect of periods and carryovers as well as blocks and treatments, whereas the randomized-blocks analysis does not take these effects into account, but confounds them with the random error term. For this reason, if a periods effect is present and sizable, as is not rare, the use of the crossover analysis will provide more powerful hypothesis tests. As you will see, however, if there is also a *sequence effect*, that analysis cannot be used.

Besides the promise of greater power, another reason for the use of the two-period crossover design is custom. The FDA suggests it in some of their Guidelines, but, on the other hand, some FDA statisticians have warned

---

[6]Cochran and Cox [11], p. 128, describe only the method using equal numbers of subjects in both sequences. Much work has been done on the two-period crossover since that book was written, however, and the use of the same randomization procedure used for randomized blocks allows the use of a randomized-blocks analysis if the assumption of no sequence effect (see what follows), implicit in the two-period crossover analysis, appears incorrect. The most detailed and complete modern summary of the randomization and analysis that I have found is that of Hills and Armitage {10}; see the crossover section of the references.

[7]For those interested, the correct analysis of a two-period crossover is a three-factor analysis of variance, preceded by a test for a so-called *sequence effect*. It is incorrect, for example, to take differences between the two responses in each block and then do a *t* test or the equivalent of these differences, as can be done legitimately if the patients constitute randomized blocks. The *t* test of differences does not isolate the periods effect, and therefore increases the error term. It is poor judgment to omit a sequence-effect test. If such an effect exists, the difference between the two treatments will vary depending upon which is given first, and may be greater for one sequence than for the other. Thus, those differences will be biased, perhaps severely.

strongly against its use. You are generally on much firmer ground when you use randomized blocks with patients as the blocks, despite the loss of power. Nevertheless, we describe the crossover here because it is still fairly widely used, and it is frequently successful if adequate care is exercised.

12.4.3 References

Before using the two-period crossover design, if your statistician has used it only occasionally, it is strongly recommended that he or she obtain and study at least some of the papers cited in the special section enclosed in braces, especially those marked with asterisks. These cover many aspects of the application and analysis of this design, and point out the pitfalls that can be encountered with it. The most important papers in the group are those by Hills and Armitage {10} and Fleiss, Wallenstein, and Rosenfeld {6}.

12.4.4 Randomization of the Two-Period Crossover

Here are details of the two methods of randomization; see also Hills and Armitage {10}. The first method produces equal sample sizes for the two sequences. The second will almost always yield unequal numbers of patients in the two sequences, but, as already mentioned, the difference will rarely be extreme enough to be important. The first method has been much more frequently used for the two-period crossover design in the past. The second is a better procedure, however, because, if you use it but then find that you cannot carry out an effective data analysis assuming a crossover design, a randomized-blocks analysis may then be done.

1. First Method

Use some valid random method of choosing which treatment is to be given in the first period, such as the procedure using odd and even random numbers described for randomized blocks in Section 12.3.4. The sample must contain an even number of subjects. Begin by assigning treatments to periods for each subject independently. As soon as assignments of one of the two configurations or sequences (D_1, then D_2 or D_2, then D_1) have been made for half of the planned number of patients or subjects, make the remaining assignments using the opposite configuration.[8] When you are done, if there are no losses of data during the execution of the trial, half of the assignments will specify D_1 first, and the other half will specify D_2. Data losses during execution of the trial that unbalance this arrangement are not a problem, because the

---

[8]That is, when half of the subjects or patients have been assigned to one of the two configurations and an equal or smaller number to the other. (When this point is reached, unless all assignments so far have been for one of the two sequences exclusively, an event of extremely low probability, you will have completed more than half the assignments.)

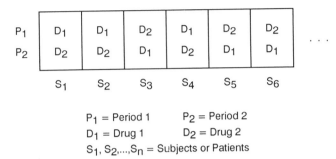

Figure 12.4 Generalized two-period crossover design.

method of analysis can take that into account. Figure 12.4 is a generic diagram of the design, and shows the randomization, which was done as just described, using a table of random numbers.

2. Second Method

Proceed exactly as described for randomized blocks (Section 12.3.4). This will usually result in two sequences having unequal numbers of subjects or patients assigned to them, as indicated, but the unbalance will rarely be extreme. This kind of randomization was illustrated in Example 12.1.

If you use the randomization method normally used for randomized blocks (method 2), the preparation for the two designs will be identical. That method is therefore the one that you should always use, because either method of analysis can then be used. See Hills and Armitage {10}. If you use method 1 instead, the crossover analysis must be used, and if trouble (a sequence effect, see Section 12.4.6) is encountered, there will be no recourse except to revert to a much less powerful analysis that probably will not show significance even if there is a substantial population difference between the two drug products. On the other hand, if you randomize with method 2, it will be correct to use either a randomized-blocks or a crossover analysis. The statistician then can plan to use the crossover analysis first, because of the likelihood that it will have greater power. Then, if there is a sequence effect that invalidates that analysis, the statistician can switch to the randomized-blocks procedure. That procedure will be less powerful, but will avoid the sequence effect problem. Of course, this procedure should be preplanned and described in the protocol, mentioning the possibility of using the RBs analysis if the crossover analysis fails. It is also advisable, when estimating the sample size, to assume that the design will be randomized blocks. This will result in a slightly greater sample size, as will be necessary if you must use the RBs analysis.

Many designs differ in numbers of ways. However, these two designs constitute perhaps a unique exception, because, if you use the second method of randomization, the only difference will be the method of analysis.

12.4.5   Representation of the Design

Despite the similarity of the two-period crossover to randomized blocks with patients as blocks, the design is conventionally represented in a different way (the "blocks" representing the subjects are joined together), perhaps to make a distinction between the two. This method of representation is that which was apparently introduced by Cochran and Cox [11] and used in both editions of their book. It is illustrated by the generalized two-period crossover design of Figure 12.4. In this illustration, six subjects, or patients, are shown, but, as the ellipsis at the right end of the diagram implies, there may be any number. In Figure 12.4, there are equal numbers of each sequence, although, as indicated, this is not necessary.

12.4.6   Carryover (Sequence) Effects

Description
A sequence effect is an interaction between treatments and orders. When such an effect is present, the difference between the two treatments varies according to the order in which the two drugs were given. When the response to a given treatment depends upon which treatment precedes it, we say that there is a carryover effect. Therefore, a carryover effect is a sequence effect. A sequence effect can also be regarded as a form of interaction between periods and treatments, because the order used is a characteristic of the period when the randomization is method 1 (equal numbers of patients with each order (drug 1 first vs. drug 2 first). However, in this book, when we refer to a sequence effect as an interaction, we will think of it as an interaction between treatments and orders.

Testing for Sequence Effects
Most users of the "standard" two-period crossover design in the past used equal numbers of subjects, although equal numbers are unnecessary. This "standard" model took the periods, subjects, and treatments effects into account, but could not compare treatment differences in the two sequences. As pointed out by Hills and Armitage {10}, the validity of that analysis, therefore, depended upon the assumption of no sequence effect, so that any difference between drugs in terms of a given response variable would be the same in both sequence groups. Yet it has been discovered by many who have worked with the design that this assumption can, not infrequently, be seriously in error. A precaution, therefore, has been to carry out a separate sequence-effects test on the data of a trial before running the standard analysis. Such a sequence-effect test, however, uses a "between-subjects"

error estimate, so that it has rather poor statistical power, considering that the trials are normally run with fairly small samples. A partial remedy is to use an alpha level of 0.10 rather than the usual 0.05 or 0.01.

If the sequence effect test is significant, the standard two-period crossover data analysis cannot be used, because the sequence effects will be confounded with the treatments information. It then becomes necessary to analyze the first period data only, which is usually unsatisfactory, as mentioned before, or to repeat the trial. On the other hand, if significance is not found in the sequence effect test, doubt as to the presence of such a problem will nevertheless remain, because the sample size is often too small for adequate power, both because of the usually small sample size in such trials and because of the use of the between-subjects error estimate.

Remedies If There Is a Sequence Effect

Because the two drugs tested in a two-treatment comparative bioavailability test will be similar in almost all cases, with the same active ingredient, it may be thought that a sequence effect is unlikely. This may be true, but the number of cases in which one is nevertheless found is sufficiently frequent to make it advisable to check and to take the recommended steps when one is found. In my experience, sequence effects occur in a surprising number of two-period crossover trials, whether they are bioavailability trials or not. They can be avoided by the use of an adequate washout period between the two drugs. However, the half-lives of the drugs are often not known accurately, and the washout may consequently not be long enough.

Recognition of the possibility of an undetected sequence effect is the principal reason that has led to the reduction in general use of the two-period crossover design outside of the field of bioavailability, although a sequence effect can be detected if the sample size is adequate. In the past, however, very few users of the crossover attempted to do so.

The test for a sequence effect and the possibility of having to repeat a trial can both be avoided by randomizing the assignments of drugs to subjects as if a randomized-blocks design is to be used, as described earlier. All things considered, this is the best compromise unless you are somehow certain that no sequence effect can exist, an unlikely assumption.

12.4.7   Example 12.3: The Two-Period Crossover Design

Discussion

This example uses the same data as those for Example 12.1. Note again that these data originated from a pilot trial. A trial with a sample size as small as this (12 subjects) is unlikely to be adequate for any purpose except those of a pilot trial, that is, it will probably not be adequate for the detection of reasonable treatment differences. This remark applies even more strongly to the detection of a sequence effect.

We will resort to our usual calculations of mean values when discussing the outcome of the trial, but the results of the actual statistical analysis will also be given. Because of their complexity, however, and because detailed statistical procedures beyond the simplest kind are not among the major purposes of this book, those procedures themselves will not be given. Interested readers will find a complete description of a generalized analysis in the appendix to the Hills and Armitage {10} paper. That analysis can be easily programmed for your computer. Most studies in this category are relatively small, so it can also be programmed on a scientific pocket calculator or a laptop computer.

This study provides a good example of some of the difficulties that can be met with in running a comparative bioavailability test. First, the sequence group sizes were unequal, which makes the study more realistic at the expense of a bit more complexity in the analysis. Second, some of the data were more scattered than had been hoped. Third, the tails of some of the curves did not return closely to the baseline, perhaps because, for some subjects, traces of the materials unexpectedly remained in the bloodstream at 24 hours. In these cases, the computation of legitimate AUC or $t_{0.5}$ values seemed impossible in some cases, and only C_{max} and T_{max} responses were available for both drugs and all 12 subjects. In some cases, reasonable values were available for only one of the two drugs for a given subject, rendering the other one useless. There are methods for "balancing" sets of data by restoring missing values, but these were not felt to be appropriate in this case. In this example, therefore, we again used C_{max} as the response to be analyzed.

Sample Size Estimation and Randomization
Although the estimation of sample size in this example was not necessary because the trial was a pilot trial, if you use a two-period crossover design in a clinical study, whether it is a bioavailability trial or not, you should, of course, estimate sample size beforehand. In comparative bioavailability studies, you will be looking for experimental assurance that the two products to be compared are indeed similar enough in bioavailability to meet your requirements as well as those of the FDA. Thus, you will usually be seeking nonsignificance, a result opposite to that for which you customarily look. You will wish to choose the *largest* difference between the two products that can be tolerated as your specification of delta, rather than the usual smallest clinically significant difference. Then, if you do not find significance, you will have assurance at probability beta that the two products differ by delta or less in their bioavailabilities. If you do find significance, you should conclude that the bioavailabilities of the two products are too different for your purposes. Therefore, with probability beta of being wrong, you may be hoping to find a difference *less than* delta regardless of its direction.

In some cases, even in comparative bioavailability testing, however, you may wish to test whether a new dosage form has *greater* bioavailability than another (peaks earlier, has greater AUC, etc.). If so, you will then be interested in the level of alpha as well as beta and the finding of either nonsignificance or significance. For example, if you are comparing a new dosage form of a drug with the old, the new product may sometimes be acceptable to you in either of two cases: (a) if the two forms are indistinguishable or (b) if the new form is superior in bioavailability, within reason. The sample size estimation for this design is described in the papers by Grizzle {7}, Lee, Kantrowitz, and Mullis {13}, Willan and Pater {16, 17}, and Willan {18} in the crossover reference section at the end of this chapter (Section 12.7.3). Also, the Borenstein-Cohen [67] program cited in the Bibliography allows the estimation of sample size for factorial designs, as does the *Design* supplement to the SYSTAT software (Dallal [66]). However, if you follow the advice given earlier and randomize the assignments as if the data were to be analyzed as a randomized-blocks design, you should estimate the sample size under that assumption also. Then, whether the statistician finds a sequence effect or simply prefers to be conservative, accordingly analyzing the data as a randomized-blocks design, the sample size will have been large enough for that design under the original specifications of alpha, beta, and delta.

An excellent approximation for obtaining the sample size for a randomized-blocks design is described in Chapter 15; see the Bratcher et al. tables referred to there. These tables are designed primarily for one-way ANOVA designs, but, as the authors point out, as a practical matter, it is easy to obtain very reasonable approximations for randomized blocks also. Because that design will usually be less powerful than the crossover (if the periods effect is substantial), the resulting sample size will usually be larger than that required for the crossover.

The randomization procedure has already been described under "Sample Size Estimation and Randomization" above for this example.

Design

Figure 12.4 in Section 12.4.5 is a generalized diagram of the design. Before a crossover analysis of the data is carried out, a sequence effect test should be run. In this example, the design is a realization of that shown in Figure 12.4, using 12 subjects. Figure 12.5 diagrams the entire experiment, with the assignments of the drugs to the periods shown for each subject. In this figure, P = periods, D = drugs, and S = subjects. The two sequence groups are (a) those subjects having D_1 in the first period and D_2 in the second, and (b) those with the opposite arrangement. Note that there were unequal numbers of patients in the two sequence groups, five who received D_1 in the first period and seven who were given D_2 first.

Data

The C_{max} data are the same as those shown in Table 12.5, but they are shown again in Table 12.6, this time separating the two sequence groups. The sequence-effect test asks whether these two groups have significantly differ-

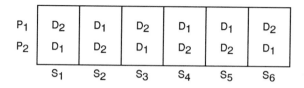

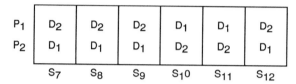

Figure 12.5 Example 12.3: Structure of two-period crossover design (randomization shown).

ent means. The table shows the C_{max} responses by subject numbers, the sequence used, and the treatments. The individual differences between treatments are included because they are related to the presence or absence of any treatments–sequences interaction.

Analyses of Data
The analyses of data as a crossover are not shown in this book, but they follow the general recommendations of Hills and Armitage {10}. This section is principally for the information of your biostatistician.

Table 12.6. C_{max} Data (Example 12.3)

Subject	Group 1 (T$_1$ in Period 1)			Group 2 (T$_1$ in Period 2)		
	T_1	T_2	D_1 $(T_1 - T_2)$	T_2	T_1	D_2 $(T_1 - T_2)$
1				37.8	21.4	− 16.4
2	15.8	13.7	2.1			
3				42.3	14.7	− 27.6
4	45.8	18.3	27.5			
5	32.5	28.5	4.0			
6				25.2	30.0	4.8
7				46.1	34.5	− 11.6
8				28.1	19.9	− 8.2
9				69.1	31.6	− 37.5
10	39.5	85.2	− 45.7			
11	50.5	49.5	1.0			
12				26.2	34.5	8.3

The data of this example were tested for a sequence effect, and none was found. Nevertheless, the analysis used when this trial was actually run was that for randomized blocks. This example of the crossover is presented only to demonstrate the preparations for and the results of such an analysis. The major steps and conclusions are illustrated by comparing means, as was done in some of our earlier examples.

For the test for a sequence effect, we recommend the use of an alpha value of 0.10, to help compensate for the expected relatively low power of this test. If a sequence effect is not found, the data may be analyzed as a two-period crossover. If there is a sequence effect, the randomized-blocks analysis should be used instead (it is assumed that the randomization was done as recommended). Some statisticians, however, will feel it desirable to use the RBs analysis in any event.

Assuming, for illustration, that the absence of a sequence effect has been satisfactorily demonstrated, the data were analyzed as a crossover for this example. This analysis was run as described in the Hills and Armitage paper {10}. There was no significant difference between the treatments ($p =$ approximate 0.25). The individual treatment means were 30.89 (T_1) and 39.17 (T_2), differing by -8.28.

12.4.8   Conclusions and Summation

The analysis of two-period crossover data can be surrounded by pitfalls. To avoid trouble, it is therefore advisable to follow the procedures outlined in the previous paragraphs. In particular, if you take the precaution of randomizing the treatment assignments using the randomized-blocks procedure and use a sample size adequate for that design, you can then either ask your biostatistician to analyze your data as randomized blocks or, at least, have that analysis to fall back upon if he or she is forced to abandon a two-period crossover analysis. If you do this, there will never be a need to discard the second period data and analyze the first period using a parallel model, as has been recommended in the past. The management of two-period changeover designs is a fine example of the need for planning ahead carefully when devising a clinical study.

12.5   OTHER CHANGEOVER DESIGNS

12.5.1   Introduction

In addition to randomized blocks and the two-period crossover, there are several other designs in which patients or subjects can be used as the blocks. The best known among these are incomplete randomized blocks, latin squares (the "l" is intentionally lower case), and Youden squares (incomplete latin squares). All three designs are rare in ethical drug trials, although Youden squares have been widely employed in antiperspirant evaluations of proprietary products (3, 4, 5). Among the latin squares, however, a particular type called a **Williams latin square** is useful when more than two materials are to be compared for bioavailability. The FDA has issued a Guideline describing the use of this design, although it does not identify it as a Williams design. Essentially, it balances the number of subjects assigned to each of several sequences, assigning equal numbers of subjects to each. For example, with four drugs, there are 24 possible sequences or permutations, but only four of them, $A/B/D/C$, $B/C/A/D$, $C/D/B/A$, and $D/A/C/B$ are needed. Using these four, and repeating the design a sufficient number of times to provide an adequate sample size, results in each drug being preceded by each of the others (excluding itself) once among each set of four subjects. Thus, any incidence of carryover effects can be controlled and isolated in the analysis of the data.

12.6   RECAPITULATION AND SUMMARY OF THE CHAPTER

12.6.1   Recapitulation

The primary purpose of this book is to present and explain the principles of experimental design and related topics for medical and paramedical professionals in the pharmaceutical industry. After the introductory material in Chapters 1 through 7, Chapters 8 through this one presented more detailed information and examples pertaining to the better-known designs used for these purposes. Part IV is much less extensive, but will supply a modicum of background in statistical analysis and will describe several simple test procedures. It is important to include this information because of the close connection between a given design and the appropriate analysis, as well as to foster understanding of the estimation of sample size. Part IV is emphatically *not* meant to equip you to carry out statistical data analyses unaided, unless you already have some experience and training in doing so.

Finally, Part V will provide a working knowledge of a few common procedures for estimating the sample size (numbers of patients) needed in a clinical study. You should have this knowledge even if the statistician does most of the estimates, and it should be used for nearly every trial you design. It is important, if at all possible, that you learn to use these procedures yourself if you have time, as they are truly an integral part of your planning activities.

12.6.2   Summary of the Chapter

This chapter has been concerned with *changeover* designs. A changeover design is one in which each patient receives more than one of the treatments. This is in contrast to a parallel design, in which each patient receives only one. In a parallel design, the patients are the experimental units. In a changeover, each patient "contains" two or more experimental units; these are the successive time periods, or plots, in which the treatments are given. We call these changeovers *temporal* changeover designs.

Changeover designs in which the plots in each block are *temporal* are the most common kind in clinical trials. However, in this chapter, we also refer to and briefly describe what we call *spatial* changeovers. In these, a set of treatments is repeated at two or more locations on a patient's body, for instance, a series of places on the skin of the back or abdomen. In earlier chapters, we have described other types of designs that involve locations, for example, designs in which a set of treatments is replicated at two or more centers. In the sense commonly used in medical statistics, however, those designs are parallel, because the blocks are not identified with patients.

After some introductory material, because bioavailability comparisons are very commonly done using changeover designs, there is a section on bioavailability testing. The remainder of the chapter is concerned with the two designs that comprise the vast majority of changeovers in clinical studies. These are randomized blocks and the two-period crossover. A third design, the Williams latin square, is briefly described, because it is widely used in comparative bioavailability trials when there are more than two treatments. Finally, several other designs are mentioned briefly, principally to indicate that many different designs of this kind exist and are used, albeit rarely, in clinical trials.

The first of the two major designs described is randomized blocks, but in which, unlike the randomized blocks designs described earlier, the blocks are the patients or subjects. This design is discussed in some detail, and an example using a small set of data representing an actual comparative bioavailability trial is included.[9] You will remember that the same design was described in the previous chapter, with the exception that the blocks were not subjects or patients.

The second important changeover design is the two-period crossover design. This structure is commonly used in clinical trials, especially in bioavailability studies, but there are difficulties, often unrecognized, in using it. One is the use of differences from baseline in each of the two periods, which is commonly done but can seriously distort the outcome of the analysis (Fleiss et al. {6}). However, this is easily remedied by avoiding that use of baseline data. A second and more serious difficulty (because the remedy is less obvious) is a possible so-called sequence effect.

---

[9]Earlier in this book, we described a difference design, which can be analyzed by a *t* test of differences (the dependent *t* test). Its analysis is described in Part IV. For this design, each of a group of patients is given two treatments, in random order. After running the trial and obtaining a response from each patient after each treatment, the difference between the two measurements for each patient is calculated and analyzed. This structure is actually a randomized-blocks design, with two treatments (blocks of two). When each block contains more than two treatments, the *t* test is no longer appropriate, at least in the ordinary way.

A sequence effect is an interaction between the *orders* of treatment of the subjects and the drug treatments themselves. It is manifested as a difference between drugs that varies with the order of their administration. It is related to carryover effects, in which a given drug is affected by the one preceding it, distorting its effect. Because "orders" cannot exist except in terms of time periods, it is also a form of interaction between periods and treatments. It is pointed out that these phenomena can seriously bias the results of a two-period crossover design unless suitable precautions are taken. A properly-designed randomized blocks study, however, although moderately less powerful than the crossover, does not possess this disadvantage because of the randomization of the orders in each block. The use of randomized blocks instead of the crossover, when possible, is therefore advised. However, in spite of the problems with the two-period crossover design, it is recognized that there are times when it may be desirable to use it. With this in mind, it is possible, using a correct randomization procedure, to arrange things so that the same structure can be analyzed as a two-period crossover or as randomized blocks.

For further study, a special set of literature references to the two-period crossover, its analysis and its problems, appears at the end of the chapter.

12.7 LITERATURE REFERENCES

12.7.1 About This Listing

The references to this chapter are divided into two separate sections. Each is numbered in a separate series. The first set, the *General References*, uses parentheses to number the items and to reference citations in the text, which is the arrangement used in most of the chapters in this book. The second set, comprising the references to the literature on the two-period crossover design, uses braces.

The second group of references to papers on the two-period crossover comprises the larger group of references for this chapter and represents a fair proportion of the literature published in English about this design up to 1988. It consists of 18 papers that are important in the application of the two-period crossover design to clinical trial work. Many of the authors are well-known, and all are highly competent in their fields. Although some of the papers will require study, I believe they are important reading if your statistician uses or expects to use this frustrating design. All the papers relate to applied work and all are relevant to the material in this chapter. Asterisks follow the reference numbers of the seven that I consider the most important. Note that many of these papers include information about analysis as well as design, and three of them discuss sample size and power.

12.7.2 General References

(1) Kligman, A. M. and W. M. Wooding, "A Method for the Measurement and Evaluation of Irritants on Human Skin," *The Journal of Investigative Dermatology*, 49, 78–94 (1967).

(2) Williams, E. J., "Experimental Designs Balanced for the Estimation of Residual Effects of Treatments," *Australian Journal of Scientific Research*, A, 2, 149–168 (1949).

(3) Wooding, W. M., and Paul Finkelstein, "A Critical Comparison of Two Procedures for Antiperspirant Testing," *Journal of the Society of Cosmetic Chemists*, 26, 255–275 (1975).

(4) Wooding, W. M., "Interpretations of Gravimetric Axillar Antiperspirant Data," *Proceedings, Joint Conference on Cosmetic Sciences* (sponsored by The Toilet Goods Association, The Society of Cosmetic Chemists and The Food and Drug Administration), 1968, pp. 91–105.

(5) Murphy, Thomas D., and Mark J. Levine, "Analysis of Antiperspirant Efficacy Test Results," *Journal of the Society of Cosmetic Chemists*, 42, 167–197 (1991).

12.7.3 References to Papers on the Two-Period Crossover Design

{1} Brandt, A. E., "Tests of Significance in Reversal or Switchback Trials," *Research Bulletin*, 234, Agricultural Experiment Station, Iowa State College of Agricultural and Mechanic Arts, 60–87 (1938).

{2}* Brown, Byron W., Jr., "The Crossover Experiment for Clinical Trials," *Biometrics*, 36, 69–79 (1980).

{3} Castellana, J. V., and H. I. Patel, "Analysis of Two-Period Crossover Design in a Multicenter Clinical Trial," *Proceedings of the Biopharmaceutical Section*, American Statistical Association, Philadelphia, PA, 1984, pp. 72–77.

{4} Chassan, J. B., "A Note on Relative Efficiency in Clinical Trials," *Journal of Clinical Pharmacology*, 10, 359–360 (1970).

{5} Chassan, J. B., "On the Analysis of Simple Cross-Overs with Unequal Numbers of Replicates," *Biometrics*, 25, 206–208 (1964).

{6}* Fleiss, Joseph L., Sylvan Wallenstein, and Robert Rosenfeld, "Adjusting for Baseline Measurements in the Two-Period Crossover Study: A Cautionary Note," *Controlled Clinical Trials*, 6, 192–197 (1985).

{7}* Grizzle, James E., "The Two-Period Change-Over Design and its Use in Clinical Trials," *Biometrics*, 21, 467–480 (1965). See also the corrections to this paper listed in {8} and {9}.

{8}* Grizzle, James E., Correction to item {7}, *Biometrics*, 30, 727 (1974).

{9}* Grieve, A. P., Correction to item {7}, *Biometrics*, 38, 517 (1982).

{10}* Hills, M., and P. Armitage, "The Two-Period Cross-Over Clinical Trial," *British Journal of Clinical Pharmacology*, 8, 7–20 (1979).

{11}* Kershner, Ronald P., and Walter T. Federer, "Two-Treatment Crossover Designs for Estimating a Variety of Effects," *Journal of the American Statistical Association*, 76, 612–619 (1981).

{12}* Koch, G. G., The Use of Non-Parametric Methods in the Statistical Analysis of the Two-Period Change-Over Design," *Biometrics*, 28, 577–584 (1972).

{13} Lee, Martin L., Julia L. Kantrowitz, and Charles E. Mullis, "Sample Size, Cross-Over Trials and the Problem of Treatment Equivalence," *Proceedings of the Biopharmaceutical Section*, American Statistical Association, Philadelphia, PA, 1984, pp. 78–80 (1984).

{14}* Louis, Thomas L., et al., "Crossover and Self-Controlled Designs in Clinical Research," *The New England Journal of Medicine*, 310, 24–31 (1984).

{15} Wallenstein, Sylvan, and Alan C. Fisher, "The Analysis of the Two-Period Repeated Measures Crossover Design with Application to Clinical Trials," *Biometrics*, 33, 261–269 (1977).

{16} Willan, Andrew R., and Joseph L. Pater, "Using Baseline Measurements in the Two-Period Crossover Clinical Trial," *Controlled Clinical Trials*, 7, 282–289 (1986).

{17} Willan, Andrew R., and Joseph L. Pater, "Carryover and the Two-Period Crossover Clinical Trial," *Biometrics*, 42, 593–599 (1986).

{18} Willan, Andrew R., "Using the Maximum Test Statistic in the Two-Period Crossover Clinical Trial," *Biometrics*, 44, 211–218 (1988).

PART IV

Basic Statistical Analysis

CHAPTER 13

Data Analysis: Fundamental Ideas

13.1 INTRODUCTION

13.1.1 Do You Need a Thorough Background in Statistical Analysis?

Not unless you expect to do some or all of your own analyses. In this book, we have assumed that you will select your experimental designs and their related procedures, such as randomization, response measurements, and sample size estimation, but that there is a biostatistician available to undertake the responsibility for the analysis of all or most of your trial data. However, as we have emphasized throughout, you cannot specify an experimental design, a randomization, a sample size estimation procedure, or a response measurement without determining or at least influencing the choice of an analysis method. Therefore, if you are to plan and be responsible to clinical studies, you must have some knowledge of the statistical methods and rationale of the data analyses. Some of that information, including the principles of hypothesis testing, has been described earlier and need only be reviewed and exemplified here. Other details, such as specific descriptions and examples of basic methods of analysis, have yet to be explained. This chapter and the next are designed to satisfy those needs.

We are aware that some readers may feel that this background is not necessary, even in the absence of any previous statistical training. Our response is that you can probably prevail without these chapters or their equivalent, but the material presented here represents a minimum that will, at the very least, be extremely helpful.

The examples in these chapters were designed to help familiarize you with the basic principles of statistical analysis in clinical work. Ideally, it would be advantageous to study and work out each one carefully yourself, being sure that you obtain the same answers as those given, and then perhaps repeating them with your own data. If you do so, do not attempt to understand everything in a first reading, but try to return to it later and read it again more closely. After a period of time, without, meanwhile, giving the matter any conscious thought, you will find that a second reading will often result in much greater illumination. Do not attempt to memorize anything. Even after a first perusal, you will retain a great deal. We purposely did not include problems for practice, because it is unlikely that you would find time for them or be inclined to use them in any event. But do study, and, if possible, carry out the examples. When information is needed later, you will then know where to find it.

13.2 STATISTICAL DATA ANALYSIS

13.2.1 Introduction

In the pharmaceutical industry, most clinical trials consist of the evaluation of drugs or drug combinations, but some are also concerned with doses, methods of dosage, supplementary treatments, or combinations of these things. Clinical trials are nearly always confirmatory, as mentioned earlier. As a rule, they are done for two purposes. First, sponsors must be sure that the drugs or other treatments are safe and effective, giving reasonable promise of becoming useful and reliable, and consequently profitable. Second, they must satisfy legal requirements with the aim of obtaining approval from the FDA to market them, accompanied by claims of efficacy and safety in accomplishing their stated purposes.

The statistical procedures described in the next chapter are confined to the simplest and most fundamental. All are commonly used in the data analysis of clinical trials. In this chapter, we try to provide the basic information needed to understand them thoroughly, and to use them if you have time and are so inclined. More complex procedures are not described in this book, although some are often needed in the analyses of clinical trial data. However, all are described repeatedly in the literature, including many of the books listed in the Bibliography. Your statistician will be, or should be, familiar with all of them, but those described here are sufficient to acquaint you with the general points of view and procedures of statistical tests. A little of this information has been introduced previously but needs reiteration and more thorough coverage. Although we will not include any further information about randomization or distribution theory, the principles of hypothesis testing need to be covered more completely, as they are basis of most the analyses done in clinical studies. We also review the kinds of measurements normally used as responses, and we discuss some other topics that have been covered only sketchily in the earlier chapters.

To summarize this introductory section, then, the purposes of this and the next chapter are as follows: (a) To provide some acquaintance with the idea of analysis if you lack training or experience with it; this will help you to avoid planning and using designs requiring statistical analyses with low statistical power or other disadvantageous characteristics. (b) To supply the background needed to enable you to use the sample size estimation procedures described Chapter 15. (c) To further clarify and reinforce some of the statistical concepts introduced earlier. (d) To help you to understand your biostatistician's jargon so that you can work with him or her effectively. (e) Finally, but not least important, to assist you in explaining the results of your trials and the reasons for your selection of particular designs to laymen as well as to the FDA in your oral and written presentations and reports.

13.2.2 The Purposes of Data Analysis

The analyses we have been referring to throughout this book and discuss here are **comparisons**. In the most obvious case, they are used to compare a new drug with a placebo to show whether it is effective or not for its intended purpose, and whether it appears to produce more adverse effects than the placebo. Or you compare it with a standard to see whether it equals or exceeds that material in efficacy or in the generation of adverse effects. In a less obvious case, the item or value you are using for comparison with your test drug(s) or treatment(s) may not be run **concurrently** with the test material or treatment. Although we have warned you about the use of historical controls or "before-and-after" tests, it is nevertheless obvious that if such tests are run, they also are comparisons, although the drugs or treatments used for comparison have been run previously, not concurrently. As a third case, frequently, you will be comparing a drug effect with a fixed value or specification as a standard. For example, in a difference trial, you may wish to know whether a difference between two drugs (usually in the form of an average or mean of several individual differences) is or is not equal to zero, or perhaps whether it is at least as great as some previously specified difference such as delta. In these cases, the sample differences are compared to zero or delta. There are still other and less obvious comparisons made in experimental work, although these three cases are the most common in clinical studies. To emphasize the point, every clinical trial is run to make some kind of a comparison. A drug or a treatment cannot be evaluated without comparing it with something.

Another point that has not been emphasized adequately up to now, because it is principally relevant to the topic of data analysis, is that most clinical trials are done for *confirmatory* rather than research (*exploratory*) purposes. This is one reason that it is so important to make and to follow an initial plan precisely. In most of the clinical trials discussed in this book, and in clinical trials in general (with the possible exception of a few Phase I trials), exploratory data analysis, in which data are examined and manipulated in various ways to discover new possibilities about the treatments tested and to generate ideas for further research, is *not* appropriate. Emphatically, the primary purpose of most clinical trials, and all clinical trials done for submission to the FDA, is to supply verification of previous results, that is, they are intended to be confirmatory experiments. Our work, therefore, can properly be classified as drug *development*, but not as new drug *research* as the term should be generally understood. This is not to denigrate its importance. In any field of science, new information obtained through research must be subjected to an extended process of verification before it is accepted or applied. And perhaps in no other field are the precision and rigor of statistical designs and analyses needed more than they are in clinical trial work.

Because, therefore, we are usually validating previously believed or suspected phenomena in our trials, it becomes practical to plan most of the details of the execution of a trial, as well as those of its data analysis, before the first dose is given to the first patient. This is good business, because no careful sponsor normally wishes to begin the very expensive clinical stages of a study without some idea of the expected safety, cost, or efficacy of a drug. But it is also good judgment, because the advocacy of any clinical trial without some information about its safety and effectiveness, particularly the former, to justify it ethically, will surely be regarded with little tolerance by the FDA when the project is initially submitted for approval. Preclinical (animal) work supplies as much of that information as can be obtained in a practical sense without clinical (human) trials before the very first Phase I trials are run. Thereafter, each new trial, beginning with very low doses and small samples of healthy volunteers (subjects), builds upon what has been learned from its predecessors. The only exceptions to the regulatory requirement of preclinical testing is in cases in which a drug has been used previously, for which there is adequate safety information, or for which the drug is now merely being tested to support a new claim.

13.2.3 Kinds of Data

Data are the basic materials with which we are concerned, so we need a brief summary of the several forms in which they occur. The kind of data that you have will often determine some or all of the analytical procedures to be used.

This is a brief review of a topic that was covered at some length in Chapter 4. Many different sorts of measurements, which we often call responses in this book, may be used in clinical trials. All of them are used as dependent variables. Like the sort of design you use, the kind of data you choose to generate is a factor in determining the sample size as well as in the nature of the analysis that must be done. The nomenclature we use here is based upon but not identical to descriptions in an early book on nonparametric testing by Sidney Siegel [45].[1]

An **ordered scale** is a scale of values representing some characteristic of the thing or event being measured, which can be arranged in the order of

---

[1] A number of citations are listed on page 30 of Siegel's book [45], cf. his reference list on pp. 241–244. This classification was not original with Siegel, but is probably the most available source today. Woolson [10], in his Chapter 2, refers to an early paper by S. S. Stevens in *Science*, 103, 677–680 (1946).

magnitude of the units of the scale, and in which such ordering conveys meaning. A **nominal scale** does not use an ordered set of numbers but a set of classifications that is either impossible to order or that is not ordered for some reason. Some scales, such as arrays of colors, can be readily used either as unordered classifications or as sets of ordered points (by using their wavelengths, saturation, or other characteristic). An example of an ordered scale is the classification of a patient's condition into none, mild, moderate, or severe. The classification of patients into black, white, yellow, and red ethnic groups is an example of a scale that cannot be ordered, that is, a nominal scale.

The points on a nominal scale cannot be ordered at all, as indicated. But there are several kinds of scales that can be ordered. We define two kinds of **integer** scales, and two that are **continuous**. All of them are basically numerical. Integer scales consist of whole numbers only. Continuous scales are those that include any number of fractional points between whole numbers, so that they can be imagined to have an infinite number of points even if they have lower and upper limits.

You can think of **integer scales** as being of two kinds—**ordinal** or **ranking**. These scales usually use numbers or can be expressed in numbers, but only in whole numbers (integers).[2] An ordinal scale is the sort we have called a "scoring" scale in this book. Most judgment scales are of this kind, and are widely used as response scales in clinical trials, because measurements such as weights, volumes, temperatures, and pressures are frequently impossible or impractical. A common example is a five-point headache pain intensity scale; none, slight, moderate, severe, and very severe. This is an *implicit* integer scale, in which the five points of the scale are expressed in words instead of numbers. Often, the statistician will substitute the integers 1 to 5 for these descriptive words and phrases, before performing an analysis. This definition and the next are not those used by Siegel.

A **ranking scale** can also be an integer scale, but it is quite different from an ordinal scale. Patients may be numbered in the order of their heights, for example. The numbers in such a scale are called **ranks**. The highest rank number actually assigned will be equal to the total number of patients or items ranked. This is sometimes true only conceptually, however, because fractional rank numbers are often used for tied ranks. To clarify the idea of ranks, think of **scoring** a disease condition as "none," "mild," "moderate," "severe," and "very severe." Given a group of patients who may have the condition, each one could be independently judged and scored by using one of these words or with the numbers 1 to 5 corresponding to them. This would

---

[2] It is obviously possible to construct an ordered scale without using numbers, but this is often clumsy and is rarely done. At times, for clarity, it is advantageous to use words or letters of the alphabet. Avoiding the use of numbers in a judgment scale is sometimes carried to extremes, however. I once encountered a published set of dermatological data expressed entirely in a cryptic scale consisting solely of combinations of punctuation marks.

result in a set of **scores** on an ordinal scale. We assume that, as is common, intermediate values such as 1.5, 2.75, etc., are not used. However, if, instead, we were be to sort the data in the order of the magnitudes of their scores, then assign the rank numbers 1 to 5 to them, we would have generated a set of ranks instead of scores. Ranks differ from scores in that they are not independent of each other. Each rank number represents the *order* of magnitude of each score. *Scores*, as well as other kinds of numeric measurements, translate an observation, such as the intensity of headache pain, into a number representing the relative intensity of the pain. The rank of such a score is its relative magnitude among the group of observations in the set. For example, in this book, we always assign a rank of 1 to the smallest item in a set of data; the highest possible rank for that set will then be equal to the total number of data. Ranks are used principally in statistical procedures designed for them. They are widely used, however, and are very useful. An example of these characteristics of ranks appears in the next chapter.

Continuous scales can be further classified into **interval** or **ratio** scales. Interval scales do not possess true zero points. For example, zero degrees on the Fahrenheit temperature scale is not the lowest possible temperature, but only an empirical point (32 degrees below the freezing point of pure water). But a ratio scale does have a true zero; examples are weight in grams or pounds, or absolute temperature (Kelvin). To say that 100° Fahrenheit is twice as hot as 50° has no meaning, but a 1-pound mass *does have* twice the mass of a half-pound mass, and 20° K *is* twice as hot as 10° K. These and the foregoing varieties of measurement scales are discussed more thoroughly in Chapter 4.

13.2.4   Randomization

This section provides a review of randomization that you should have at this point to remind you of its relationship to data analysis. Randomization in clinical trials refers to the random assignment of treatments to patients. In clinical studies, we almost never select patients randomly from their populations, because, although that would be desirable, in most cases, it is highly impractical or impossible. As a result, in nearly all clinical trials, we must content ourselves with the assumption that the samples we choose are adequate representations of certain predefined parent populations, accepting that assumption on logical and scientific grounds, unaided by the use of any statistical sampling procedures. See Chapter 2, Section 2.2.3, for a detailed discussion of this point. Despite this, it is generally recognized that random assignment is essential in most clinical trials.

There has been much discussion of the methodology of random assignment in this book, but we have not as yet discussed its purposes sufficiently. That is, so far we have not ventured beyond discussions of its obvious ability to distribute the assignments of treatments in an unbiased fashion among patients with a variety of different characteristics. There are schools of thought among some statisticians that question the need for randomization, but these ideas have not been accepted by practitioners of applied statistics in clinical work. For that matter, the FDA does not accept trial data based upon nonrandomized treatment assignments as primary evidence of efficacy. In clinical trial studies, then, we endorse the idea that random assignment is essential, and that without it, no statistical hypothesis test or confidence interval (such as those to be described in the next chapter) can be known to be valid.

This is not to say that in some areas, usually noncommercial or where "proof" of efficacy or safety need not be presented to a regulatory body, other kinds of evidence may not be acceptable. Even for clinical studies, the FDA may accept *supplementary* evidence of efficacy and safety, such as nonrandomized or nonrandomizable survey data. Primary evidence, however, must be supplied in the form of randomized, controlled clinical trials. There are some few exceptions to this, in cases where, for one reason or another, randomization is impossible or unethical. And in some noncommercial areas, rather than abandon any statistical analysis at all when randomization is not possible, many competent statisticians feel that the best option may often be to use such tests, although with reservations about the conclusions drawn. Of course, it often happens that such studies turn out to have led to the correct conclusions. However, this does not validate the use of statistics in these cases.

An example is the study on smoking and health in the United States, which resulted in the Surgeon-General's report. The evidence against smoking was overwhelming, but was based principally upon scientific reasoning and observation of the data, rather than statistical hypothesis tests. Such tests were done, but were regarded by the statisticians involved as supplying only weak corroboration. Another example is the National Halothane Study. In both of these nonexperimental studies (and there are many others), it was impossible or utterly impractical to randomize. Nonetheless, statistical hypothesis tests were used. However, the statisticians involved (all of outstanding competence and candor) apparently felt that the use of these procedures was merely the only reasonable course open to them, and that the results should be accepted merely as corroboration.

To summarize, in clinical studies, there is *no* really satisfactory alternative to random *assignment* beyond the adoption of statistical philosophies that are not widely accepted among clinical biostatisticians, would not be accepted as primary evidence by the FDA, and, to my knowledge, are never used in industrial clinical studies.

There is a very logical reason why random assignment of treatments is necessary to validate hypothesis tests. It is this: The use of statistics as a tool of data analysis includes the assumption that random assignment has been used. If the null hypothesis is true, random assignment assures that differences among patients, investigators, or measurement procedures or devices will be equally likely to be associated with each of the treatments, at random, in a trial. Therefore, any rejection of the null hypothesis can be accepted as legitimate if differences between the mean responses of the patient groups are sufficiently great to rule out such miscellaneous variation as their sole source.

13.2.5 Probability

This is a very brief review of this topic. It is necessary because the use of probabilistic concepts are the very basis of hypothesis testing, not to mention of statistical analysis in general.

Mathematical probability is a numerical concept. We speak of the probability of various **events**. If an event is impossible, its probability is zero. If it is certain, the probability is one. The probability of an event can lie *anywhere* between 1 and 0, although certainty or impossibility may characterize theoretical events only.

Probability is never expressed as a percentage. We might say that the odds or the chance of some event is 80%, but 80% is not a probability. The corresponding probability is 0.8, a fraction.

In the next paragraphs, we speak of alpha and beta, the two "risks" we have spoken of many times previously. Both are probabilities of events.

13.2.6 Hypothesis Tests and Related Procedures

Introduction

In the previous chapters, we "analyzed" the data in some of our examples by calculating treatment means (for example) and comparing them visually. Using such procedures, we had no method of estimating the probability that any observed differences between the means really reflected actual population differences (i.e., actual treatment effects), rather than, instead, merely random variation, or "error." We now examine methods for testing such treatment differences with stated probabilities relating to the conclusions drawn. These probabilities are specified by you, and can have any value less than one and more than zero.

Up to this point, hypothesis (significance) testing has been mentioned repeatedly, but has not been described in detail. It is widely misunderstood among nonstatistical professionals, partly because we statisticians rarely explain it very clearly. In addition, to one unfamiliar with the kind of formal logic used, it can appear strange and antiintuitive. However, even if you never analyze a single set of data, it is important that you understand it fully, because a thorough grasp of this most basic concept is necessary when you select a trial design, as well as when you estimate sample size.

All the preparation you will need to understand this section is supplied in Chapter 5, in which sample size, power, and the concept of frequency distributions are introduced. All of these are closely related to hypothesis testing. A review of that chapter at this time may help you here, in the remaining sections in this chapter, and in Chapter 15. On the other hand, if you are sure that you have a good command of the material in this section, you may wish to skip it.

Hypothesis testing is not difficult to comprehend, although it is easy to misunderstand it. To further cloud the issue, there is disagreement among many competent statisticians about its theoretical forms and use, and many wish there were a better way to accomplish its purposes. But in clinical work, in particular for assuring compliance with FDA regulations, such a way has not been discovered. Therefore, it is most important that you fully understand it during the planning, analysis, and reporting of clinical trial data, even if you never personally run any analyses at all.

The important concept of hypothesis testing and related ideas in our field involves the **Neyman-Pearson** procedure; see references (2), (3), and (4) at the end of Chapter 15. You specify alpha and beta risks, postulate a value of delta, estimate the sample size using these specifications and an estimate of sigma, and consider the power function for your statistical procedure. In a typical simple test using these ideas, you would wish to conclude whether there is a difference, delta, of a magnitude you consider important, between two sample groups of experimental units (patients or plots within patients), one treated with each of two drugs of interest. The test will lead to one of two conclusions: (a) that a difference, **delta** (δ), exists between the means of the populations represented by the two sample groups, with a risk, **alpha** (α), of being wrong, or (b) that there is no difference, with a risk, **beta** (β), of being wrong if, in fact, the difference is delta. The value of $1 - \beta$ is called the **power of the test**.

We describe two hypothesis-testing procedures in the following sections. The first (*simplistic*) procedure to be described was formerly widely used, but it is not the Neyman-Pearson procedure and it has serious limitations. It is described here *only* because it makes for an easier understanding of the second procedure—that of Neyman and Pearson. It is *not* recommended except in the case of certain tests of the parametric assumptions and similar procedures, to be described later in this chapter.

The "Simplistic" Hypothesis-Testing Procedure

To carry out a hypothesis test in its simplest form, you must construct two hypotheses *before* the data to be tested are available for examination. These are called the **null** and the **alternate** hypotheses. Each time you plan a trial, you may wish to write these hypotheses down in the context of that particular study. If there is to be a statistical section or addendum to the protocol, as there should be, they should become part of it. They need not be expressed in symbols in the protocol; words will do.

The null and alternate hypotheses are mutually exclusive; only one of them can be true in a given case. The hypothesis test supplies the means for arriving at a decision. In the simplistic test, you do not specify beta, and you can never *accept* the null hypothesis. Instead, the simplistic test can have one of two outcomes: *rejection* of the null hypothesis with probability alpha of being wrong, or *failure* to reject it, with *no* stated probability. In concrete terms, if you are comparing two treatments, you will either conclude that they derive from two populations having different means or you will be unable to claim that a difference exists. *You cannot claim that there is no difference, only that a difference has not been shown.* You do have the power to specify alpha (although you cannot specify zero or one), provided that you do so before the data are available. In the simplistic test, the sample size is not estimable statistically in a satisfactory way, and you cannot specify delta. There well may be a population difference that is large enough to be important to you, but your trial may be too small to detect it. Alternatively, if your sample size is large, the test may be *more* sensitive than is desirable, and you may detect a population difference that is too small to be clinically important.

Example 13.1: Simplistic Hypothesis-Testing Procedure

Let's say, as an example, that you are planning to run a parallel trial with two drugs. Assume that you expect to run some test of significance, such as the t test described in the next chapter, when the data are available. Let's assume that you will have arranged to randomly assign two drugs to two groups of patients, one drug (T_1 or T_2) to each. You set up a null hypothesis, which is written as follows:

$$H_0: \mu_1 = \mu_2 \qquad\qquad (13.1)$$

Later, you will either reject this hypothesis in favor of the alternative hypothesis described in what follows or you may *fail to reject it* (this does not imply that you will accept it). Next, you set up an alternative hypothesis. At the time of the test, you must accept this if the null hypothesis is rejected. The test lets you determine whether to reject H_0 and accept H_1, or not to reject H_0. If you accept the alternate hypothesis, you are said to have found *significance* (two-tailed test):

$$H_1: \mu_1 \neq \mu_2 \qquad\qquad (13.2)$$

The symbol $\neq$ means "is not equal to." These two hypotheses may appear so simple as to be trivial. But wait. The symbols H_0 and H_1 stand for the null and alternative hypotheses, respectively. The Greek letters μ_1 and μ_2 refer to the means (parameters) of the two populations that you actually wish to compare, although you will have only estimates of them in the forms of the means of the two treatment groups, $\overline{T}_1$ and $\overline{T}_2$. Switching from the algebraic to the English language, Equation (13.1), the null hypothesis, states that the two *populations* are identical, that is, they have the same means—we are assuming that the other parameters, the variances, are also identical. Equation (13.2), the alternate hypothesis, states that there are two populations with different means. Obviously, only one of these two hypotheses can be true. Note that we are concerned with the *population means*, not the means of the two treatment groups, but that we have only the latter to use as guides, because the population means (the parameters) can only be estimated.

We assume that the populations or distributions with which we are concerned are normally distributed and, as just mentioned, that they have the same variances. If H_0 is really true and H_1 is false, both means are identical, and, because of the assumption about the variances, there is really only one population.[3] If H_0 is actually false and H_1 is true, one of the two population means is larger than the other, that is, our sample means are telling us that there are really two different populations, differing in their means (we say their **locations** are different). Because the test is two-tailed, if the observed difference is large enough to cause you to reject the null hypothesis, you will do so regardless of its direction. That is, you will be interested in a significant result whether it indicates that μ_1 or μ_2 is the larger of the two means.

You use a *t* test to estimate the probability that the observed difference between the two sample means could be as large as that observed if it were due only to random variation, rather than to a treatment difference. If that probability is less than your prespecified value of alpha, you have found significance and you should reject the null hypothesis as untrue. However, if the probability yielded by the *t* test is equal to or greater than alpha, you should not reject the null hypothesis; it *may* be true. If significance is found, examination of the two means will tell you which is the larger.

Whether the test is one- or two-tailed depends, in this case, upon the nature of the *alternate hypothesis* formulated beforehand. In a one-tailed test, for example, you may wish to discover whether μ_2 is greater than μ_1 but not the opposite. You may believe that the opposite situation is impossible. Perhaps one of the two treatments is a placebo and you are certain that there can be no "placebo effect." If so, assuming that μ_1 is the placebo, the test will then be constructed to show that μ_2 is or is not greater than μ_1. Sometimes, however, a one-tailed test may be used simply because the experimenter is interested only in one of the two ways the treatments can be different, even if both are possible.[4]

---

[3]Remember that a normal distribution has only two parameters: the mean, μ, and the variance, σ^2.

[4]There is a disagreement even among statistics textbooks as to whether this justification for the use of a one-tailed test is acceptable. However, you should be cautious in its use, whatever your beliefs, because in clinical test submissions, the FDA tends to look at one-tailed tests with a jaundiced eye. This is reasonable, because the value of alpha for a one-tailed test is just half of that needed when a two-tailed test is run. This means that for a given alpha value, a finding of significance is possible when a smaller treatment difference exists than is needed when the test is two-tailed. To some applicants with questionable honesty and a low opinion of the astuteness of the FDA statisticians, this at times results in the use of a one-tailed test simply to increase the probability of a convincing submission. This caution does not apply if it is obvious to anyone that the test can come out in only one way. Such a result is rare in clinical studies, however, even when one of the "treatments" is a placebo.

Certain specialized tests, such as those for testing normality and homogeneity of variance referred to later, do legitimately use the simplistic procedure. Estimation of sample size in these cases would be inconsistent with the estimates made upon the basis of the principal response, and so usually cannot be done. Thus, delta and beta are not usually specified for these tests.

Note that in the simplistic procedure, it is possible to legitimately claim that there is a difference between two populations if significance is found, but *impossible* to claim that there is *no* difference if significance is *not* found. The simplistic hypotheses—Equations (13.1) and (13.2)—and the associated procedures are undesirable not only because of this, however, but also because they do not require prespecified values of beta or delta and thus do not make a reasonable sample size estimate possible. If you cannot accept the null hypothesis when significance is not found, but only claim that it has not been rejected, your conclusion will be a weak one. But if you have specified beta and delta *and* used an appropriate sample size, and *then* do not obtain significance, you can accept the conclusion that no difference greater than delta exists (with your chosen risk, beta, of being wrong, of course). If you use that procedure, you should remember, however, that prespecifying alpha, beta, and delta and obtaining an adequate prior estimate of sigma, without using an adequate sample size, is meaningless. In such a case, if you find upon postcomputing delta that your trial was too small, you will not know whether significance would have been found had the sample size been great enough.

Of course, regardless of which hypothesis testing procedure you use, if you find significance, you will know that the sample was large enough to give significance even if you did not estimate it beforehand. But even then, it would be desirable to postcalculate delta upon the basis of the assumption of a reasonable value of beta—perhaps 0.10 or, at most, 0.20. You might find that your trial was sensitive only to quite a large difference in the treatment means of the two populations, and that may stimulate you to specify and correctly apply a smaller beta or delta value in a subsequent trial. Or, worse, you may find that delta was very small because the trial used a sample size much larger than would have been necessary to detect a "clinically significant" difference.

The "simplistic" procedure has been described first not only because it provides a clear introduction to the topic, but also because it illustrates the serious disadvantages inherent in this very commonly used form of hypothesis testing. I cannot stress strongly enough that if you use it and fail to find significance, you cannot *accept* the null hypothesis, but must merely conclude that you have failed to reject it. But if you recall the outline of the estimation of sample size in Chapter 5, you know that it is possible to arrange things so that you *can* accept the null hypothesis if significance is not found. You can also estimate an adequate sample size for your trial. To accomplish these things, you must prespecify alpha as before, but you must also prespecify beta and delta. An estimate (not a specification) of sigma will also be needed.

Neyman-Pearson Hypothesis-Testing Procedure
To gain these advantages, the Neyman-Pearson procedure is available to you. The recommended forms of the hypotheses are shown in what follows. They lead to data analyses that are substantially more revealing and useful than the simplistic ones. For example, they make it possible to use sample size estimates on a logical basis. When the sample size is approximately that required for the specified values of alpha, beta, and delta, and is based upon a reasonably adequate estimate of sigma, any study provides much more information about the treatments and their interactions than otherwise.

The following null and alternate hypotheses are suitable for a two-tailed test:

$$H_0: \mu_1 - \mu_2 = 0 \tag{13.3}$$

$$H_1: |\mu_1 - \mu_2| = \delta \tag{13.4}$$

The null hypothesis is still Equation (13.3), the null hypothesis shown before for the simplistic procedure. But, as you can see, the alternate hypothesis is *not* the same as that of Equation (13.2) (it is more specific). The simplistic alternate hypothesis in this case would be $H_1: \mu_1 > \mu_2$ or $\mu_2 > \mu_1$. Equations (13.3) and (13.4) are suitable for use in the Neyman-Pearson procedure that follows.

Example 13.2: Neyman-Pearson Procedure
Let's look at a trial similar to the kind just described, but using the hypotheses of Equations (13.3) and (13.4) instead of the simplistic hypotheses.

We again postulate a two-tailed test. Let's say that you have run a parallel design using two treatments. You have your data and are now comparing the treatment means. If your statistical test shows significance, you can conclude that the observed difference between the treatment means reflects *a population difference of delta* (with a probability of being wrong that is less than the value of alpha, which you may have specified to be, say, 0.05). If you do not obtain significance, you can conclude that there is no population difference (i.e., you accept the null hypothesis), with a probability, beta, or being wrong of, say, 0.10. This means that the power of the test will be $1 - \beta$, or 0.90, that is, you will have a "90% chance" of detecting an absolute difference larger than delta ($\delta = |\mu_1 - \mu_2|$), if one exists in the population. We will assume that you are now at the point where you have already estimated the sample size and run the trial.

Let's go through this again in more detail. There are several statistical tests that you may use; a few of the most common are explained in the next chapter. In all of them, however, the underlying concepts are similar. We assume that the samples of patients (the two treatment groups) are from two hypothetical populations. The tests make it possible for you to find the probability that the difference between the two *sample* means could be as large as that observed, if the difference between the means of the two *populations* represented by the samples is really zero—that is, if the means are equal (H_0 true). If this probability is less than the specified value of alpha (say, 0.05), you will then *reject H_0* and accept H_1, concluding with risk alpha that the population difference is equal to delta. So far, this procedure is exactly the same as that of the simplistic procedure, except that the alternate hypotheses are different.

Now, instead, suppose that your calculated probability turns out to be equal to or greater than alpha. In this case, you will *accept* the null hypothesis, concluding that the *population* difference is zero. Notice that the way the null and alternate hypothesis have been set up reflects the fact that you are not concerned with population differences less than delta, whether or not they are zero. If you do not obtain significance, concluding that the difference is zero will have the same consequences as if it lay between zero and delta, inclusive, namely, the conclusion that the difference does not exceed delta. Only if the difference exceeds delta will you react differently. Now, the beta risk comes into play, because it is possible that *this* conclusion is wrong, and that you should have accepted the alternate hypothesis. The probability of your making this error by incorrectly accepting H_0 is beta.

The parameters that can be compared using various kinds of hypothesis tests need not be limited to means. As one example, you can also use them to compare standard deviations or variances. Nor do you need to confine yourself to the normal distribution and its two parameters (μ and σ).[5] But even if you are comparing means, there are other forms of the hypothesis tests. You might test single quantities, asking if they are different from some postulated "standard" value. A common example is the test of a mean difference to see whether it could be zero or not at a stated probability level.

Confidence Intervals

Nature of Confidence Intervals

Hypothesis tests and confidence intervals are closely related, but whereas the former are used for a single purpose (significance testing), the latter, although they can be adapted to that purpose, have broader applications. Confidence intervals calculated from experimental data consist of upper and lower bounds and a probability. Their meaning is that in the long run, some

---

[5]This does not imply that distributions other than the normal do not possess means or standard deviations.

parameter will be included between those bounds with a stated frequency or probability.[6]

For example, suppose you have run a drug trial and have averaged all the results for one response and one drug. This single average is an estimate of a parameter—the mean of the distribution of which your data for that drug constitute a sample. How precise[7] is your estimate? What are the limits of the interval within which, with a given probability, the parameter will be included? Putting it another way, if you run the same trial repeatedly, how often will these bounds enclose it?

If your concern is with a mean or a mean difference, one way to answer these questions is to calculate the 95% confidence interval about that mean. *Before the trial*, you may state that in 95 out of 100 such trials, the parameter (the mean or the mean difference in this instance) will be located within the calculated interval. You have then described the precision with which you know the parameter, the width of the interval, and the frequency within which your parameter will be enclosed in the stated interval, all in one statement. But after you do one trial and calculate the interval, you will not know for that specific case whether the population mean is included or not. This sounds like a quibble, but it is not. It is meant to show that these notions apply only before an experiment is done and a confidence interval is calculated. After the current experiment, you *will* know, as you did initially, that about 95% of such trials will include the population mean. You will not know whether your trial is among the 95%. But you will now know something else. Because 95% of such experiments will yield intervals containing the parameter, there is a probability of 0.95% that the parameter lies in the one you just calculated. You may use other intervals instead of 95%, if you wish. If you use a higher value, such as 99%, the interval will be wider; with a lower

---

[6]To the majority of applied statisticians, a frequency is the equivalent of a probability. If an event is expected to occur 500 times in 1000 instances, its expected probability is 500/1000, or 0.5. For example, if you toss a fair coin, spinning it in a random fashion, you would anticipate getting a head about 50% of the time. If you toss it 100 times, you expect to get about 50 heads, because heads and tails are equally probable. The frequency of heads will be about 50/100, and the probability of a head in any one toss will be 0.5. Note that these statements all concern the state of things *before* an event occurs. After you toss a coin once and observe the result, considering the probability of a head is meaningless, because you *know* the outcome. These ideas apply to finite populations and samples. When a theoretical distribution (population) is defined as being infinite, a different approach to the ideas of probability is needed.

[7]A reminder: In this book, *precision* means the reproducibility of a quantity when it is measured or determined repeatedly. The related term *accuracy* refers to bias. A biased statistic is one that, if recomputed and averaged cumulatively and repeatedly, does not tend to approach its parameter more and more closely, but "misses" it. For example, an arithmetic mean, m, is said to be an unbiased estimate of mu. Everyone believes that if it is recalculated with increasing sample sizes without limit, it eventually becomes equal to mu. This is not true of the standard deviation, s, which does not become sigma in the limit. This is one reason for the wide use of variance, the square of the standard deviation, which is unbiased.

value, it will be narrower. What you are doing here is estimating the *precision* with which you know a parameter, such as the mean.

Practical Application

You may find the previous paragraph confusing because it is easy to become lost in the unfamiliar paths of formal logic. However, after you calculate a confidence interval about the average difference between two treatment means in your current trial, it is reasonable to treat it as an approximate statement of the precision of the calculated mean difference, and to state that about 95% of any future trials will yield confidence intervals that contain it. Just remember that this process applies in the long run, not in any one particular experiment. And after all, the long run is the important consideration. When you later generalize the results of a trial, you will be speaking of the long run, not the results of that one trial.[8]

A final point to emphasize is that although confidence intervals about the mean are more common than other kinds of intervals in clinical work, a confidence interval may be calculated for any parameter. For example, you can calculate one about the variance, although this is not discussed in this book.

It is meaningless to state, as is frequently done, that a measured value is so and so, plus or minus a stated quantity, with no further information. This kind of statement is widely used in the chemical literature, and frequently in clinical trial work. First, in a statement such as "the mean is 25.34, plus or minus 5," the reference *must* be to a *parameter*, not to the statistic just calculated. But that is not clear. You *know* the exact value of the measurement you just made (within the number of decimal places you have used). You can *see* whether it lies between any specified limits. What you cannot see is whether or not that interval contains the corresponding value of the parameter, because you *do not* know the latter. The real interest lies in the parameter—the value of the mean of the distribution, μ—because the object is usually to extrapolate your conclusions to future situations, not to the results of a single experiment, if they are to be at all useful. Second, the previous statement lacks specificity because it does not state *how often* (i.e., the probability) the value will lie within the interval given.

Although standard errors are defined in the next chapter, here is a brief definition to help clarify my complaints in the next two paragraphs. Let us assume that the population of concern is the normal (Gaussian). Then, simply defined, in terms of the population mean, the standard error of the mean defines the approximately 0.68 confidence interval (one sigma) about the mean. That is, it defines the limits between which an unknown population mean may be included, with a "chance" of about 68% (a probability of about

---

[8]But, to repeat, you can also relate your work to the current experiment by remembering that because 95% of the experiments will produce intervals containing a given parameter, the probability is 0.95 that *any one of them* will contain it.

0.68). As you can see, there is thus a "chance" of 32% that the mean lies outside that interval.

A common misuse of statistics related to the subject of confidence intervals is the incorrect or, more often, correct but vague use of the standard error. It is commonly used in the literature to give an idea of the precision with which a measurement has been made. But although the standard error of the mean may have been correctly calculated, (a) it assumes that the data consist of a representative sample from a normal distribution; (b) given that assumption, it defines a rather narrow interval beyond which it would be quite common to find some measurements in a set; and (c) although the concept of a standard error is simple and easily understandable by almost anyone, many readers, editors, and authors of the medical and clinical literature have not bothered to discover its correct meaning.

Other Uses of Confidence Intervals

We mentioned that confidence intervals have broader uses than do hypothesis tests. In the previous illustration, you might describe the use to which the confidence intervals were put as estimating the precision of a statistic, such as a single mean. But you can also use confidence limits as hypothesis tests.

For example, you can use the confidence limits about a mean difference as a hypothesis test of the difference between two treatment means. If the limits do *not* include zero (i.e., do not extend from a negative value to a positive one), it may be concluded that the population difference is greater than zero, with a probability of $(1 - c)$ of being correct (c is the "size" of the confidence interval such as 0.95). Furthermore, such a procedure can easily take beta and delta into account. It thus can be made to serve a purpose identical to that of a conventional significance test. On the other hand, a common but questionable way of using confidence intervals is the display in many of the bar charts used in business and financial literature of upper and lower confidence intervals above or below the bars, illustrating either mean (or individual) quantities. These are upper or lower confidence bounds, and they tend to be used, usually incorrectly, as implicit hypothesis tests, although they are rarely described as such. When they are used in this way, the exercise is incorrect if there are more than two bars unless it takes the inherent multiplicity into account (see Section 13.4, "Multiplicity," which follows). In addition, these intervals are usually based upon the assumption that the data are samples from normal distributions with equal variances. There is much statistical analysis and graphics software on the market that encourage the misuse of confidence intervals in this manner.

To summarize, confidence intervals may be calculated about any statistic. They require the same raw materials as standard hypothesis tests (a specification of alpha, and, preferably, specifications of beta and delta, and estimates of sigma and sample size). They are more informative than statistics such as standard errors. Because confidence intervals are sometimes used for the estimation of the precision of a statistic as well as for hypothesis testing, they may often be more useful than a conventional significance test. It is often helpful to report both. Their calculation is not given in this book, but many of the statistics texts and professional books listed in the Bibliography give complete details.

Least Significant Difference (LSD)

We consider here only least significant differences based upon the normal distribution. Like the other fundamental concepts listed in this section, a method of calculating them, with an illustrative example, will be given in the next chapter. A least significant difference is analogous to ordinary hypothesis tests or confidence intervals; in a way, it is a *t* test in disguise. It is the critical difference between, say, two sample means, which must be exceeded before you can claim that the means are significantly different. But after setting up a null and an alternate hypothesis, you can calculate an LSD at some specified alpha level. If the LSD is exceeded by the difference between the sample means, the difference between the two means will be significant. The LSD is therefore subject to the same limitations and caveats as any other significance test, as you would expect. But if you wish to apply it repeatedly to pairs of means from a trial in which there are more than two treatments, you must first solve certain multiplicity problems (see Section 13.4, "Multiplicity," which follows).

Significance Testing Specifics

Nature of the Statistic Tested

We use the term *statistic* here to refer either to an individual measurement or to a quantity derived from an individual or group of measurements. A statistic is an estimate of a parameter of a distribution (population). For example, it could be a treatment mean or the difference between two treatment means. A parametric hypothesis test such as a *t* test compares a statistic like this with another statistic, using an estimate of the experimental error applying to it, also estimated from the data. The sample mean estimates the distribution mean, mu (μ). The error estimates the distribution standard deviation or variance, sigma (σ) or sigma squared.

Hypothesis tests are *comparisons*. In one very common kind of test, the **t test** (a parametric test), we obtain a quantity, *t*. This is calculated from the ratio of a difference between two treatment means to an estimate of the error of that difference. Then, referring to a **t table**, we find the probability that *t* would have a magnitude as great as that just calculated if the difference tested were due to chance and did not reflect a population difference. If this probability is less than a prespecified value, alpha, we say that the difference between the means is **significant**. A difference this large would occur only rarely if it were due to chance alone. A simple application of this kind of test is to the comparison of two drug treatments in a single-factor parallel trial with two patient groups, with one of the drugs assigned to each.

In another common case, a mean of several data or derived quantities, such a mean response from several patients receiving a single drug, or, more often, a mean of a set of differences between two treatments, is tested. In these cases, the comparison is to some postulated value (not derived from the data); for the mean difference, this value is zero.[9] If such a claim can be made, it is said that the mean difference is **significant**, or that **significance** has been found. The result is expressed as a probability that must be less than alpha to claim significance. When significance is claimed, as you know, there will be a risk alpha that the null hypothesis is nevertheless true. If significance is *not* found and you have used the Neyman-Pearson ideas as recommended, you can claim that any presumed population difference is less than delta, with risk beta.

Interpretation
There are differences of opinion in the literature regarding whether, to claim significance, the probability found in a significance test must be *less than*, or *equal to or less than* alpha. Practically speaking, the question is trivial, because, if you require that the probability found in a significance test must be less than alpha, *any* probability less than alpha, however small the difference, will force you to claim significance. For conservatism, in this book, we use the rule that the probability must be less than alpha. Our interpretation with regard to delta is that a significant difference means that a difference of delta exists in the population, as is stated in the alternate hypothesis.

Independent and Dependent Tests
A parallel design, in which each patient receives a treatment consisting of only one level of a factor, requires a hypothesis test for so-called *independent* data to compare treatment levels. A changeover design, on the other hand, in which each patient receives both levels of a two-level factor (two drugs, for example), requires a test for *paired* or *dependent* data. The difference between the two test procedures lies in the derivation of the experimental errors. When testing a difference between the means of two different groups (an independent test), the error is a function of the differences *between* (among) the patients within each treatment group. In a paired test, on the other hand, it is based upon the differences between plots *within* patients. The errors within patients must logically be equal to or smaller than the between-patients variation, because they are included in the latter (ignoring random variation in the estimates).

There are other designs involving pairing that are not changeovers, although they are rare in clinical trials. For example, studies of twins are used

---

[9]Note that the mean difference (the average of a set of differences between pairs of treatment data obtained from a changeover test) is *not* the same as a difference between two group means obtained in a parallel test.

in psychological experiments, and the use of littermates in designs such as randomized blocks is frequent in preclinical drug work.

One- and Two-Tailed Tests

The difference between one- and two-tailed tests lies in the formulation of the hypotheses and the interpretation of the outcomes. In a one-tailed test, the investigator or the statistician asks whether treatment T_1 produces either a *higher* or *lower* average response (not both) than T_2. In a two-tailed test, the question is whether T_1 and T_2 could be *different*, regardless of the direction of the difference. The principal difference between these two is in the formulation of the null and alternate hypotheses.

Suppose an investigator believes that two treatments, T_1 and T_2, both possess equal efficacy, or, if not, that T_1 *must* be more effective. In this case, although the null hypothesis is unchanged, Equation (13.4) is no longer appropriate. The null and alternate hypotheses are now those shown as Equation (13.3) (as before) and Equation (13.5), which is not the same as Equation (13.4); compare it with Equation (13.4):

$$H_1: \mu_1 - \mu_2 = \delta \qquad (13.5)$$

In the two-tailed test, Equations (13.3) and (13.4) are concerned with *absolute* differences. The null hypothesis, Equation (13.3), states that any difference in the populations is equal to zero, whereas the alternate hypothesis says that the difference is equal to delta, *regardless of sign*. There would be equal interest if H_0 were found to be false, whichever population mean were the larger.

On the other hand, in the one-tailed test represented by Equations (13.3) and (13.5), although the null hypothesis is unchanged, the alternate hypothesis, Equation (13.5), states that the *signed* difference between the means is zero. In this illustration, there is interest if H_0 is false and the difference is equal to delta, but *only* if μ_1 is the *larger* of the two means, so that the difference is positive in sign. In other cases, μ_1 might be postulated to be the smaller of the two, but only one of these alternatives would be assumed in a given one-tailed test.

Relationships between Variables

Sometimes the object of a study is not to compare means of treatments, but to study the variation in a response as some independent factor is changed. Dose-response studies, in which the object is to estimate the nature of the response curve when a dose is varied systematically, are of this type. More rarely in clinical work, there might be interest in studying the degree to which two (or more) variables follow one another, that is, to what degree they are *correlated*. If there is a high degree of positive correlation between two kinds of response measurements, one might choose to eliminate one of them from a proposed trial because it conveys almost the same information as the other (the information would not be exactly the same unless the correlation was perfect).[10] When concern lies with the correlation between or among variables, which variable is dependent and which independent are questions of no interest.

Questions like these, involving the quantitative search for a pattern of variation between two variables, can be investigated with the use of *correlation* and *regression*. These techniques are not discussed further in this book. You can find information about them in Dixon and Massey [33], Draper and Smith [34], Mandel [36], Neter et al. [37], Snedecor and Cochran [38], and several other books listed in the Bibliography. For statistical applications, Draper and Smith [34] is the de facto standard on this topic.

Parametric and "Nonparametric" Tests

In general, most of the discussion here is concerned with the manipulation of data that can be assumed to derive from approximately normal distributions. These are called the **parametric methods**.[11] A test of this assumption is described in the appendix to Chapter 14. The reason for the emphasis on the normal distribution in this and many other professional books and texts on statistical analysis are these: First, much measurement data is approximately normal. Second, there are greater numbers and varieties of procedures available for manipulating normally distributed data than there are for any other kind. Third, in many cases, nonnormal data can be transformed in ways that make them suitable for use with parametric tests. And, fourth, many parametric tests are quite **robust**, that is, they give reasonably accurate results even when the data are somewhat nonnormal. Despite all of this, there are many sets of data that appear to come from distributions that are far from normal. Therefore, two widely used kinds of tests that do not assume normality are also described in the next chapter.

13.3 ASSUMPTIONS

13.3.1 Nature of the Assumptions

There are several **assumptions** underlying the correct use of most statistical procedures. They are often called the **parametric** assumptions, but, strictly

---

[10]The correlation between two variables can be positive or negative. When positive, as one variable increases, the other tends to increase also. When negative, as one variable increases, the other tends to decrease.

[11]We are using the common and casual terminology, in which **parametric** is taken to mean methods based upon the normal distribution. This usage is not really correct, because the term actually refers to a method based upon a distribution, but not necessarily the normal. The opposite term, **nonparametric**, supposedly refers to a method that does not depend upon any particular distribution for its validity. However, "nonparametric" is also widely misused. The only truly nonparametric tests of which I am aware are the randomization tests, such as the Fisher Exact Test [39, 43, 44, 45] or the tests described by Edgington (1, 2).

speaking, they include assumptions that, although they are possessed by normal ("parametric") distributions, are also necessary for the correct application of nonparametric methods. These have been mentioned previously, but we delve more deeply here because concern with the assumptions is essential for reliable and informed statistical hypothesis testing and related procedures. In this section, we will describe the important "parametric" assumptions. Moderate to reasonably large samples of data can be tested to learn whether the necessary assumptions are reasonable. Some of these tests are described briefly in the next chapter. Although, as mentioned, many statistical hypothesis tests are **robust** to some violations of the assumptions, a safe and conservative approach is good science, does not entail much additional work, and allows you to feel more secure in the conclusions you draw from your tests. We therefore strongly advocate a knowledge of the assumptions and the use of methods of testing their validity whenever your trial involves the expenditure of any appreciable amount of time and resources.

The correct use of Student's t test and other hypothesis testing procedures, as well of confidence intervals and LSDs, requires familiarity with these assumptions. And, especially in the planning and analysis of clinical trials, for good or ill, hypothesis tests have become a necessity. The t test is one of these, and is described in detail in the next chapter. The analysis of variance (ANOVA) is another kind of hypothesis test, but it is beyond the scope of this book. These two procedures are probably the most widely used statistical tests in the world, not only in clinical studies, but in most other fields. They both require an assumption of normality, but they are based upon several additional assumptions. These assumptions and the consequences of their violation are most clearly and succinctly described in Chapter 10 of Scheffé (3), still the basic work on the analysis of variance.[12] They are also reviewed in Snedecor and Cochran [38], Chapter 14, pages 259–260, and Chapter 15, pages 274–297, where some remedies for their violation are described. We summarize them in this section.

There are other parametric as well as nonparametric tests that require one or more of these assumptions for their correct use, but the two parametric tests just mentioned are probably the most important of all.

Many parametric procedures are quite **robust** to violations of some of the assumptions, particularly that of normality (see what follows). But in any particular case, unless your knowledge of the degree of violation and its effect is thorough and you believe it to be minor, the safer course is to assume the worst and to take whatever steps are necessary to eliminate or reduce the severity of the problem. Fortunately, much work has been done both upon tests of the assumptions and remedies for their violation. Today, most tests of the assumptions are simple and rapid, and in most cases, there are reasonably effective and easy remedies when there are violations.

---

[12]Scheffe's book is not included in the Bibliography because it is a somewhat advanced work.

After describing the assumptions here, we will devote some space to a summary of the better-known tests for their violation. The procedures for two of them will be discussed further in the next chapter. We also include descriptions of some remedies for the many cases in which you will find that the assumptions are not met. With the exception of some procedures that have come into use recently, we will not cover the subject exhaustively, because many of the references, such as Snedecor and Cochran [38], provide much more information.

The Assumptions

The first assumption that follows is applicable only to the analysis of data when there is more than one factor in the design. The other three refer to the normal distribution and apply to multifactor ANOVAs, the t test, multiple regressions, and many other procedures. The last two also apply to some nonparametric tests. They can be summarized as follows:

1. *Additivity.* The effects of the factors are additive.[13]
2. *Normality.* The distribution (population), of which the data and their errors are assumed to be representative samples, is normal (Gaussian).
3. *Homoscedasticity (Homogeneity of Variances).* The errors of the measurements (the data), when they come from different distributions (populations), are the same. That is, in the t test, for example, when the mean values of the two treatments to be tested come from different distributions, the **variances** of these two distributions (and therefore also the standard deviations, which are the square roots of the variances) are assumed to be the same.
4. *Independence.* In tests of data from parallel designs, the errors of the measurements in the two or more treatment distributions sampled by the treatment groups are independent random variables. In difference tests and similar single-statistic tests, the differences are assumed to come from a single population of differences.

13.3.2 Testing the Assumptions

There are many tests for nonnormality and heteroscedasticity. We mention some tests here with literature references, but do not describe the proce-

---

[13]The assumption of additivity means that there are no interactions between factors. But some interactions depend upon the kind of measurement scale being used. These may wholly or partially disappear if the scale is transformed to another type. Simple examples are transformations of the data to their logarithms or square roots. Interactions that weaken or disappear upon some transformation are thus at least partially artifacts of the scale used. But interactions that do not behave in this way are of serious interest, or should be, because they are characteristics of the way two or more factors affect the response.

dures. Two recommended methods are described in the appendix to Chapter 14.

If there are sufficient data, all the assumptions can be tested successfully. The number of data needed depends upon the method of test, the kind of violation tested for, and its severity. In most cases, the *simplistic* hypothesis-test procedure described earlier, in which only alpha is specified beforehand, can and usually must be used. The reason for this is that it is critical that the sample size in any trial (and the values of delta and beta) be based only upon the responses and significance tests planned to try to answer the questions posed by the objectives of the study. Therefore, there may not always be sufficient data to allow reliable conclusions to be drawn from the tests of the assumptions. On the other hand, there will be times when the number of data available will exceed that required. In the first case, unfortunately, conclusions about violations will be weak or nonexistent. In the second, less important contingency, the tests will detect deviations that may be too small to be important. However, testing the assumptions and attempting to remedy any violations found will make your work substantially more reliable in the long run.

Nonadditivity

We will not be concerned with nonadditivity (certain types of interactions), because this book does not describe the *analysis* of multifactor studies, although we have described the design of the important ones. However, the biostatistician who analyzes your data will be familiar with the correct procedures when they are needed. If you are interested, Snedecor and Cochran [38] describe the best-known procedure, **Tukey's test for nonadditivity**, in their Chapter 15, Sections 15.8 and 15.9.

Nonnormality

The second assumption, that of normality, applies only to the parametric tests, obviously. It is the least important of the four, because most such tests are not strongly affected by nonnormality, especially when sample sizes are equal. However, tests of this assumption are easy and require the smallest sample sizes; often a sample of 30 to 50 data is adequate (sometimes less if the condition is severe). It is therefore recommended that you be certain that the statistician tests any set of trial data for normality unless you are quite certain that any nonnormality is trivial.

Tests for nonnormality are rife, and are described in many of the references in the Bibliography. They include tests of **skewness**, and **kurtosis**. A **positively skewed** distribution is shown in Figure 13.1. Compare this with a normal distribution, such as that shown in Figure 5.4 in Chapter 5. The distribution of Figure 13.1 is a **log-normal** distribution. This means that if the logs of the data were plotted, instead of the original data, the distribution

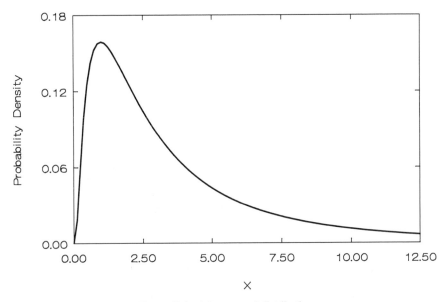

Figure 13.1 A log-normal distribution.

would be normal. Many data distributions are approximately log-normal, and may be **normalized** to an approximate but adequate degree by this means.

Kurtosis is a characteristic of data that produces distributions that are flatter, with higher tails than the normal (**platykurtic**), or more peaked, with lower tails (**leptokurtic**).

Other nonnormality tests include the **Shapiro-Wilks** test (4), the **Lilliefors** (5), **Dallal and Wilkinson** (6), **probability plots** (see Dixon and Massey [33], for example, for a good discussion, and **Michael's** (7) and **Nelson's** tests (8). The latter two are described briefly in the next chapter.

Unequal Variances
Testing the third assumption, homogeneity of the errors (homogeneity of variance or heteroscedasticity) may often require a larger sample, at least 50 to 100 items. Unfortunately, violation of this assumption can have more serious consequences than violation of the normality assumption. However, when your groups sizes are equal and the lack of homogeneity is not great, the consequences are usually not crucial. It is desirable to do these tests using residuals (error estimates for each individual datum), and this is necessary for multifactor designs. Procedures can be carried out easily on any desktop, mini, or mainframe computer with any of several statistical packages. Residuals are treated in a number of references; four of them are Anscombe and Tukey (9), Haberman (10), Daniel and Wood (11), Draper and Smith [34], and Wooding (12). It is strongly recommended that you

ensure that your statistician test for this violation, because it can be serious in many cases.

Well-known tests for inequality of variances include **Hartley's Maximum F Ratio** test (13), **Bartlett's** test (14), **Levene's** test (15), and the **Siegel-Tukey** test (16). Hartley's test is suitable only for the case of two variances (two groups) because of the danger of multiplicity otherwise. Bartlett's and Levene's tests can be used for any number of variances. The Siegel-Tukey test is a rank test. Hartley's and Bartlett's tests are very sensitive to nonnormality, and are not dependable in such circumstances. If your statistician has done a test for nonnormality and found little or no problem, or if you have used a transformation of scale to normalize the data, rechecking afterward with a nonnormality test, these tests are then reliable. Otherwise, the Levene test is the best choice. This test is described briefly in the next chapter.

Independence

The fourth assumption, independence, can generally be assumed to hold if the experimental design is one in which correlation of the errors could not easily come about. However, there are some methods of detecting lack of independence if it is necessary, although they are not described here.

13.4   MULTIPLICITY

13.4.1   The Meaning of Multiplicity

In clinical studies, the word *multiplicity* has come to mean the *repeated use* of hypothesis tests in an incorrect manner. When multiplicity exists in a study, serious errors in the interpretation of your data will be made if you do not use adequate corrections. The true probability, alpha, will be greater than that specified when planning your study; sometimes much greater.

13.4.2   Illustration

Let's say that you are doing a t test to examine a difference between just two treatment group means. You calculate a value of t from your data and compare the result with a tabular (standard) value at the alpha probability that you specified a priori. You then claim significance for the difference being tested if the value of t that you calculate exceeds the tabulated value at probability alpha. Alpha was specified under the assumption that you planned to compare only two treatments, and to use the significance test on the same pair only once, and that is what you have done. You have used the test correctly.

But suppose that your trial consisted of *three* treatment groups, and you wished to compare each of them with each of the others, making a total of three comparisons. You are now introducing multiplicity. Without employing any method of compensation such as the Bonferroni procedure, you repeat the *t* test for each of the three comparisons. Alternatively, suppose, having two or more treatment comparisons you wish to make, you compare one pair of treatments several times (once for each of several different responses) or you use the significance test repeatedly on data obtained at several different times during the trial. Or you may perhaps perform a combination of two or more of these procedures. All of them are incorrect.

To do a *t* test, you calculate a value of *t* from your data and then compare the result with a tabular value. If there is multiplicity, the *correct* tabular *t* value will be *smaller* than the one that you find in the *t* table, and this smaller value will be associated with a larger value of alpha than the one you find. To put it another way, in the long run, you will then incorrectly reject H_0 and claim significance too often. The larger the value of *t*, the smaller the probability that the observed difference could occur if H_0 were really true, other things being equal. Thus, if there is multiplicity, the true alpha probability will not be that originally specified, but a larger value, and your conclusion that a difference delta exists between the treatment group populations may be incorrect.

The reason for this is easy to see. Suppose you have specified an alpha value of 0.05 during the planning stage. This is the probability of claiming significance incorrectly (when H_0 is true). But if you based that specification upon the expectation of the use of a *t* test (which is designed for a single pairwise comparison), but you then make one or more *additional* comparisons, the true alpha value will be substantially greater than 0.05, so that your risk of incorrectly claiming significance will be greater. An alpha value of 0.05 means that you will be wrong in claiming significance about 5% of the time. But if there is multiplicity, you will be wrong considerably more often.

Misuse of Hypothesis Tests
Several sources of multiplicity are mentioned or discussed in some of the references in the Bibliography, for example, Feinstein [21], Friedman et al. [2], Inglefinger et al. [23], Pocock [4], and Shapiro and Louis [5]. Pocock ([4] pages 228–233) provides a particularly complete and well-organized section on the subject. The kinds of multiplicity discussed here are mentioned in these references and others, but should be reiterated here. This kind of misinterpretation of the use of significance tests could hardly be more serious an error, because it can completely change the conclusions you may draw from a clinical study. And this error is quite common in industrial clinical work, especially in smaller houses where a large or easily available statistical department does not exist. Some tests, such as the *t* test, seem simple and straightforward, and hence are frequently done without consulta-

tion with a biostatistician. The introduction of uncompensated multiplicity into clinical trial designs and analysis is so widespread in industrial clinical studies that there cannot be too much emphasis upon the problem.

13.4.3 Compensation for Multiplicity

Fortunately, compensation for multiplicity is easy if the problem is foreseen and appropriate measures are taken at the planning stage. It is frequently necessary to introduce some form of multiplicity into your data-analysis procedures. There will be no untoward effects if you provide appropriate compensation. When there must be multiplicity, it should be taken into account during planning, and a suitable remedy arranged for at that time. The most suitable form of such corrections is to arrange for a suitable sample size when planning a trial. If multiplicity is foreseen, the sample size will be greater than otherwise. When the sample size cannot be adjusted in this way, there are other methods to avoid incorrect claims of significance, but they are less satisfactory.

In this section, we consider the three most frequent ways (mentioned briefly earlier) that multiplicity is introduced into a clinical study. The words "test" and "comparison" in the following refer to hypothesis tests. Multiplicity can occur if (a) **more than one comparison** is made in a trial, either by repeating tests of the same two treatments, or by testing more than two treatments, that is, making more than one comparison, using a test valid for only one; (b) **several different kinds of response measurements** are made and tested in the same clinical study; or (c) one or more **interim tests** are done using data obtained before the final response measurements are made, in addition to those done with the final data. One or more of these problems is usually present when *any* clinical study is run, and should always be compensated for.

Increasing the sample size during planning is the best remedy for each of these problems, and of course this may increase the cost or time required to complete a trial. If additional costs or a longer trial associated with increased sample size cannot be tolerated, perhaps the design can be rethought—using two treatments instead of more than two, or fewer responses, or foregoing the analysis of some of the intermediate data, or eliminating other interim testing arrangements.

Compensation for multiplicity in the common cases is described in what follows. These procedures are most useful when you can anticipate a problem before your trial is begun, and adjust the sample size accordingly. However, there are some less satisfactory solutions that can be used without preplanning.

When There Is No Multiplicity

First, let's consider a trial in which there will be no multiplicity at all. Suppose that you plan a study of rheumatoid arthritis using two groups of patients, each patient having been randomly assigned to one of two drugs and treated over a period of time. You are concerned with ESR measurements (erythrocyte sedimentation rate). Assume that you will not be using any other response in the data analysis, you will not analyze any data except for baseline and final measurements on each patient, and you plan to calculate and test differences from the baseline, so that each patient will yield one datum at the end of the trial. You will have set up alpha and beta risks (say, 0.05 and 0.10, respectively), specified a value for delta, obtained an estimate of sigma, and used these quantities to estimate your sample size.

After the trial, you do a two-tailed t test of your data to compare the two population mean differences from baseline.[14] (This and other significance tests will be described in detail in Chapter 14.) If you find significance, you will conclude that the difference between the two drugs (in the population) is delta, and that the probability of being wrong because the null hypothesis is really true, is alpha. The strength and validity of that conclusion will be functions of the sample size (which you are satisfied is adequate), the specified alpha and delta, and the care with which your trial was planned and carried out (which you are also satisfied is adequate). If you do not find significance, you will conclude that the null hypothesis is true. The probability of being wrong (because the null hypothesis is really false) will be beta. In a word, you will have done everything *right*.

More Than One Treatment Comparison

Suppose instead that your trial had consisted of *three* groups, testing *three* different drugs. You might now proceed to use t tests to compare each pair of drug groups in turn (T_1 vs. T_2, T_1 vs. T_3, and T_2 vs. T_3). If you use the same value of alpha and the same sample size as before, and you find significance, say, with a p value just under 0.05, for one or more of the three comparisons, what will you conclude? In fact, your tests, taken as a group, will not have been done at the 0.05 alpha level at all. Use of the Bonferroni inequality (Chapter 5), for example, although it is a little conservative, would have shown that you should have tested each of the pairs at the 0.05/3, or the 0.016, level of alpha, at most, to ensure that the *experimentwise error rate*, that is, the alpha value for all three tests taken together, was less than 0.05.

The reason for this is as follows: If you use an alpha value of 0.05 in comparing a single pair of treatments, and if the population difference is really zero (i.e., if the null hypothesis is true), you would nevertheless find significance (i.e., a p value less than 0.05), on the average, about 5% of the

---

[14] The t test is used here merely as a paradigm. The remarks in this section about the multiplicity introduced by repeated use of the t test apply equally strongly to other significance tests intended for comparing just two treatments, including rank tests or other procedures. Of course, there are differences in the use and applicability of various tests, including the lack of need for the normality assumption when using some tests. The next two chapters will include information on the conditions necessary for the valid use of each of several common procedures.

time that such tests were done, because 0.05 is your chosen error rate. On the other hand, if there is really a population difference greater than delta, p values of less than 0.05 will usually occur *more often* than 5% of the time.[15]

However, when you test more than one pair of means by repeating the t test procedure for each pair, this procedure is no longer valid. Suppose that the null hypothesis is really true, and there is no difference among the three groups other than random error. If you make, say, three comparisons (such as the means of group A vs. B, A vs. C, and B vs. C), using an alpha value of 0.05, *each* of those three comparisons will have an alpha value of 0.05. You will incorrectly conclude that there is significance for one or another of the three comparisons more often than 5% of the time. With three treatments instead of two, and thus three comparisons rather than one, the rate of occurrence of false significances will no longer be 5% (5 in 100 tests); there will be about 14 in every 100 tests.[16]

How can you compensate for this kind of multiplicity? You already know part of the answer. You must not use the ordinary t test or other procedure designed for one comparison only; rather you must use a multiple-comparisons test. The one we have recommended is the Bonferroni method. This procedure takes the multiplicity into account, and your *experimentwise* error rate, which applies to the group of three comparisons, taken together, will now be 0.05, your specified value of alpha. But if you have not increased the sample size to a value appropriate to your specifications of alpha, beta, and delta, and to your estimate of sigma, assuming three t tests are to be made, although the use of a multiple-comparisons procedure will ensure, on the average, that the *alpha* level will be approximately that intended, *beta, delta,* or *both will increase.* Therefore, if you are going to make more than one comparison at the end of your trial, you must increase the sample size per treatment accordingly during planning, *and* use a multiple-comparisons test.

---

[15]This is not merely theory. It can be demonstrated easily, even on a desktop computer using a BASIC program, by means of a Monte Carlo study. Pairs of sets of random normal deviates (random normal numbers) of a given sample size, with the population mean kept constant, are repeatedly generated. These are taken to represent repeated samples of two treatment groups from identical populations. Tests using Student's t at 5% alpha are done on each pair. It will be found that as the number of repetitions increase, the percentage of significances found approaches closer and closer to 5%.

[16]The reason that the error rate (for all three treatments taken as a group) is now about 14% rather than 5% is easy to show. Let's assume that you have run a trial in which there are three possible paired treatment comparisons, and let's further assume that the null hypothesis is true. Suppose that you were to test one of the three pairs of treatments repeatedly, using 100 identical tests. You would get about five incorrect positives and 95 correct negatives. When you repeat this with the second pair, the 95 correct tests remaining would be further reduced by an expected 0.05×95, which is a substantial additional number, 4.75. Finally, when you apply the test the third time, calculating the number in the same way, there would be 4.5125 further false significances expected. Thus, if you used the t test at the 0.05 alpha level three times instead of once in the same experiment, your *true* total experimentwise error rate would not be 5% but $(5 + 4.75 + 4.5125)\%$, or about 14.26%.

More Than One Response

Although multiplicity stemming from the use of several different kinds of response measurements is very often ignored in clinical trials, this can have just as serious an effect upon the significance level (and thus also upon beta) as the testing of more than two treatment contrasts in an unprotected manner. It is therefore recommended (a) that the sample size be adjusted during planning to correct for whatever multiplicity remains if there are several responses, and (b) that the number of responses be kept as small as possible to avoid the expense of excessive increases in the sample size.

Intermediate Measurements

This is another frequently encountered kind of multiplicity. It often occurs in one of two forms. The first and less common is the use of so-called *interim* testing. This may be planned a priori, but is sometimes decided upon after visual examination of ongoing data during a study. It may become important for either ethical or economic reasons to discontinue a study early (before the originally planned period has elapsed). If the visual examination of the data seems to show superiority for a test drug (versus a placebo, for example), the patients may be examined and an intermediate response (or set of responses) obtained and analyzed. If significance is found in favor of the test drug, the trial may be stopped prematurely. Of course, if the "interim" tests then become the final tests because the trial has been discontinued, there will be no multiplicity. Such a procedure is not advisable, however.

The second and more common use of intermediate measurements occurs when a study must run for a long period of time, perhaps because of the nature of the disease, because the drug(s) are anticipated to require some time to achieve full effect, or a combination of these two. Suppose that you are working with a parallel design that uses drugs at two levels (i.e., a test drug versus a standard or placebo) as the only factor. Suppose the disease is one requiring continuous medication, such as hypertension, a cardiac condition, dyspnea, or one of the varieties of arthritis. The trial may need to be run for a long period because regular treatments cannot be discontinued without pain or discomfort for the patients. Any benefits of the test treatments are then partially masked, and, in addition, some weeks of continuous dosing with the study drugs may be required before they can become fully effective. In such a case, if for no other purpose than the necessity of good supervision of the trial, repeated response measurements may be desirable, perhaps every 2 weeks or every month. Suppose that the trial is to run for 12 weeks and measurements are made every 2 weeks. In such a case, there will be a series of six data recorded for each patient, and if these data are to be analyzed and the results used to draw conclusions about the drug, serious multiplicity will exist.

To compensate satisfactorily for the multiplicity, any intermediate measurements should be preplanned, because it is necessary that the a priori sample size estimate take them into account. Alternatively, if a series of such measurements is taken as a routine, "for the record," with no intention of doing significance tests, using them to influence the final conclusions, or determining whether to stop the trial, there is no problem. But if the intermediate data are to be tested and the results used for one of those purposes, without preplanning, the specified values of alpha, beta, or delta, or all three, will not be what they seem. In other words, the effect of interim or intermediate significance tests will be exactly the same, in principle, as an increase in the number of comparisons, as discussed earlier.

Special Problems and Remedies

In addition to the use of an a priori sample size estimate that takes the expected multiplicity into account, testing a series of measurements taken throughout a trial requires special techniques when the analyses are done.[17] Unfortunately, such techniques are frequently neglected. The data are often analyzed by the use of a series of t tests, without the use of a procedure such as the Bonferroni to compensate for the multiplicity. Multiplicity is introduced because of the repeated measurements of the same treatment groups, even when there are only two treatments. But in this situation, there is still another effect: the probability that there will be autocorrelation of the errors of the successive measurements on each patient. If there is a large enough set of data, this kind of lack of independence of successive measurements can be detected if it exists, but a large enough set is uncommon. The independent form of the t test is not designed to be used in such a case, and if such dependence exists, a series of analyses of successive responses will give incorrect results. Taking the measurements as a group, the result will be nonconservative because the estimate of sigma made during the test procedure will be too small. That is, even if the treatments are not really as different as that specified by delta, the probability of the test indicating significance will nevertheless be greater than planned.

Linear regression analyses,[18] even when they are the appropriate kind to use, will give similarly misleading results in the presence of autocorrelation. This problem is discussed thoroughly and clearly in Mandel [36], Chapter 12, especially pages 295–310. If there is autocorrelation, its effect in this case is

---

[17]It may occur to you that a bioavailability trial does just this—it uses a number of data based upon blood samples collected throughout the trial. However, there is no multiplicity in such a trial except for that introduced by the use of four different kinds of response (this, of course, should be compensated for). The blood-concentration values accumulated during the test are used to create just four derived responses, and these are the responses that are tested. In the same way, in a comparison of analgesics, for example, the sum of pain intensities (SPI) and the sum of pain intensity differences (SPID) are single derived responses based upon a series of primary responses (pain intensities) that, however, are not analyzed per se.

[18]As mentioned earlier, regression analysis is not described in this book, but excellent references include Draper and Smith [34] and Snedecor and Cochran [38].

to produce an incorrectly small estimate (often very much too small) of the error of the slope, although the estimate of the slope itself will not be biased. However, if the regression can be assumed to be linear, there is a simple solution, as described by Mandel.

Sometimes recurrent measurements are not planned, but there is a temptation to extend the trial if an effect has not appeared.[19] Such abandonment of the plan laid down by the protocol is obviously bending the design to get a desired result. Besides the capacity for self-deception that this procedure entails, it is one of the most effective ways to invite rejection of a study by the FDA.

Please note that we recognize that you must make interim measurements and consider whether to discontinue a trial, or you may plan to complete a trial but nevertheless include one or more intermediate measurements. These things can be done, but they must be *planned* to be done properly if significance tests are to be run. There are some easy ways to avoid the effects of multiplicity without increasing the sample size. One of these is to do the analysis using the data of the final period only, or perhaps the difference between this and a baseline measurement (a better way, instead of using such differences, is to use an ACOVA with baseline data as the concomitant measurement[20]). Another solution is to analyze averages of the measurements made in the last two or three periods. Unlike simply compensating for the additional measurements by increasing the sample size, these procedures also eliminate any effects of autocorrelation of successive measurements.

If the foregoing procedures seem unsatisfactory, and you wish to emphasize the variation in responses throughout a trial, the biostatistician can perform a rough test for treatment-related trends. This can be done by assuming a linear model, even if the data do not appear to be linear (but not if they form a peak or depression, because that would reduce or eliminate any evidence of an overall trend). To do this, a straight line is fitted (linear regression) to the data for each patient. The slopes found for these lines are then used as data for comparing treatments. Such calculations will often display useful information about the rate and nature of changes in a response during the course of a trial.

---

[19]Sometimes, instead, without planning, a trial is discontinued prematurely, even if there is no danger or inconvenience to the patients, if an interim significance test is positive before the planned endpoint. This mistake is as serious as extending the trial in an unplanned way. Continuing a fixed sample size design beyond the time and sample size originally planned, or discontinuing it before all the patients have been entered or maintained in the study for the planned period is wrong, and will lead to incorrect interpretation of the data. Of course, there are times when patient welfare may require such action, but, if so, the temptation to analyze the data and draw anything but tentative conclusions from them should be resisted.

[20]The procedure for running an ACOVA (analysis of covariance) is not described in this book, but is covered in Snedecor and Cochran [38], Chapter 18 and in several other books listed in the General Statistics section of the Bibliography.

13.5 SUMMARY OF THE CHAPTER

After an introductory section, there is a major section on the basic ideas underlying a statistical analysis of data from a clinical study. This includes a section that discusses the purposes of data analysis, and one describing the several kinds of **response data**. The nature of a data analysis can be highly dependent upon the kind of data to be analyzed. For example, methods for the analysis of dichotomous (two-valued) data are very different from those suitable for continuous response data, such as blood pressures, weights, volumes, or temperatures.

There is a section concerned with **randomization** and **hypothesis testing**. Some aspects of these topics have been discussed earlier, but because of their fundamental importance in clinical trial work, we treat them here at some length. In the same section, the related topics of confidence intervals and the use of the **least significant difference** are discussed briefly. A short examination of several other topics related to analysis follow.

A brief discussion of **probability** follows, to foster understanding of the section on hypothesis testing.

The section on basic ideas concludes with a detailed discussion of **hypothesis testing**. Some of these ideas were discussed in Chapter 5, in which the estimation of sample size was introduced. Here, the topic is reviewed and substantially expanded.

The second major section is concerned with the **parametric assumptions**. Most statistical hypothesis tests and related procedures make certain assumptions about the distributions or populations from which the samples of patients are assumed to have come. Methods for testing the validity of these assumptions are discussed further in Chapter 14.

A final section is concerned with managing multiplicity.

13.6 LITERATURE REFERENCES

(1) Edgington, Eugene S., *Randomization Tests*, Marcel Dekker, New York, 1980.

(2) Edgington, Eugene S., *Randomization Tests*, 2d ed., Marcel Dekker, New York, 1987.

(3) Scheffé, Henry, *The Analysis of Variance*, John Wiley, New York, 1959.

(4) Shapiro, S. S., and M. B. Wilk, *Biometrika*, 52, 591–611 (1965).

(5) Lilliefors, Hubert W., *Journal of the American Statistical Association*, 62, 399–402 (1967).

(6) Dallal, Gerard E., and Leland Wilkinson, *The American Statistician*, 40, 294–296 (1986).

(7) Michael, John R., *Biometrika*, 70, 11–17 (1983).

(8) Nelson, Lloyd S., *Journal of Quality Technology*, 21, 213–215 (1989).

(9) Anscombe, F. J., and John W. Tukey, *Technometrics*, 5, No. 2, 141–160 (1963).

(10) Haberman, Shelby J., *Biometrics*, 29, 205–220 (1973).

(11) Daniel, Cuthbert, and Fred S. Wood, *Fitting Equations to Data*, John Wiley, New York, NY, (1971).

(12) Wooding, W. M., *Journal of Quality Technology*, 1, No. 3, 175–188 (1969).

(13) Hartley, H. O., *Biometrika*, 37, 308–312 (1950).

(14) Bartlett, M. S., *Journal of the Royal Statistical Society*, 4, 137 (1937).

(15) Levene, H., *Contributions to Probability and Statistics*, Stanford University Press, Stanford, CA, 1960, p. 278.

(16) Siegel, S., and J. W. Tukey, *Journal of the American Statistical Association*, 55, 429–444 (1960). There are corrections in ibid., 56, 971–976 (1961).

CHAPTER 14

Data Analysis:
Basic Statistical Procedures

14.1 INTRODUCTION

As you know, the primary goal of this book is to help you understand the elements of experimental design and some related topics needed in preparing for industrial clinical trials. The most important related topic is the analysis of the data from your clinical trials. Although, perhaps, your statistician may perform the necessary analyses and you may never analyze any data, it is almost impossible to design a clinical study or estimate sample size without some understanding of the principles of applied statistics.

Prior to the preceding chapter, we presented very little discussion of statistical analysis. This material appears near the end of the book because the basic principles of applied experimental design must be more thoroughly and extensively explained than those of analysis, providing, as we assume, that professional statistical help is available to you. Nevertheless, the design of most clinical trials requires familiarity with some of the basic procedures of data analysis. Furthermore, a clear understanding of the purposes of randomization and of the methods of sample size estimation is impossible without some basic knowledge of statistical analysis.

As was pointed out in the preceding chapter, all or nearly all the statistical procedures used in the analysis of data from clinical trials involve hypothesis testing. These procedures include the various forms of the t test, equivalent rank tests, contingency table tests, tests involving the binomial distribution, the many forms of analysis of variance, and many others. The statistical literature abounds with these tests, both from theoretical and applied points of view. In this chapter, we present descriptions of five of them: two t tests, two rank tests, and a simple contingency table procedure. You are not expected to use these in your work; you will probably leave that to the biostatistician. However, if you have time to work through the examples, you will develop a greater appreciation and a better understanding of clinical studies, overall, than you could acquire otherwise.

I do not wish to discourage you from trying some of these statistical procedures in your trials; in fact, you are encouraged to do so, if you wish. But if you do, check your work with the statistician. Do not fall into the trap of believing that even if you are aware that you do *not* fully understand a statistical procedure, you can nevertheless run it on the computer without help because you possess a good statistical software package. No package can make this possible, the advertising of some to the contrary. It is essential that you understand a statistical procedure and its background, whether you are using a computer, a pocket calculator, or just paper and pencil. This degree of understanding can only be obtained by acquiring some knowledge of the theoretical bases of the methods you wish to use. You should also have actually done a number of examples by hand (i.e., with paper, pencil, and a pocket calculator). After reading a description and an example, it is easy to *think* we understand a procedure until we try it and must stop to consider points that were not clear after all. In summary, the purpose of these two chapters is to help you to design studies, not to teach you very much statistics. Nevertheless, you *can* learn from them, and that knowledge will help you to design better trials.

14.2   ESTIMATING ERROR

14.2.1   Introduction

Every hypothesis test requires an estimate of the error (precision) of the data to be tested. If you are using data from continuous distributions, and parametric test procedures, the error estimate should almost always be calculated from the current data. The rank tests and contingency table tests are based upon the distribution of ranks and upon the binomial distribution. In these cases, too, error estimates are used, but they are often inherent in the procedures, and need not be explicitly calculated.[1]

14.2.2   Estimating Variance and Standard Deviation

Nomenclature
In Chapter 5, the standard deviation, sigma, of a normal distribution curve was discussed and defined geometrically as a measure of the distance between either inflection point and a perpendicular line at the center of the curve (i.e., the "width" of the distribution; see Figure 5.4 in Chapter 5). At that time, however, methods of estimating sigma from the data, although mentioned, were not described in detail.

---

[1]In certain **normal approximation** procedures for both rank and contingency table tests, error estimates must be calculated. These procedures are not described here, but they are not difficult to use. One of them is incorporated in BASIC program AP.2 for the Wilcoxon Rank Sum test in the Appendix to this book.

Table 14.1. Symbols for the Standard Deviation

σ	Standard deviation or sigma (parameter)
σ_{yi}	Standard deviation or sigma (parameter)
$\hat{\sigma}$	Estimated sigma (statistic)
$\hat{\sigma}_{yi}$	Estimated sigma (statistic)
s	Estimated sigma (statistic)
s_{yi}	Estimated sigma (statistic)
S	Estimated sigma (statistic)
S_{yi}	Estimated sigma (statistic)

The terms **standard deviation** and **sigma** refer both to a parameter and to its estimate, a statistic. The distinction will always be unambiguous when we use mathematical notation, as we will always use the Greek *lowercase* letter sigma (σ) for the parameter, and a capital or lowercase "S" for the statistic (i.e., the estimate of the parameter). In other cases it will be made clear. Some texts symbolize the statistic as **sigma hat** ($\hat{\sigma}$) rather than as s. The "hat," or circumflex, implies that the quantity is a statistic. Appropriate subscripts will usually be used. If there is no subscript, you may assume, unless the text indicates otherwise, that the quantity of concern is the basic one, the **standard deviation of single items from the mean**. Sometimes we will call this quantity the **standard deviation of single items**. We may say sigma or **standard deviation** for short. There are other kinds of standard deviations. Forexample, there is the **standard deviation of the mean** (also called the **standard error of the mean**, or the **standard error** for short), and the **standard deviation of a mean difference**, also called the **standard error of a mean difference**, to mention two of them. When we have occasion to use any of these, which one is meant will be apparent. For the moment, we are concerned only with the standard deviation of single items.
items.

The symbols for the standard deviation of single items have a variety of forms. Table 14.1 shows some of the more common ones, some or all of which we may use in this and the next chapter.

14.2.3   How to Calculate the Estimated Standard Deviation

Method 1

This and the method described next may appear somewhat difficult at first glance, especially if your algebra is a bit rusty. If you follow the explanation and the example carefully, however, you should have no trouble.

One of the phrases just mentioned, *the standard deviation of single items from their mean*, suggests an approach to calculating an estimate of this quantity from a set of data. This approach is more obvious when we use a more complete description—**the square root of the sum of squares of deviations from the mean, divided by the degrees of freedom**. We will call this procedure Method 1 and explain it in what follows, and then illustrate it with an example. Method 1 illustrates the nature of the quantity s_{y_i} most clearly. Method 2, which we will explain later, is easier to use with hand calculations and some pocket calculators.

Let's assume that you have 16 data representing the height in centimeters (to the nearest 0.1 cm) of a patient, taken over a period of time. For this illustration, the data were obtained by taking a random sample of 16 from a population of so-called random normal deviates (normally distributed random numbers) having a mean of zero and a standard deviation of one.[2] The value 175 was arbitrarily selected as the population mean and was added to each random number. In this way, a sample was constructed that was known to have been taken from a normal population with a known mean (175) and standard deviation (1). Our knowledge of the parameters of the distribution that was sampled will later allow us to observe the precision of our estimates of the standard deviation and mean. Differences from these parameters will be principally due to sampling variability.

The calculations for Method 1 are done as follows. This description is followed by an example.

1. Prepare a table with three columns. Label the first column y_i, the second $y_i - \bar{y}$, and the third $(y_i - \bar{y})^2$.

2. Place your data in the first column (y_i). The subscript i in the column label represents the number of each datum, that is, y_1, y_2, etc.

3. Calculate the sum of all of the data (symbolized as $\sum_i y_i$) and write it below the first column. Under that, write the number of data, N, and, finally, in the third row under that column, write the **mean** (i.e., $\bar{y}$, which is the sum divided by N).

4. Calculate the difference between each datum in the first column and the mean of all of the data (in either direction but consistently) and place these differences in the second column. In the example that follows, the mean is subtracted from each datum, as indicated by the column label $y_i - \bar{y}$. Although we are going to square these deviations, so that their signs will not matter, record the signs anyway. They may be useful in some circumstances during an analysis. Add this second column and place the sum underneath it. The sum should be zero, but because of decimal rounding error, it rarely is. However, after dividing that sum by the number of data in the column, if you have used sufficient decimal places in your calculations of each difference and their averages, the result should be very small relative to the magnitudes of the individual values in the column. If it is not, you should check your work or use more places.

5. Square each deviation (difference) and place the squares in the third column.

---

[2] For example, see Beyer [47], pp. 484–493.

6. Add the third column, putting the sum below the column. This is the **sum of squares of deviations from the mean**, and can be written as follows: $\Sigma_i(y_i - \bar{y})^2$. This step completes the table.[3]

7. Calculate the **degrees of freedom** (the number of data minus 1) and divide the sum of squares by it. This is the variance of single items from the mean.

8. Take the square root of the result. This is the estimated **standard deviation of single items from the mean**.

For reference, we will identify these steps by a series of algebraic formulas based upon these definitions. These summarize the previous process more succinctly.

First, calculate the degrees of freedom for the standard deviation and variance. This is one less than N, the number of data, and is symbolized by df:

$$df = N - 1 \tag{14.1}$$

Next, calculate the estimated *variance of deviations from the mean*, often called just the *variance* and symbolized by $S_{y_i}^2$. This is done by calculating the sum of squares (i.e., the sum of squares of deviations from the mean) and dividing it by the degrees of freedom:

$$S_{y_i}^2 = \frac{\Sigma_i(y_i - \bar{y})^2}{df} \tag{14.2}$$

Finally, take the square root of the result to obtain the estimated standard deviation of single items from the mean, S_{y_i}:

$$S_{y_i} = \sqrt{S_{y_i}^2} \tag{14.3}$$

[3]There are various common ways to symbolize a summation. A simple one is that used here (Σ_i). It represents the addition of the numbers represented by y_i, with i beginning with one, representing the first datum, and increasing by one as each successive value is taken. Sometimes the summation sign, capital sigma (Σ), is used with no subscript when the expression being summed is obvious. The forms conveying the most information, however, are $\sum_{i=1}^{N}$ or $\Sigma_{i=1}^{N}$. Here, N symbolizes the total number of data, and i becomes successively the number of each as the addition proceeds, so that $i = 1, 2, \ldots, N$ ("i goes from 1 to N"). When a summation sign is followed by a subscripted (numbered) variable such as y_i, as in ($\Sigma_{i=1}^{N} y_i$), it is read, "The sum of the values of y sub i (or the sum of y sub i), from $i = 1$ to $i = N$." Sometimes, the starting point will be a number other than 1.

All of this can be summarized in a single equation, as follows:

$$S_{y_i} = \sqrt{\frac{\Sigma(y_i - \bar{y})^2}{N - 1}} \qquad (14.4)$$

Example 14.1, which follows, illustrates these calculations, following the previous steps.

14.2.4   Example 14.1: Calculating SS, S^2, and S

Table 14.2 comprises the sample of the 16 patients' heights in centimeters, and was created following steps 1 through 6 and the previous equations. The sum of the second column is shown in order to make a point. Note that this sum is almost zero. It would be exactly zero except for the rounding error in the division used to calculate the mean and in the rounding of the results of the subtractions. I used two decimal places in calculating each deviation from the mean to reduce this error, although the precision of the original data suggest that only one should be used.

The remainder of the procedure (steps 7 and 8) is as follows: The df is $N - 1$, or 15, from Equation (14.1). Using Equation (14.2) (dividing the sum

Table 14.2. Data and Initial Steps in Calculation of Variance and Standard Deviation Using the Deviations Method (Method 1)

	y_i	$y_i - \bar{y}$	$(y_i - \bar{y})^2$
	173.7	-1.51	2.2801
	176.3	1.09	1.1881
	175.6	0.39	0.1521
	175.7	0.49	0.2401
	175.1	-0.11	0.0121
	173.6	-1.61	2.5921
	174.4	-0.81	0.6561
	175.1	-0.11	0.0121
	176.4	1.19	1.4161
	176.2	0.99	0.9801
	175.8	0.59	0.3481
	174.1	-1.11	1.2321
	174.2	-1.01	1.0201
	175.0	-0.21	0.0441
	177.6	2.39	5.7121
	174.6	-0.61	0.3721
Sum	2803.40	0.04	18.2576
N	16	16	16
Mean	175.21	0.0025	

of squares of deviations from the mean by this df), we obtain the variance:

$$S^2_{y_i} = \frac{\Sigma_i (y_i - \bar{y})^2}{df} \qquad (14.2)$$

$$= \frac{SS_{y_i}}{df}$$

$$= \frac{18.2576}{15}$$

$$= 1.2172$$

Taking the square root of the variance according to Equation (14.3), we then obtain the estimated standard deviation:

$$S_{y_i} = \sqrt{S^2_{y_i}} \qquad (14.3)$$

$$= \sqrt{1.2172}$$

$$= 1.1033$$

The result was rounded to two decimal places, giving 1.10 for the final estimate of sigma. As you see at the bottom of Table 14.2, the sample mean, which is an estimate of the population mean, mu, is 175.21. You will recall that the sample was randomly selected from a population with a known sigma of 1 and a known mean of 175. The differences between the values we have calculated and these known parameters are results of sampling error. In this case, the errors are reasonably small (the estimated sigma is 1.10, about 10% higher than the [known] parameter and the mean is very close). Note that the numbers in the third column of the table are all positive regardless of the signs of the differences in the second column, because they were squared. Also, you should be aware that *every* sum of squares of deviations from the mean of any set of numbers is always positive or zero, never negative. Furthermore, they are zero only if there is no variation among the original numbers. Therefore, if you ever calculate a sum of squares of deviations and get a negative number, try again; there will be an error in your calculations. If you get zero, check to see that all the numbers in the set are the same. Of course, if this is true, you need not make the calculation at all, because it will be obvious that there is no variation among the data. But if you do encounter such a set of data, you should become very skeptical. In this imperfect world, measurements made without error are very rare, to put it mildly.

If you need only standard deviations, variances, or means, you can do all the previous calculations rapidly with any of several different pocket calculators (e.g., various Hewlett-Packard, Texas Instrument, and Casio models). If you are going to use the data or the results in further calculations, the statistician will probably wish to do them instead on a desktop computer or a mini or mainframe, using one of the several available statistical program packages such as SYSTAT [66], or a program you or your statistician have written yourselves.

Method 2

The method just described is the fundamental procedure for calculating estimated sigma, and is always appropriate. However, to use it, you must first calculate the mean of the data. If you use a calculator, unless you enter your data twice, it must have enough memory to store all the data, because you will need to use the set of data twice, first to calculate the mean and then to obtain the deviations. However, for writing a computer program (or a calculator program if the calculator has adequate memory), Method 1 is better, as it minimizes the rounding errors, and it is easy to provide for initial input and storage of the data. On the other hand, Method 2 is faster with a calculator than with a computer if you do not have many data. With small sets of data, the method can be used even with simple desk or pocket calculators, although a scientific calculator having a simple summing and squaring procedure makes the process easier. When you use Method 2, you should be sure that you carry plenty of decimals, rounding only at the end of the entire process (four to eight decimal places are not too many). Most scientific pocket calculators do this internally and automatically, to even more places than this (10 to 14), rounding results only for the display.

Like Method 1, Method 2 also requires the initial calculation of the sum of squares, SS, but it uses a different expression. The result, however, is the same quantity as that shown in the numerator of Equation (14.2). This result is then divided by the df, as before, yielding the variance, and the square root is finally extracted. The process is illustrated by the three equations that follow. Equation (14.5) yields the sum of squares, Equation (14.6) the variance, and Equation (14.7), the standard deviation. The variance is calculated separately here both because it simplifies understanding of the process and because it will be used alone later in this chapter. As you can see, the difference between Methods 1 and 2 lies in the calculation of the sum of squares; the remaining steps are the same in both cases. Note carefully that in Equation (14.5), the first term is the sum of the squares of y_i, that is, each datum (each value of y_i) is first squared and then all the squares are added. But the second term is *the square of the sum* divided by N. In this case, all of the y values are first added, and then this sum is squared and divided by N.

$$SS = \Sigma_i y_i^2 - \frac{(\Sigma_i y_i)^2}{N} \qquad (14.5)$$

$$S_{y_i}^2 = \frac{SS}{N-1} \qquad (14.6)$$

$$S_{y_i} = \sqrt{S_{y_i}^2} \qquad (14.7)$$

You may wish to try Method 2 using the data of Table 14.1, and see that it gives the same result as Method I.

14.3   THE t TEST FAMILY

14.3.1   In General

Except in special circumstances, the procedures described in this section are intended to be used to compare two treatments only. Special procedures are available when a trial involves more than two. These are called **multiple-comparisons tests**, and are described in Section 14.6.

The t test methods of this chapter have been mentioned several times in earlier chapters, but until now we have not given specific details for using them.

All forms of the t test use the Student (W. S. Gosset) t distribution. Student's t was the first so-called parametric **small-sample statistic**. Its discovery by Student led the way to the design and analysis of experiments pioneered by Sir Ronald A. Fisher in the 1920s and 1930s. Prior to Student's and Fisher's work, large sample sizes were necessary to obtain reasonably precise comparisons based upon experimental data. In one famous case, Charles Darwin asked Francis Galton, a famous English statistician,[4] to make such a comparison for him using some of his botanical data. To accomplish this, very large numbers of observations were necessary. Today, the use of the t distribution often makes it possible to draw reliable conclusions from samples as small as 15 to 30 experimental units, provided that the samples are representative of their populations and the necessary sigma values are of reasonable magnitude.

The calculation of t is used as the basis of a hypothesis test, to "compare" two statistical quantities (and, in the absence of special procedures, only two, as mentioned before).[5] These quantities are usually arithmetic means, but one of them is sometimes another statistic, such as the slope of a line fitted to data, or some other quantity to be compared with a specified constant or known value. The t test asks whether an a priori null hypothesis that refers, for example, to two population means is reasonable in the light of statistics calculated from sample data. In other words, it tests whether an observed difference between means or from a standard value could reasonably be of the magnitude found if H_0 were true.

---

[4]To give Galton due credit for his versatility, he was also a noted geographer and meteorologist, and a Fellow of the Royal Society. In later life, his principal interests lay in genetics, statistics, and psychology. He is well known in statistics for his work in regression and correlation.

[5]In the past, the t test has been often misused, especially in industrial data analyses. The misapplications have included comparing multiple pairs of means from data comprising more than two groups, its use to analyze designs that call for multifactor analyses of variance (such as the two-period crossover), its use without checking the assumptions, its use for tests of grossly nonnormal data, and more.

14.3.2 Varieties of *t* Tests

Independent and Dependent t Tests

There are two major kinds of *t* tests, as well as some related procedures that can be considered to be part of the family. One of these two is used to compare independent groups (often called *independent t* tests), such as occur in two-treatment parallel designs. The other is a test for comparing a single value of interest, such as a mean difference obtained from a set of response data, with a standard value (perhaps a postulated population value), such as zero or some other specified quantity. For instance, a *t* test of a set of differences between two treatments, obtained from a changeover trial in which each of several patients receive both treatments in random order, could be run. The result would answer the question of whether the mean of a population of treatment differences could be equal to the standard quantity, zero, in view of the observed difference and the calculated sigma value. This is often called a *dependent t* test because the original data are not expected to be independent, as in a parallel design, but correlated in pairs, as in a changeover study. Other uses of the so-called one-sample *t* test are similar, in that they compare a single quantity with a standard value. That quantity need not be a difference, for example, it can be a single mean. The standard value might then be a postulated population mean. However, aside from difference tests, dependent *t* tests are rarely used in the analysis of clinical trial data.

To further clarify the difference between the common uses of an independent and a dependent *t* test, consider the following: The independent procedure tests whether two treatment group means coming from a *parallel* study could both come from the same population of *individual response values*. If not, the conclusion will be that there are two independent populations from which the two means arise. The difference procedure tests whether the mean of a population of *differences*, one from each patient *in a paired study*, is zero. If that mean is not zero, the two treatments are significantly different.

LSDs and Confidence Intervals

In addition to the *t* tests, there are two common and related procedures in the *t* test family that you should know about. These are least significant differences (LSDs) and confidence intervals (CIs). LSDs are not commonplace in clinical studies, but CIs are ubiquitous (and, like *t*, have been widely misused).

Other Considerations in Using t Tests

There are other features and characteristics of the use of *t* that will vary from one study to another depending upon the exact type of *t* test or related method planned. These include the necessity for a decision as to whether to use a one- or two-tailed test, as well as noting whether the test will use equal-sized patient groups (if it is an independent test). The use of the Neyman-Pearson procedure (the establishment of specifications for alpha, beta, and delta; the prior estimation of a value for sigma; and the use of these quantities to establish a sample size for the trial) should virtually always be a part of your trial plan.

14.3.3 Independent *t* test

This is the most common kind of *t* test, and is intended for use when there are just two independent samples (i.e., from a parallel study). For example, an independent *t* test would be appropriate when

(a) You have data from a trial of two drugs, each having been randomly assigned to a separate group of patients.

(b) When your object is to estimate whether the two treatments are different in their effects, that is, to compare the population means represented by the two groups (samples), using data comprising a single response related to efficacy or safety.

(c) When the errors of the data come from a distribution reasonably close to normal.

(d) When you expect that whether or not the samples come from two distributions with different means (as when the two treatments have different effects upon the response), the distributions represented by each of the two samples nevertheless have the same or nearly the same variances.

To use this procedure, you need an estimate of the standard deviation, which you can calculate from your data. After you do so, you will need to modify the result to get a new variety of estimated standard deviation—that of the difference between two independent means, which is the comparison you will be making. The means about which you will be making an inference are u_1 and u_2, the means of two independent *populations or distributions*. The *t* tests uses the observed difference between the two *sample* means and the estimated standard deviation of that difference to estimate whether there is a population difference. As long as you can safely assume that the variances in the two distributions are equal or nearly so, you can and should use the data from *both* groups for the calculation of the estimated standard deviation. As shown in what follows, to avoid the result being influenced by any differences between the means of the two groups, you calculate a *pooled* standard deviation.

Before performing the *t* test, you need to decide whether it is to be one- or two-tailed. It is important that this be settled when the trial is planned. You must also note the number of patients in each group, because you will use these sample sizes in your calculations. In addition, unless previous work with the same kinds of data and experimental designs have established reasonable normality and homogeneity of variances, the conformance of your data to these assumptions should be tested. Tests of the assumptions are referred to in what follows. They can be done by the statistician, but if you are interested, descriptions of two recommended procedures are given in the Appendix to this chapter. Finally, you should note from the experimental design and your trial procedure whether they could reflect any lack of **independence.**[6]

14.3.4 Example 14.2: *t* Test for Independent Groups (Small Sample)

Outline of the Trial

This study is intended to model many actual trials, but the data were fabricated from random normal deviates, because, as is true for most of the examples of this book, suitable industrial data are rarely in the public domain or available for publication. The sample size used was small to clarify the explanations, and the two treatment groups were unequal to reflect a common situation and to make the example more general. The usual small trial of this kind might use perhaps two or three times the number of patients we use here.

This experiment simulates the comparison of two wide-spectrum antibiotics, using patients with moderately severe throat infections. We assume that the nature of the infections was not verified beforehand by any microbiological procedures, although plate counts were run during the trial, as noted in what follows. The study was a preliminary trial, done at an industrial organization. A new drug, T_2, was thought to be more rapid in its action (although no more effective) than the previous drug of choice, T_1. As patients became available, one of these two drugs was randomly assigned to each of them using a double-blind arrangement, until the smaller of the two groups consisted of seven patients, the minimum number required on either treatment. As it happened, at that point, 10 patients had been assigned to the T_1 group, and the assignments were therefore concluded. The dosages were the same for both drugs, as the two were closely related chemically and pharmacologically, and preclinical work had indicated that the use of equal doses was appropriate.

Complete details of the protocol were read by each patient. Each who agreed to take part in the study was then given a one day supply of his or her assigned medication, and was instructed in its use. Each drug, in capsule form, was to be taken in a specified dose b.i.d. until the end point was reached for each patient, as described in what follows. Each patient was to continue participation until released by the investigator.

---

[6]Independence of the errors of the data from one observation to the next might be strained if similar instrument or observer biases could have been imposed when the data were taken, if no randomization or a faulty one were used, or the like. It is unlikely that you will be able to successfully test this possibility in a small experiment. However, if the experiment is well-conducted and the randomization properly done, there is unlikely to be an independence problem.

Execution and Data Collection

The patients were interviewed twice daily, and throat swabs were taken once a day. Plate counts based upon the daily throat smears from each patient were run, incubating them for 3 days but viewing them after 1, 2, and 3 days. After the first interview each morning, the patients were instructed to take the first of that day's doses of the assigned drug. The second dose was to be taken in the evening. This process was continued daily until the last plate count showed the infecting organisms to be reduced below a specified count. If there was no sign of reduction of the infecting organism after 4 days, a patient was to be dropped from the trial and switched to another treatment. As it happened, no such cases occurred. At each of the two daily interviews, each patient was asked whether his or her throat pain had disappeared completely. If it had, he or she was asked to estimate when this had occurred, to the nearest half hour, if possible. In cases of uncertain memory or failure to take notes, the interval was taken as the nearest number of full hours between the beginning of dosage and interview time. For each patient, the trial was continued until he or she reported no further throat pain, but in any event until 3 days after the last plate count showed no abnormal numbers of infectious organisms. This example will use the reported time intervals as the response.

The data (hours to disappearance of throat pain) are given in Table 14.3. The number of patients in each group, group means, sums of squares,

Table 14.3. Antibiotic Comparison in Throat Infection:
Hours to Disappearance of Subjective Symptoms,
Measured to Nearest Half Hour (Two-Treatment Parallel Design) (Example 14.2)

	Drug T_1	Drug T_2
	49.5	47.5
	48.0	48.5
	52.5	40.5
	46.5	43.5
	52.0	49.0
	48.5	43.5
	40.0	42.0
	50.5	
	46.0	
	46.5	
Sum, $\Sigma_i y_i$	480.0	314.5
Number of data, n_i	10	7
Mean, h., $\bar{y}$	48.00	44.93
Sum of Squares, SS_{y_i}	117.5000	68.2143
Variance, $S_{y_i}^2$	13.0556	11.3690
Std. Dev., S_{y_i}	3.6132	3.3718

variances, and standard deviations, all calculated as described earlier, are shown below each column of the table.

Checking Assumptions

Assumption Checking in General

The parametric assumptions were described in Chapter 12. With some exceptions, checking data for conformance to the assumptions is not a topic that has been strongly emphasized in the literature of clinical studies. Furthermore, that step has not infrequently been omitted in industrial clinical studies.

Convenient testing procedures are available for the two most important of these assumptions, when running single-factor trials (normality and homogeneity of variance). These procedures have been mentioned before, and their use for single-factor trials is described in detail in the Appendix to this chapter for anyone interested. Your statistician will be familiar with them or with equivalent tests. They are Michael's and Nelson's test for nonnormality, and Levene's test for heteroscedasticity. Both require the use of residuals, and the calculation of these for simple designs is also described in the Appendix to this chapter. References are given for the calculation of residuals in more complex designs. A third procedure that can be very useful, is easy to do, and will increase your confidence in your results is Tukey's nonadditivity test. This is not described in this book, however, but it is cited in what follows. It is not needed for single-factor designs.

We recommend very strongly that you ensure that tests for nonnormality and heterogeneity of variance be used routinely before analyzing any trial data, using these two procedures or their equivalents. In addition, if the design has more than one factor, so that interaction(s) are possible, it is desirable to run Tukey's nonadditivity test to determine whether a transformation will eliminate an apparent interaction. See Snedecor and Cochran [38], pages 283–285 or Tukey's paper (1). Finally, you should also consider whether there is any question of independence. The Tukey procedure will give information regarding the validity of any interactions and the desirability of transforming the responses before a final analysis is done (transformations are discussed in Snedecor and Cochran [38], Chapter 15. Independence can often be checked by an examination of the design, the randomization procedure, and the presence or absence of multiplicity. The amount of labor required, including that needed to find and test a transformation, is not great, and is certainly justified in light of the amount of time, effort, and money invested in almost any trial.

Normality

A number of parametric statistical tests are robust to nonnormality, but this robustness is reduced when there are unequal group sizes. As you have no doubt frequently observed, unequal group sizes are common in clinical studies, especially in those of long duration, even when they are initially equal (because the probability of noncompleters increases with the length of a study). Furthermore, many common responses, such as judgment scales, are likely to be inherently nonnormal. For these or other reasons, every so often the examination of a set of data will suggest that more severe nonnormality exists than can be compensated for adequately by the assumed robustness of your statistical tests. Of course, on the other hand, you cannot expect perfect normality in any real-life data.

Variances

In addition to the assumption of normality, the use of the t test implies the assumption that the variances of the populations represented by the two treatment groups being compared are the same.[7] Violation of this assumption is more serious than lack of normality, especially when cell or group sizes are unequal, and we recommend *always* testing for heteroscedasticity (nonhomogeneity of variances), even if the statistician decides that normality testing is unnecessary. One of the best and most reliable procedures for this purpose is Levene's test, mentioned before. It is described in the Appendix to this chapter, and in Snedecor and Cochran [38] (pp. 253–254 in Chapter 13), and is not very laborious. See Scheffé (3), Chapter 10, for more information about the effect of unequal variances.

The Assumptions in Example 14.2

In this example, as shown in the Appendix, the data could not be shown to be either nonnormal or heteroscedastic (alpha = 0.05). Although the sample size is smaller than would normally be used for most trials of this kind, for purposes of illustration, we will assume that the tests for these characteristics were satisfactorily powerful. We therefore proceed, using Student's t test. But, first, the appropriate standard deviation must be calculated from the data.

Standard Deviation

The error estimate used in a t test must be expressed in a form that is appropriate to the quantity being tested. In this case, a statistic derived from the basic form of the standard deviation, called **the standard deviation of the difference between two means**, is calculated. To do so, we use all the data (from both groups) in order to obtain the maximum available precision. This procedure is called **pooling**. We begin by calculating the **pooled variance**, which is calculated from the sums of squares of the two groups. This quantity

---

[7]There are well-known parametric tests that do not assume that the two treatment groups are derived from populations with the same variance. They are somewhat more complex than the t tests, and are not described in this book. The simplest was originated by Satterthwaite and is an approximation procedure. It is described both in his original paper (2) and in Snedecor and Cochran [38], pp. 97 and 98.

will then be used to calculate the necessary standard deviation of the difference.[8]

The pooling was done and will be described in a moment. The corresponding standard deviation, which will apply to the difference (or the sum[9]) between the two means, is obtained by multiplying the pooled variance by the factor $[(1/n_1) + (1/n_2)]$, then taking the square root of the result. This factor can be reduced algebraically to a single term, $[(n_1 + n_2)/(n_1 n_2)]$. The symbols n_1 and n_2 refer to the two sample sizes. When they are the same, this expression reduces to $2/n$, where n is the sample size of each group. This is the standard deviation of the difference between two means, sometimes called the standard error of the difference between the two means (note carefully that this is not the same standard error as that of a mean of a group of differences, such as is used in the dependent *t* test described in the next section). This standard deviation is the one needed as long as the variances of the two populations represented are independent, and as long as they can be safely assumed to be the same, or nearly so. The equations given in what follows are then applicable whether or not the two sample sizes are equal.

The two group sums of squares and variances have already been calculated, and are shown at the bottom of Table 14.3. The pooled variance and standard deviation are obtained using Equations (14.8) and (14.9), as described in what follows:

1. Obtain the **pooled variance of individual items from the mean** by obtaining the total sum of squares and dividing this total by the sum of the degrees of freedom for the two groups:

$$S^2_{\text{pooled}} = \frac{SS_1 + SS_2}{(n_1 - 1) + (n_2 - 1)}$$

$$= \frac{117.5000 + 68.2143}{15}$$

$$= 12.3810 \tag{14.8}$$

2. Calculate the **standard deviation of the difference between the group means** by multiplying the pooled variance by a fraction consisting of the

---

[8]A common error is to *average* the variances. Averaging gives the same result as pooling if each variance has been computed from the same number of data, but not otherwise. A pooled variance is a **weighted average** of the individual variances, which compensates for the difference between the numbers of data, so that a variance based upon a smaller number of data will influence the result less than one from a larger group. The greater the discrepancy between the group sizes, the greater the difference between a simple average and the pooled value will be. In a trial having more than two treatments, the same principles apply.

[9]If you ever need the variance or standard deviation of a sum rather than a difference, remember that the error of a sum is the same as that of a difference, because errors are additive in either case.

sum of the two sample sizes divided by their product and taking the square root of the result:

$$S_{\bar{d}} = \sqrt{S_{pooled}^2 \frac{n_1 + n_2}{n_1 n_2}}$$

$$= \sqrt{12.3810 \frac{10 + 7}{(10)(7)}}$$

$$= 1.7340 \qquad\qquad (14.9)$$

Completing the Two-Sample (Independent) t Test

In this example, the t test will be two-tailed because it is possible for either drug to show a larger or smaller response mean. Once you obtain the standard deviation of the difference, Equation (14.9), completing the test is very simple. You divide the difference between the two group means by the standard deviation of the difference, obtaining a calculated value of t. You then compare this value with a critical value obtained from Table A.1 in the Appendix at the back of the book. To find the critical value, first find the row giving the df for error $[(n_1 - 1) + (n_2 - 1)]$ in the first column, and then use the alpha value you specified during planning to select the column intersecting with that row. The critical value is found at that intersection.

For this example, the error df is 9 + 6, or 15, and you prespecified a value of 0.05 for alpha. The critical value is therefore found in the row labeled 15 and the column labeled 0.050; this value is 2.131. You compare this value with that which you calculated. If the calculated value is *greater* than the critical value, you can claim significance at the 0.05 level of alpha, that is, you can reject the null hypothesis and state, with a risk no greater than alpha of being wrong, that the two population means are different. On the other hand, if the calculated value of t is *equal to or less than* the critical value, you should conclude that significance was not found. Supposing in this case that you had used Neyman-Pearson, specifying some value for delta and a beta risk of, say, 0.10, you could then conclude that the difference sought was zero (less than delta), with a risk no greater than beta of being wrong.

The calculated value of t in this example is

$$t = \frac{\bar{T}_1 - \bar{T}_2}{S_{\bar{d}}}$$

$$= \frac{48.00 - 44.93}{1.7340}$$

$$= 1.7705 \qquad\qquad (14.10)$$

Since this value is less than the tabulated value, the treatment difference was not significant.

When the t Test Should Not Be Used

To emphasize some of the points made earlier:

If you plan to use a *t* test, you should first be sure that the relevant assumptions are reasonably satisfied. Independence is usually obvious from the design of your trial, and should have been kept in mind during planning (probably the most important of the several items to consider with respect to independence is that a correct randomization has been done).

If there is significant nonnormality, the statistician should calculate the residuals, plot them versus the fitted values, and consider a transformation before using the *t* test (see the Appendix to this chapter), or use a rank test such as the Wilcoxon Rank Sum test described later. Your statistician will understand that if he or she tries a transformation, the tests of the assumptions also described in the Appendix must be repeated, and this process iterated until as close an approach as possible to conformance to the assumptions is achieved. Unhappily, often a transformation giving adequate normality may not reduce heteroscedasticity adequately. When a choice is necessary, the latter should be considered the more critical. As long as you obtain equal or nearly equal variances, if the errors are not normal, the rank sum test can always be used, is only trivially less efficient than the *t* test, and is not influenced at all by nonnormality. There are also some modified *t* tests with which the statistician will be familiar, which are quite insensitive to unequal variances. These include the Satterthwaite modification of Student's *t* test, and the Fisher-Behrens test. Fisher-Behrens is described in many sources, for example, see Snedecor and Cochran [38], page 97, which mentions it and cites references. The Satterthwaite test, however, is easier and more convenient, and although it is an approximation, it is quite satisfactory. Details of this test are also given in Snedecor and Cochran [38], pages 97–98, as well as in Satterthwaite's original paper (2).

14.3.5   Example 14.3: A Larger Example (Independent Groups)

We used the previous small data set to clarify the procedure. For this example, we will use a larger and more realistic set of data (58 patients as compared to 17). The data are given in Table 14.4. The same data will be used again later to illustrate the Wilcoxon Rank Sum test. The data are joint tenderness index (jti) values obtained in the comparison of two antiinflammatory drugs at one of several sites in a multicenter trial. We noted when describing a similar trial earlier that a rank test was probably more suitable than a *t* test because of the nature of the responses. The data are sums of whole numbers, so that it is theoretically impossible for the underlying populations from which the two groups were assumed to be sampled to be perfectly normally distributed, because the scale cannot be continuous. However, a long scoring scale (nine or more points, if all of the points are used) will often work in an analysis with a parametric method, especially when the sample sizes are equal and the method is known to be robust. We nevertheless checked for both nonnormality and heteroscedasticity using

Table 14.4. Joint Tenderness Index Values (jti) (Example 14.3)

A_1 (Drug 1)		A_2 (Drug 2)	
Patient No.	jti	Patient No.	jti
3	5	1	19
4	18	2	17
5	15	9	15
6	15	10	20
7	13	12	15
8	5	16	25
11	9	17	20
13	12	18	18
14	19	21	11
15	18	23	12
19	16	24	12
20	8	25	14
22	8	26	14
27	12	28	20
31	14	29	19
34	17	30	18
35	17	32	15
37	13	33	23
40	14	36	13
44	10	38	19
46	10	39	19
47	22	41	14
48	8	42	18
49	15	43	26
50	5	45	9
51	13	52	22
55	17	53	25
56	6	54	17
58	11	57	17

Michael's and Levene's tests (see Appendix to this chapter), and looked at the residuals before doing the t test. We present these results for your reference.

Normality and Heteroscedasticity Tests
These tests were applied to the previous data, using the procedure described in the Appendix to this chapter, Section 14.9. An alpha value of 0.05 was

used, and the actual probability found was well above that level, so that no nonnormality was detected. The results were similar with the Levene test, so that it was assumed that there was unlikely to be any severe violation of either of these two assumptions.

Michael's Test for Nonnormality

For the convenience of readers interested in details of Michael's method as described in the Appendix to this chapter (Section 14.9), we give the results of this test here, based upon the data of Table 14.4. Some may wish to skip this section, after noting that the test did not detect nonnormality. For a complete understanding of these results, interested readers should refer to the Appendix. We include the output of the BASIC program used to implement the method, but we do not show the probability plot. Michael's probability plots are displayed and the method of constructing them is described in the Appendix.

The test was done using residuals calculated from the response data. Alpha was specified as 0.05. Table 14.5 is a copy of the output of the BASIC program. The greatest absolute difference between X' and Y' was 0.045 (it occurs twice), and as shown at the bottom of the table, the critical value needed to claim significance at a probability less than alpha was greater than 0.083, so that the test gave no evidence of nonnormality.

Levene's Test for Heteroscedasticity

In the same way, we give here the results of Levene's test for this example. Interested readers may consult the Appendix to this chapter, Section 14.9, for details of the procedure. Others may wish to skip this section also, after noting that no evidence of unequal variances was found.

The original jti values and the absolute deviations from the group means are shown in Table 14.6. Sums and means of the jti values and of the deviations were calculated and are shown at the bottom of the table. The latter furnish a visual indication of the sample difference in variance between treatment groups. As you can see, these means are quite similar.

Following the procedure described in Snedecor and Cochran [38] and in the Appendix to this chapter, to test whether the two treatment groups were likely to have originated from two distributions having different variances, a one-way analysis of variance of the two groups of absolute deviations was done. A one-way ANOVA is equivalent to a *t* test when there is only one factor at two levels, as in the present case.[10] We do not describe the ANOVA procedures in this book, but it is described in detail in virtually every book on applied statistics, including most of those listed in the Bibliography. The

---

[10]Although the example here uses only two treatments (two levels of the factor, drugs), Levene's test is used in an exactly analogous way when there are more than two. The ANOVA would then be testing more than two treatment groups. A rank test may be used instead of the ANOVA. When there are more than two treatments, an appropriate test would then be the Kruskal-Wallis test or the adaptation of the Wilcoxon Rank Sum test for the case of several treatments, which is somewhat more convenient to use. See Wilcoxon and Wilcox [46].

Table 14.5. Michael's Test for Nonnormality: BASIC Program Output (Example 14.3)

Residual	X'	Y'	$|X' - Y'|$	Residual	X'	Y'	$|X' - Y'|$
− 8.45	0.059	0.104	0.045	0.41	0.505	0.524	0.019
− 7.59	0.103	0.130	0.027	0.55	0.516	0.532	0.016
− 7.59	0.133	0.130	0.003	0.55	0.527	0.532	0.005
− 7.59	0.158	0.130	0.028	0.55	0.539	0.532	0.007
− 6.59	0.180	0.165	0.015	1.41	0.550	0.582	0.032
− 6.45	0.199	0.170	0.029	1.41	0.561	0.582	0.021
− 5.45	0.217	0.211	0.006	1.55	0.572	0.590	0.018
− 5.45	0.234	0.211	0.023	1.55	0.583	0.590	0.007
− 4.59	0.250	0.250	0.000	1.55	0.595	0.590	0.005
− 4.59	0.265	0.250	0.015	1.55	0.606	0.590	0.016
− 4.59	0.280	0.250	0.030	2.41	0.618	0.638	0.020
− 4.45	0.294	0.257	0.037	2.41	0.630	0.638	0.008
− 3.59	0.307	0.300	0.007	2.41	0.642	0.638	0.004
− 3.45	0.321	0.307	0.014	2.55	0.654	0.646	0.008
− 3.45	0.333	0.307	0.026	2.55	0.667	0.646	0.021
− 3.45	0.346	0.307	0.039	2.55	0.679	0.646	0.033
− 2.59	0.358	0.353	0.005	3.41	0.693	0.691	0.002
− 2.59	0.370	0.353	0.017	4.41	0.706	0.742	0.036
− 2.45	0.382	0.360	0.022	4.41	0.720	0.742	0.022
− 2.45	0.394	0.360	0.034	4.41	0.735	0.742	0.007
− 2.45	0.405	0.360	0.045	4.55	0.750	0.748	0.002
− 1.59	0.417	0.408	0.009	5.41	0.766	0.787	0.021
− 0.59	0.428	0.466	0.038	5.41	0.783	0.787	0.004
− 0.59	0.439	0.466	0.027	5.55	0.801	0.793	0.008
− 0.45	0.450	0.474	0.024	6.41	0.820	0.829	0.009
− 0.45	0.461	0.474	0.013	7.55	0.842	0.869	0.027
− 0.45	0.473	0.474	0.001	7.55	0.867	0.869	0.002
0.41	0.484	0.524	0.040	8.55	0.897	0.899	0.002
0.41	0.495	0.524	0.029	9.41	0.941	0.921	0.020

Alpha = 0.05   Critical value = 0.083
Alpha = 0.01   Critical value = 0.097

Table 14.6. Levene's Test (Example 14.3)

	Original Data		Absolute Deviations	
	T_1	T_2	$|T_1 - \bar{T}_1|$	$|T_2 - \bar{T}_2|$
	5	19	7.59	1.55
	18	17	5.41	0.45
	15	15	2.41	2.45
	15	20	2.41	2.55
	13	15	0.41	2.45
	5	25	7.59	7.55
	9	20	3.59	2.55
	12	18	0.59	0.55
	19	11	6.41	6.45
	18	12	5.41	5.45
	16	12	3.41	5.45
	8	14	4.59	3.45
	8	14	4.59	3.45
	12	20	0.59	2.55
	14	19	1.41	1.55
	17	18	4.41	0.55
	17	15	4.41	2.45
	13	23	0.41	5.55
	14	13	1.41	4.45
	10	19	2.59	1.55
	10	19	2.59	1.55
	22	14	9.41	3.45
	8	18	4.59	0.55
	15	26	2.41	8.55
	5	9	7.59	8.45
	13	22	0.41	4.55
	17	25	4.41	7.55
	6	17	6.59	0.45
	11	17	1.59	0.45
Sum	365	506	109.23	98.55
N	29	29	29	29
Mean	12.59	17.45	3.7666	3.3983

two-tailed probability found was 0.587, far greater than the 0.050 we specified for significance, leading to the conclusion that there was no evidence of unequal variances.

A Wilcoxon Rank Sum test, as well as the analysis of variance just mentioned, was also run for comparison. The two-tailed probability obtained was 0.629, quite similar to that obtained with the analysis of variance and again far from significance.

Examination of Residuals

The residuals for this example were calculated using the method described in the Appendix. For one-way data as we have here, these values are the same as the absolute values of the deviations except that the appropriate signs are now used. The signs were those that occur when the group means were subtracted from each individual datum. The subtraction can be done in either direction as long as you are consistent.

In this particular example, in view of the results of the normality and heteroscedasticity tests, it was probably not necessary to examine the residuals beyond, perhaps, making a plot of them vs. the fitted values, such as is shown in Figure 14.2 later in this section. We do so here for completeness only. It will be useful to you to have some knowledge of residual testing if you are not already familiar with it. However, this section may also be skipped by those not interested without detriment to the continuity of the example.

The analysis of residuals is a most convenient technique for the examination of the conformance of your data to the so-called parametric assumptions, and should be made a regular part of your statistician's data analysis routines. It is very widely used in experimental work in chemistry, engineering, and much applied product research and development, but is more rarely used in clinical trial work, at least in facilities lacking large statistical staffs.

The idea is to examine your residuals in various ways, looking for evidence of nonrandomness, nonnormality, heteroscedasticity, trends with time, patient numbers or treatments, etc. The particular kinds of examinations you should employ often depend upon the nature of the design. For example, in a multicenter design, any differences among centers would be of interest and should be investigated. Trends with time within any center would also suggest that something may be wrong. Unusually large residuals often result from an error in recording data. Some of the methods of computing and examining residuals are described in the literature by Anscombe and Tukey (4), Daniel and Wood (5), Daniel [13], Draper and Smith [34], Searle (6), and Wooding (7), and may be of interest to you or your statistician. None of these is oriented specifically to clinical trial data analysis, but they are useful for work in almost any scientific field.

The examination of residuals as just described is a simple technique, but, to repeat an earlier reminder, the complexity of the calculation of residuals from data is related to the complexity of the experimental design. In the case of the present one-way parallel design with two treatments, the computation is very simple. You merely calculate the mean for each drug group and then subtract it from each of the individual data in that group. In the case of multifactor designs, the calculation of the residuals can be much more complex, and is different for each cell, because you must remove the effects of all factors, leaving only the estimates of error for each response measurement. Some common examples are shown in the literature just cited.

To use residuals successfully in a simple design like the present one, the two treatment groups should have been handled uniformly, and all other procedures, including the sampling of patients, should have been the same for both treatments. Under these circumstances, if the variances of the two distributions from which the two treatment groups were taken are the same, then subtracting the means in this manner will give two groups of residuals that should be virtually indistinguishable from each other. To test this, you can first plot the *original data* separately, but on the same graph, for the two treatments. The observations can be plotted on the Y-axis and the two treatments placed at two arbitrary points on the X-axis. Figure 14.1 shows such a plot, using the two groups of 29 jti values from Table 9.2 in Chapter 9. The column of points for the T_2 group is higher on the ordinate scale than that for T_1, presumably because of differences in the effects of the treatments.

Now construct a similar plot of the two sets of residuals. These are the same data after any effect of treatments has been removed by subtracting the

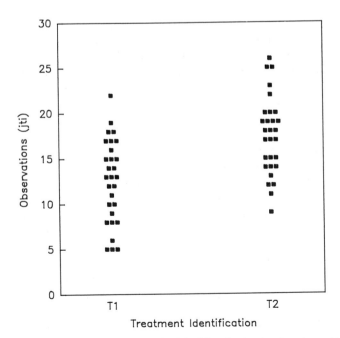

Figure 14.1   Example 14.3: Plot of original data for two treatment groups.

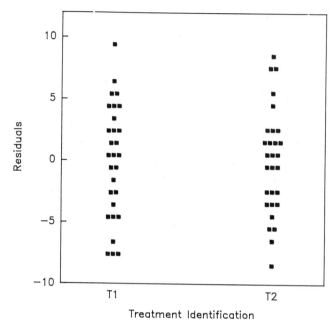

Figure 14.2   Example 14.3: Plot of residuals formed by removing effects of the treatments from the two groups.

appropriate treatment mean from each datum. This plot is illustrated in Figure 14.2. It is no longer possible to distinguish any clear-cut difference in the vertical locations of the two columns of points; there now appears to be no marked influence that affects the vertical locations of the two samples differently. Furthermore, the points appear to have approximately the same spacing, just as in Figure 14.1, also suggesting that the sample variances of the two groups are similar.

If you wish to investigate the residuals further, you might plot them against the order of their measurements (if you have randomized in the manner suggested in this book, the patient numbers will reflect this). Any differences between plots for the two groups of residuals, or any trend with time, may indicate some kind of nonrandomness and suggest investigation. Examples of some of these effects are shown in several of the references just cited. When there is more than one factor, and/or several levels, you can plot the residuals (preferably on the Y-axis) against their "fitted values," the portions of each observation estimated to be due to all effects *except* error (see the references cited). In the present case, the fitted values are the two means. Be suspicious of any unusually large (or small!) residuals. But note that it is normal for the residuals to occur in correlated pairs, although this is not true of the errors in the parent distribution. If the data are homoscedastic, the residuals should be found to form a cloud without discernible trends or unusually high or low values.

For brevity, we will content ourselves with the two cases just given, calculating the residuals of this example and plotting them versus their fitted values. For your trial data, however, you may find it safer and more profitable, in addition, to plot them in at least two ways—by patient numbers, as well as by treatment groups, and by centers, if the trial is a multicenter study.

The subject of the examination and interpretation of residuals is a large one, and can be given no further space here. Nevertheless, again, you should be sure that your biostatistician does examine the residuals before completing the analyses. This may be especially important in large multicenter trials, where the degree of control and supervision of the various stages of the trial may not be as rigorous as is possible in smaller studies. It is common, for example, to detect errors such as the incorrect transcription of data through the examination of residuals.

Doing the Independent *t* Test

This test is performed in exactly the same way as that of Example 14.2. A standard *t* test can be used because we appear to have approximate normality, and the Levene test has indicated that the variances of the two populations represented by the treatment groups appear to be similar. The two sample variances can thus be pooled to take advantage of all the data. The pooled variance is calculated as shown by Equation (14.8). The standard deviation of the difference between the two means is calculated using Equation (14.9). Finally, with Equation (14.10), *t* is computed by taking the difference between the two group means in either direction (you may ignore the sign) and dividing it by the standard deviation of that difference.

The calculated value of *t* is compared with a critical value obtained from Table A.1 in the Appendix. To get the critical value, you need the df, the degrees of freedom associated with the difference, and its standard deviation. As long as you used both groups of data to calculate the standard deviation, as you should have if the two variances were not shown to be different, the df will be equal to the sum of the number of data used to calculate each mean, after 1 is subtracted from each, that is,

$$df_{1,2} = (n_1 - 1) + (n_2 - 1) \qquad (14.11)$$

where

$$n_1 = \text{sample size for group (treatment) 1}$$

$$n_2 = \text{sample size for group (treatment) 2}$$

Because n_1 and n_2 are each equal to 29 in this example, the total degrees of freedom associated with the standard deviation is 56. Equation (14.8) gives

19.7180 for the pooled variance. Using Equation (14.9) gives 1.1661 for the standard deviation of the difference, and dividing the difference between the means by this standard deviation yields a calculated t value of 4.1695. At an alpha value of 0.05, the tabulated two-tailed critical value of t in the Appendix t table (Table A.1) is about 2.004 (by linear interpolation; the value at 40 df is 2.021, and that at 60 df is 2.000). Because the calculated t value is greater than this, we conclude that the difference between the two means is significant. The actual probability from Table A.1 in this case is substantially less than 0.001 (symbolized as $\ll 0.001$).

14.3.6 One-Sample t Tests

Varieties

One-sample t tests can be thought of as having two subspecies, closely related but different in their purposes and the uses to which they are put. Only one of them, however, is likely to have very frequent use in clinical studies.

The first and less often used kind compares a single mean with a standard or known value. Suppose the population is represented by a sample of patients who have been dieting. The response might be patients' weight gains, with the sample responses to be compared with an ideal value or standard. Another example might utilize the diastolic blood pressures of a single sample of patients taken after treatment with a test drug for a period of time, asking the question, "Does the mean diastolic pressure exceed 90 mm?" Here the group mean is the sample statistic, and the value of 90 mm is the standard.

The second kind of one-sample t test is a difference test, which is frequently used in connection with paired (i.e., changeover) trials. Instead of testing a mean of a group of observations, such a test uses a mean difference calculated from a group of individual differences. The differences are calculated individually and then averaged, and the error estimate used in the test applies to that average. In a clinical trial of this kind, each single difference originates from a patient or subject who has been given two different treatments, each at a different time. Some response is measured, and the data to be tested consist of differences between the responses for the two treatments for each patient. The mean difference is the average of such a group of individual differences. You will recognize the design as randomized blocks, with the patients as the blocks, each with two plots, that is, a changeover design. A typical study that could be analyzed using the t test of a mean difference is the randomized-blocks changeover trial using two drugs described in Chapter 12 (Example 12.2).

In the difference test, the order of administration of the drugs is randomized for each patient (we are *not* referring to the two-period crossover design, which can use the same kind of randomization, but must be analyzed in an entirely different manner; see Chapter 11, Section 11.4). The data to be tested are differences between two treatments, usually taken, for convenience, in a direction that makes the majority of the differences positive. The *t* test can be used to decide whether the mean difference is great enough to be statistically significant and of clinical importance. That is, you can use it to test the null hypothesis that the mean population difference is zero, against an alternate hypothesis that the difference is delta.[11]

Testing a Mean Difference

For clarity, we will use a small set of data in the following example, and because the tests of the assumptions have already been illustrated (see the Appendix to this chapter), we will presume that a test for nonnormality has been done and that you are satisfied that the distribution of your set of differences is reasonably close to normal. A variance test is irrelevant, because there is only a single group of data—the differences.

Example 14.4: t Test of a Mean Difference

Equations

EQUATION FOR THE *t* TEST. The only new equation necessary for the one-sample *t* test is the following:

$$t = \frac{\overline{D} - \mu}{S_{\overline{D}}} \tag{14.12}$$

In Equation (14.12), $\overline{D}$ represents the mean of your set of differences. Mu symbolizes the population mean and is zero under the null hypothesis for a difference test (or a standard value otherwise). The value of $S_{\overline{D}}$ is the sample standard deviation of the mean of the differences, that is, the **standard error of the mean difference**.

CALCULATING THE STANDARD ERROR. The standard error of the mean difference is most easily calculated by first obtaining the standard deviation of single items (i.e., single differences), and dividing that by the square root of the number of items in the mean. Or, more simply, by dividing the *variance* of the individual differences by the number of differences and then taking the square root of the result, as shown in Equation (14.13), which follows. The variance of individual differences is calculated in the same way as that for individual measurements, and was explained in Section 14.3. You simply use the individual differences, d_i, instead of the individual measure-

---

[11]Delta should have been prespecified as a value equal to a population mean treatment difference large enough to be clinically and/or economically significant in the opinion of the monitor or investigator.

ments, y_i. You then calculate the standard error of the mean difference as follows:

$$s_{\bar{D}} = \sqrt{\frac{s_{D_i}^2}{n_i}} \tag{14.13}$$

The Trial

In an early trial of a new drug, an investigator wished to compare the effects of the drug with an existing treatment in a group of patients having a restrictive lung condition. Each patient was *randomly* assigned either to the regular treatment or to the test drug for a month, returned to whichever of the two treatments had not yet been used, and then followed for another month. The study was double blind. Any patient who felt that the assigned treatment was ineffective was free to resume his or her regular medication, but was dropped from the study.[12] All patients were informed of this provision beforehand.

Fourteen patients were entered into the trial. The assignment procedure was followed. A washout period at the start of the test or between treatments was not used, as this would have left the patients without treatment. The investigator had sufficient information regarding the half-lives of the drugs, however, to assume with some confidence that any carryover effect from either drug would be eliminated during the first week after changeover. It was therefore planned to use no data gathered during that period, although measurements would be made. In the event, to minimize error, only the fourth-week data were used in the analysis.

Several responses were used in this trial, but in this example, we refer to only one of them—FEV_1. This is a pulmonary function measurement, forced expiratory volume, equal to the number of liters of air that a patient can discharge in 1 second after inhaling as deeply as possible. A normal patient's FEV_1 is approximately 4.0 liters. The data in Table 14.7 show measurements made at the end of the fourth week of each period.

Data Analysis

For each patient and each drug, the fourth-week FEV_1 for drug T_2, the old drug, was subtracted from that for T_1, the new one, and the difference recorded. Taking the differences in this direction meant that higher values represented greater FEV_1 values for the new relative to the old drug. Thus, if the average of the 14 differences were shown to be significantly *greater* than zero, the conclusion would be that the new drug was more effective than the regular medication, with a probability of at least alpha of being wrong. If it

---

[12] Even if they were not used in the final data analysis, however, the data for such patients up to the time they were dropped should be submitted to the FDA along with all other data, if the study is being done for regulatory purposes.

Table 14.7. Data for t Test of Differences (Example 14.4)

Patient	T_1	T_2	$T_1 - T_2$
1	2.9	3.9	-1.0
2	4.0	3.9	0.1
3	3.4	3.3	0.1
4	3.2	4.3	-1.1
5	3.8	3.2	0.6
6	5.2	3.5	1.7
7	3.9	2.7	1.2
8	3.9	2.4	1.5
9	2.5	3.6	-1.1
10	6.5	2.1	4.4
11	5.5	4.0	1.5
12	4.0	3.9	0.1
13	5.3	4.0	1.3
14	4.3	2.3	2.0
Sum	58.4	47.1	11.3
N	14	14	14
Mean	4.17	3.36	0.81

were significantly *less*, superiority of the old drug would be indicated, with the same value of alpha applying. If significance were not found, it would be concluded that the population difference was less than delta, with probability beta of being wrong. The value of delta specified was equal to a difference that the sponsor considered clinically important. The data, their differences, and their sums and means are shown in Table 14.7.

The variance of the individual differences in the fourth column of Table 14.7 was calculated using Equations (14.5) and (14.6), substituting the individual differences, d_i, for the data, y_i. The standard error of the mean difference was then calculated using Equation (14.13). The value found was 0.3962.

Next, t was calculated using Equation (14.12); the mean difference was simply divided by its standard error. This yielded a value of 2.037 for t. The critical value, taken from Table A.1 in the Appendix (i.e., $t_{0.05}$ at 13 df), is 2.160. Because the calculated value of t did not exceed this, the null hypothesis was not rejected, and it was concluded that the population difference between the two treatments was less than delta.

14.4 LEAST SIGNIFICANT DIFFERENCE (LSD)

The least significant difference (LSD) was discussed briefly in Chapter 13, but its calculation was not given there because we had not introduced the necessary prerequisite procedures. A least significant difference is most useful when considering the difference between two means, as is done in studies that are appropriate for the independent t test. An LSD is a difference that must be exceeded in order to reject the null hypothesis. Like the other parametric tests, normality and equal variances are assumed. It is calculated as follows, assuming two uncorrelated means of equal size, n:

$$\text{LSD} = t\sqrt{\frac{2s^2_{\text{pooled}}}{n}} \tag{14.14}$$

The value of t in Equation (14.14) is obtained from the t table at probability alpha and $(n - 1)$ df. The pooled variance, s^2_{pooled}, is calculated as shown for the t test in Example 14.2.

We include the LSD here for completeness, but it is merely another form of the independent t test, Equation (14.10). Because this is the case, it is *not* applicable to multiple comparisons except under special circumstances, which are treated only briefly in this book.[13]

14.5 CONFIDENCE INTERVALS

The idea of confidence intervals or confidence limits was introduced in Chapter 12, but again without details of the necessary calculations. Like the LSD, confidence intervals are closely related to the t test when concern lies with procedures based upon the normal distribution, but they have a somewhat broader range of applications. Although we do not discuss them in this book, appropriate confidence intervals can also be calculated for nonnormal data, such as binomial responses, ranks, and the like.

There was adequate discussion of the uses of confidence intervals for the normal distribution in the preceding chapter, and here we merely present a method of calculation of a parametric confidence interval about a mean:

$$(\text{CI})_{1-\alpha} = \bar{y} \pm t_\alpha S_{\bar{y}} \tag{14.15}$$

In Equation (14.15), $(\text{CI})_{1-\alpha}$ stands for the confidence interval with probability $1 - \alpha$ of containing the population mean. The symbol $\bar{y}$ stands for the sample mean, t_α is the value of t at probability alpha and $(n - 1)$ degrees of freedom, obtained from a t table such as Table A.1 in the Appendix, and $s_{\bar{y}}$ is the sample standard deviation of the mean, $\bar{y}$. The latter is obtained by dividing the variance of single items found using Equation

---

[13]That is, the use of the LSD after a finding of significance in an analysis of variance (ANOVA) as described by Fisher [16]. Fisher called it the *protected* LSD when used in this way for multiple comparisons. It was also described in a reference to Carmer and Swanson (8) and Bernhardson (9), who showed the validity of the procedure by Monte Carlo trials.

(14.2) or (14.5) and Equation (14.6) by n, the number of items used to calculate the mean, and then taking the square root of the result. If you wish to compute the confidence interval about some other kind of mean, substitute the appropriate value and its standard deviation. For example, a confidence interval about a mean difference (where the data are a set of differences from a paired test) would use the mean difference instead of the mean of a set of original observations, and the appropriate standard deviation, as in Equation (14.16):

$$(CI)_{1-\alpha} = \overline{D} \pm t_\alpha s_{\overline{D}} \qquad (14.16)$$

14.6   RANK TESTS

14.6.1   Introduction and Principles

Rank tests begin by substituting rank numbers of the data to be tested for the data themselves. Sometimes ranks instead of other types of responses are assigned directly at the time of the trail, so that the ranks comprise the original data. Rank numbers or ranks are numbers representing the *relative magnitudes*, the *order*, of the data.[14] The statistical tests are done using the ranks, ignoring the original data. A marked advantage of testing ranks instead of the data is that the distribution of ranks and the estimation of its parameters are well-known. You therefore *know* the distribution of the population represented by your sample, in contrast to the situation when you use the original data. The test procedure is one appropriate for samples from a distribution of ranks. Thus, the assumption of normality is no longer of importance, although that of equal variances still applies when you are comparing independent groups.

Data are usually ranked from the smallest to the largest, and we assume throughout this section that that has been done. Suppose you have a set of observations, for which the kind of distribution is unknown, such as the following:

2.35
1.68
8.92
9.36
3.02

[14]There is sometimes confusion between the terms **order statistics** and **ranks**. In the most common usage, order statistics are sets of numbers such as observations or responses that have been arranged in order, for example, from the smallest to the largest. Ranks are the *numbers* of the ordered values in a set of order statistics, that is, their ordinal numbers, such as the first (rank number 1), the second (rank number 2), etc. It could be said that if a set of ranks comprised original data rather than being generated from a set of random variables arranged in order, then the ranks themselves would be order statistics.

These numbers are assigned the following ranks, with a rank of 1 assigned to the smallest value:

2
1
4
5
3

If there are ties, they can be handled in several ways, but the most common and convenient method is the following: Suppose the data to be those shown in the following left-hand column. Their ranks are shown next to them:

Observation	Rank
2.35	2
1.68	1
8.92	3.5
8.92	3.5
9.36	5

The two values, 8.92, would have received ranks of 3 and 4 if they had not been the same. Because they are equal, each received the average of the two rank numbers 3 and 4, or 3.5. This "used up" these two ranks, so that the next one assigned was 5. When there are more than two tied data, the same principle is used, averaging all the tied ranks and then continuing to rank using the next available unused rank.[15]

Although rank tests are called **nonparametric**, if that term is taken to mean that the ranks used have no distribution, or that their distribution is not important, the term is a misnomer. As just explained, the ranks have their own distribution, which is known. Tables needed to find the appropriate probability of an observed result under H_0 in a rank test are available. There are many different kinds of rank tests. The most common serve as substitutes for the t test or various forms of the analysis of variance (ANOVA). In the common forms, the sums of the ranks for the treatment groups are calculated and referred to a table to obtain the probability needed for comparison with alpha. Two of these tests are described and exemplified in what follows.

Some truly nonparametric tests exist, for example, Fisher's exact test (mentioned later in the section on contingency tables) and those described in Edgington (10).

---

[15]If there were more than about 10% ties, hypothesis tests using ranks become noticeably conservative, that is, they yield significance probabilities that are incorrectly high. The literature gives some methods of compensating for ties (see Conover [39] or Siegel [45]).

14.6.2 The Usefulness of Rank Tests

Why substitute a set of nonnormal numbers, like ranks, for the original data? Rank tests used to be called "approximate"[16] or "quick-and-dirty" tests, although in a sense they are less approximate than other hypothesis tests, because the parent distribution is known. Before the easy availability of computers, their major purpose was as convenient and fast "pencil-and-paper" procedures. Today, they are most useful for occasions when you suspect that the data are not normal, and you either cannot transform the data to make them more normal, or do not wish to do so. Few data are truly normal, and despite the robustness of the common parametric tests, unless you are quite sure that the nonnormality is sufficiently minor to cause no trouble, you may often be better off using a rank test.

There is a small penalty for using some rank tests. If the original data are really perfectly normal, the rank tests described here, in the long run, will be about 95.5% $[100(3/\pi)]$ as efficient as a standard t test would have been. This means that in such a case, the t test will require about 95 patients compared to 100 for the rank test.[17] But most data are not normal, and some are far from it. When this is true, the efficiency of the rank test can soar to very high values (often greater than 100%). Then, the rank test will require *fewer*, perhaps many fewer, patients than a t test (of course the t test should not be used in such cases in any event).

Another possible problem is the presence of unusual numbers of ties. The presence of ties makes either of the two rank tests described here more conservative, that is, the p values you obtain will be *larger* than the correct values. Wilcoxon stated that this effect can be ignored if there are less than 10% ties. The literature contains some procedures for compensation in such cases—see Conover [39], pages 215–223. The program for Wilcoxon's Rank Sum test given in the Appendix to this book (Program AP.2) does not include such a routine.

We will describe two rank tests here. You will find them applicable to a fairly large proportion of your work. This being so, you might ask, "Then why worry about t tests or parametric confidence intervals?" The answer is that clinical trials, as well as being very expensive, often involve inconvenience or risk to your patients, and hence it is important to make any trial as informative and dependable as possible. The use of t tests or confidence intervals is simple and direct under normality, but this is not so when the data are not normal. It is not much trouble to use a parametric as well as a rank test before drawing your conclusions, and each will contribute to the

---

[16]Hence the title of Wilcoxon and Wilcox [46]. The first edition of this was published by Wilcoxon in the late 1940s.

[17]This is the so-called asymptotic efficiency of the tests, a common measure. An approximate definition of this—Conover [39] (p. 89) calls it the A.R.E., or asymptotic relative efficiency—is that it is the long-run sample size needed with the t test to get the same power at the same alpha level as a rank test of the same data.

reliability of your work. If the rank test results differ substantially from those obtained with a t test, it may be that the data are sufficiently nonnormal to affect your results within the t test, and you should therefore favor the rank test. Of course, you should remember that any heteroscedasticity will affect either test.

14.6.3   Rank Analogues of the Common t Tests

The two rank tests to be described here, and their parametric analogues, are the following:

Rank Test	Equivalent Parametric Test
Wilcoxon Rank Sum test	Independent groups t test
Wilcoxon Signed Ranks test	Differences t test

There are many other rank tests. These two are designed for comparing two groups only, just as is the t test. They are actually comparisons of medians rather than of means, but this is a technicality that is not important unless your data are substantially skewed. In such cases, medians are somewhat more accurate than means for comparing the "locations" of distributions, although the mode (which, unfortunately cannot be calculated simply) is the really correct measure of centrality for skewed distributions.

The **Wilcoxon Rank Sum test** is used for comparing two independent groups, like the independent groups t test. Another independent groups rank test, published about 2 years after Wilcoxon's paper, is called the **Mann-Whitney U test**. The procedure for the Mann-Whitney is a bit more complex than that for the Wilcoxon test, but its use persists, especially among workers in the social sciences, although it leads to exactly the same conclusions. You should keep in mind that although the assumption of normality need not be made for either of these tests, like the independent t test, their results can be strongly affected by heteroscedasticity. Consequently, if the population variances of the two groups being tested are not the same, both tests will give incorrect results. If you have any doubt about the homogeneity of the variances, you should be sure to precede either the independent t test, Wilcoxon's Rank Sum test, or the Mann-Whitney test by a variance test such as Levene's, and then find a transformation if there is significant heteroscedasticity.

The **Signed Ranks test** is used to test differences, and is the rank analogue of the dependent or one-sample t test. In this test, as in the case of the dependent t test, the possible existence of different variances in the two groups is both unlikely and, in any case, irrelevant. The presence of excessive ties among the difference data tested, however, has the same conservative effect as for the Rank Sum test.

Both of these rank tests will be illustrated using the data we used for the corresponding t tests.

14.6.4 Example 14.5: Wilcoxon Rank Sum Test

In this example, we employ the data originally used in Example 14.4, Table 14.7, to illustrate the independent groups t test in this chapter. Although the group sizes are equal in this case, the Rank Sum test, like the t test for independent groups, can also be used when they are not. The method comprises ranking all the data, obtaining rank sums, and making a comparison with a critical value. In doing this test, the critical value can be obtained from tables in Wilcoxon and Wilcox [46] or from the Appendix to Snedecor and Cochran [38] (Table A10). Alternatively, it can be obtained using a normal approximation. We have compared results from Wilcoxon's tables with the normal approximation using several sets of data of various sizes. They agree well when the total sample sizes are 8 to 10 or greater and the group sizes are equal or nearly equal (see the example that follows), at significance levels of 0.010 to 0.100. Wilcoxon's tables, the largest available in the reference given, extend only to a size for the smaller group of 25. They have been extended elsewhere, but the normal approximation is quite satisfactory for such cases.

In this example, we demonstrate the use of a BASIC program given in the Appendix to this book, which uses the normal approximation procedure with a moderately sized set of data. In the next example, Example 14.6, we show the procedure using tables for the more "exact" method, which is more suitable when the sample size is very small.

The BASIC program is Program AP.2.[18] It ranks the data and does the necessary calculations for a Wilcoxon Rank Sum test, and then prints the ranks and the original data, one- and two-tailed probabilities, and other information, using normal approximations. The program is written in GW-BASIC so that it will run on most IBM PC, PC/XT, and PC/AT clones, on 80386 and 80486 machines, and on most IBM machines, which use

---

[18] In the BASIC program, *two* normal approximation procedures are used. The first, described in Snedecor and Cochran [38] and elsewhere, is used to obtain the rank equivalent of Z, the normal abscissa point. By using Z, the p value can be obtained from a normal table, but in the program, a logistic approximation is used. For the latter, see Page (11) and Tiemstra (12). Both the approximation of Z and that of the probability are satisfactory in the ranges normally used. This second procedure adds a small additional degree of approximation to the estimation of the p value. As a result, the program is most accurate when 10 or more data exist for each of the two treatments. This is not a severe handicap, because the principal advantage of the use of the program is its performance of the slow and error-prone process of ranking when the sample size is large, and the use of a normal approximation when exact tables are not available. For small samples, it is usually equally fast to use hand calculations (i.e., a scientific pocket calculator). Three methods are compared in Example 14.6, which follows; the use of Wilcoxon's tables of rank totals, the hand calculation of the approximate value of Z, followed by the use of a normal table of areas to get the p value, and the use of the program.

Table 14.8. Data and Ranks, Wilcoxon Rank Sum Test (Example 14.5)

	A_1 (Drug 1)		A_2 (Drug 2)	
	Data (jti)	Rank	Data (jti)	Rank
	5	2	19	47
	18	42	17	36.5
	15	29.5	15	29.5
	15	29.5	20	51
	13	19.5	15	29.5
	5	2	25	56.5
	9	8.5	20	51
	12	15.5	18	42
	19	47	11	12.5
	18	42	12	15.5
	16	33	12	15.5
	8	6	14	24
	8	6	14	24
	12	15.5	20	51
	14	24	19	47
	17	36.5	18	42
	17	36.5	15	29.5
	13	19.5	23	55
	14	24	13	19.5
	10	10.5	19	47
	10	10.5	19	47
	22	53.5	14	24
	8	6	18	42
	15	29.5	26	58
	5	2	9	8.5
	13	19.5	22	53.5
	17	36.5	25	56.5
	6	4	17	36.5
	11	12.5	17	36.5
Rank Totals		623		1088

a version of BASIC called BASICA.[19] If you copy it to your computer, instructions will appear on your screen when you use the command "RUN," after typing "BASIC."

Table 14.8 shows the data and their ranks for this example. The ranking was done by Program AP.2. There are 29 data in each group, which exceeds the maximum sample size provided for in any of the commonly available

---

[19]An excellent reference to many of the current forms of BASIC, with examples, is David Lien's *BASIC Handbook* (.3).

tables. We therefore used the normal approximation procedure. If you use the program, all the ranking as well as the calculations will be done for you. However, you may wish to try one or two examples "by hand" (with a pocket calculator) to gain familiarity with the process. If you do this, it is easiest to practice with small samples, like the one given in the next example. Any data sets as large as that of this example are quite tedious and error-prone when ranked by hand.

Program AP.2 gave a two-tailed probability of 0.0003 for the data of Table 14.8. The t test of these data showed a probability of less than 0.001, obtained from the t table in the Appendix. Thus, the two tests led to the same conclusion, viz., that the two means very likely derived from populations with two different medians.

14.6.5   Example 14.6: Wilcoxon Rank Sum Test (Small Sample Size)

Introduction
Example 14.5 did not explain the steps in the Rank Sum test, but merely gave the results obtained by using Appendix program AP.2. This is the more practical procedure for the use of the Rank Sum test, when there are moderate to large numbers of data, for several reasons, including (a) the tables necessary to run the test without using the normal approximation may not be available in such a case; (b) the ranking procedure, when done "by hand," is quite tedious and error-prone when the sample size is large.

In this example, we describe the steps needed to carry out the "exact" procedure for the Rank Sum test, using Table A10 in Snedecor and Cochran [38]. We use a new set of data, created for the purpose and made very small for clarity. This time we will carry out all of the steps using a pocket calculator when needed, but no other electronic aids, but we will also compare the results with those given by program AP.2. We will make the comparison as a matter of interest. However, you may well find, after a little practice, that for small samples, it is faster to do the test with a calculator ("by hand") rather than to use the computer. The tables necessary for this procedure are given in Snedecor and Cochran [38], (Table A10, pp. 475–476), but similar tables are available in other references in the Bibliography; see Hollander and Wolfe [43] or Wilcoxon and Wilcox [46]. There are also other references that describe the test as the Mann-Whitney test, referred to earlier.

Sample Size
To use this test with the tables in Wilcoxon and Wilcox [46], the smaller of your two samples must consist of at least three data. This is the smallest sample size per treatment given there. The smallest sample size used in the Snedecor and Cochran [38] table referred to in what follows, however, is two. Of course, you will be quite unlikely to use such small samples if you do a

sample size estimate when planning a trial, because in such cases, you would detect only differences that are quite large. Furthermore, it is very doubtful whether agreement of the tabular values with those obtained by the normal approximation procedure in the program given in the Appendix will be satisfactory in such cases. In the following example, however, as you will see, with sample sizes of 5 and 6 for the two treatments, agreement is not bad. Your rule should be that when there is disagreement, the results using the table rather than the normal approximation should be used.

Method

1. Copy the data into two columns, one for each group. Leave space for a rank number next to each datum.

2. Rank *all* the data in a single series of ranks, disregarding the separation of the data into the two groups. As explained previously, use average values of the ranks for tied data. Assign the ranks in ascending order, beginning with 1. If there are many data, as there were in Example 14.5, keep track of the rank numbers you have used as you go along, to avoid errors.

3. Add the ranks for the two groups separately.

4. Check your work by adding the two rank sums. The total should be equal to $N(N + 1)/2$, where N is the total number of ranks, starting with 1, in both columns. In Example 14.5, the rank sums of the two groups of 29 rank numbers were 623 and 1088, and their total was 1711. The equation verified this total (N was 58): $(58 \times 59)/2 = 1711$.

5. If the groups are equal in size, refer the smaller rank sum to Table A10 in the Appendix to Snedecor and Cochran [38]. If the group sizes are not equal, you must follow the procedure given in step 7, which follows, or on page 145 of Snedecor and Cochran to find a value called T. In this case (see Table 14.11), T happens to be equal to the rank total for the smaller group, 17, but this is not always so. Compare T with the critical value in Snedecor and Cochran's table. If T is less than the tabular value, the two population medians are different at the tabulated probability.

6. Instead of using the table, or when one or both of your sample sizes exceed that in the table, you may use the BASIC program. This procedure becomes less accurate as the sample sizes become smaller.

7. (a) To find the value of T: Let T_1 = the rank total for the smaller group. Let m equal the size of the smaller group and n that of the larger. If the groups are equal in size, let T_1 = the smaller rank total and let $m = n$, the size of either group. If the rank totals are equal, you will know already that there will not be significance.

Table 14.9. Wilcoxon Rank Sum Test Data (Example 14.6)

	A_1 (Drug 1)		A_2 (Drug 2)	
	Data	Rank	Data	Rank
	1	1	4	4.5
	2	2	5	6.5
	3	3	6	8
	4	4.5	7	9
	5	6.5	8	10
			9	11
Rank Totals		17		49

Whether or not the groups are equal, calculate T_2:

$$T_2 = m(m + n + 1) - T_1 \qquad (14.17)$$

Then, define T:

If T_1 is less than T_2, let $T = T_1$.
If T_2 is less than T_1, let $T = T_2$.
If T_1 and T_2 are equal, then $T = T_1 = T_2$.

(b) If you wish to use the "hand" method, refer T to the table in the Appendix of Snedecor and Cochran [38] (Table A10, pp. 475–476).

(c) The simplest way to use the normal approximation is to use the BASIC program. Remember that the result will not be accurate when the samples are small.

The data for this example are shown in Table 14.9.

Here are the steps just described, using the data of Table 14.9. The ranks have already been assigned and are shown in the table.

1. Copy your data into two columns (see the table).
2. Rank the data (see the table), ignoring the division into two columns.
3. Add the ranks. The rank sum for column A_1 is 17, and that for A_2 is 49, as shown in the table.
4. Check the rank sums. There are 11 rank numbers. Using 11 for N in the formula $N(N + 1)/2$, we obtain $11(11 + 1)/2 = 66$. Because $49 + 17$ also equals 66, we have a check that the total of all ranks is correct.
5. Find T as just described. In this case, it will be 17. Using T, in Table A10 in Snedecor and Cochran, pages 475 and 476, find the critical small rank total for $n_1 = 5$ (the smaller sample size) and $n_2 = 6$ (the

larger). For alpha = 0.05 (page 475), this value is 18, and for alpha = 0.01 (page 476), it is 16. Because the rank total we found for the smaller group was 17, lying between these two critical values, we conclude that the probability is between 0.01 and 0.05, in the neighborhood of 0.03. Hence, if we had selected a value of 0.05 for alpha when the trial was planned, we can claim significance.

6. To carry out the normal approximation procedure, run the BASIC program. The probability found was 0.0176 (0.02 to two places). Within the two-place limits imposed by the table, the agreement is good. To be rigorous, you should accept the hand-calculated value of about 0.03. However, either method, in this case, leads to the same conclusion.

14.6.6   Example 14.7: Wilcoxon Signed Ranks Test

This test is the "nonparametric" analogue of the one-sample t test. It is most often used as a test of differences between treatments in a paired experiment. In this example, we will use the same data that were used to illustrate the t test of differences in Example 14.4. We repeat the data table for that example as Table 14.10, but with an additional column showing the signed ranks of the differences (the explanation follows).

Table 14.10. Data and Ranks for Wilcoxon Signed Ranks Test (Example 14.7)

Patient	T_1	T_2	$T_1 - T_2$	Rank
1	2.9	3.9	-1.0	-5
2	4.0	3.9	0.1	2
3	3.4	3.3	0.1	2
4	3.2	4.3	-1.1	-6.5
5	3.8	3.2	0.6	4
6	5.2	3.5	1.7	12
7	3.9	2.7	1.2	8
8	3.9	2.4	1.5	10.5
9	2.5	3.6	-1.1	-6.5
10	6.5	2.1	4.4	14
11	5.5	4.0	1.5	10.5
12	4.0	3.9	0.1	2
13	5.3	4.0	1.3	9
14	4.3	2.3	2.0	13
Sum	58.4	47.1	11.3	
N	14	14	14	
Mean	4.17	3.36	0.81	

The Wilcoxon Signed Ranks test of the differences in Table 14.10 is done as follows:

1. Calculate the differences, as for the *t* test, and as shown in Table 14.10 in the fourth column.
2. Rank all the differences, beginning with a rank of 1 and averaging ties as described for the Rank Sum test. Rank the absolute values, that is, ignore the signs. *If any differences are zero, ignore them and do not rank them.* Reduce the count (*n*) by one for each zero. The ranks of the differences are shown in the fifth column of Table 14.10.
3. After ranking, *assign the signs of the differences to the ranks.* Thus, in the fifth column of Table 14.10, there are 14 ranks, with the first, fourth, and ninth ranks then given minus signs because their differences were negative.
4. Add the ranks with negative and positive signs separately and consider the *absolute* values of the sums. In this example, the absolute value of the negative rank sum is 18 and that of the positive sum is 87. These add to 105. As a check of your ranking, calculate the total value of the ranks from 1 to 14, as for the Rank Sum test. This total is also 105, showing that the correct ranks have probably been assigned.
5. Call the *smaller* rank total, 18, *T*. Look up T_0 in Table A9 of Snedecor and Cochran [38], page 474. In this table, *n* is the number of pairs (here, *n* = 14; it would be less if any differences had been zero). For 14 pairs, T_0 for a *P* value of 0.05 is 21, and for *P* = 0.02, it is 16. Our value of *T* is less than 21, so the probability is less than 0.05, but it is greater than 0.02, so *P* lies between 0.02 and 0.05.

Unlike our example for the Rank Sum test, you will note that we obtained significance in the rank test but not in the *t* test. Looking at the *p* values, however, we see that for the rank test, it lies between 0.02 and 0.05, whereas for the *t* test, it is just over 0.05. Thus, the two values are not very far apart, and the difference might have been considered small if both probabilities had been on the same side of the 0.05 point.

We will not include a description of the normal approximation procedure in this case. If you wish to use this method instead of the tables, or to write your own program using it, you will find the equations and a description in Snedecor and Cochran [38], page 142. The calculations are similar but not identical to those described for the Rank Sum test.

14.7 CONTINGENCY TABLE TESTS

14.7.1 Introduction

There are many variations of this kind of test that are useful in analyzing clinical trial data. We describe only the simplest and most common here. If

Test Result	Physician's Diagnosis		Totals
	(+)	(-)	
(+)	agree	disagree	
(-)	disagree	agree	

Figure 14.3   Contingency table schematic for comparing diagnoses with test results.

you wish to study the topic in more detail, other procedures are explained in Fleiss [41], Freeman [42], and Snedecor and Cochran [38]. For contingency tables, the word "data" refers to counts or proportions[20] of experimental units, for example, numbers of patients. In clinical work, these counts are the responses. The independent variables or categories are the usual kinds of factors and levels. In this book, we discuss only single-factor designs, in which the factors may have any number of levels. Thus, you can often think of these two sets of variables as independent and dependent, as you do in general for factors and responses. You should be aware, however, that in certain situations, the two variables can take the same role. For example, in Figure 14.3, either the rows or the columns could be called responses.

In Figure 14.3, the results of a diagnostic test are compared with a physician's opinion. If we are using counts, the words *agree* and *disagree* in the table would be replaced by the number of patients in each category for whom the test result and the physician's diagnosis agreed or disagreed. The count (number of patients) for whom both the test result and the physician's opinion were negative would be placed in the upper left-hand corner of the body of the figure (the first row and first column). The count for which both were positive would be placed diagonally opposite, in the second row and second column. Analogously, the count of patients for whom the test was negative but the physician's opinion was positive would be placed in the first row and second column. Finally, if the disagreement was in the other direction, that is, if the test result were positive and the opinion negative, the count would be placed in row 2 and column 1. The row and column totals would be placed as shown, and the grand total should appear in the space below the row totals and to the right of the column totals.

---

[20]The examples here use counts as responses, that is (in the simplest case), the number of patients responding to a treatment vs. the number who do not respond. Such counts can be converted into proportions responding to a given treatment by dividing the number responding by the total count for that treatment. For example, if 90 patients are given a particular drug and 61 of them improve whereas the remaining 29 do not, the proportion improved is 61/90, or 0.678. We usually use counts rather than responses when calculating the chi-squared value for a contingency table, but proportions can be used. The equations in that case, however, will be slightly different.

14.7.2 Constructing Contingency Tables

When used as described, the table of Figure 14.3 would contain information that can be used to answer the following questions. Note that although we are using counts, the results will generally be expressed in terms of proportions:

1. What proportion of the patients shows agreement between physician and diagnostic test?
2. What proportion does not agree?
3. Are these proportions significantly different in the populations?

We will not discuss the kind of table illustrated in Figure 14.3 any further, because it is quite rare as a tool for the analysis of industrial drug trials. We will be concerned, rather, with tables in which a factor and a response are clearly distinguishable. Suppose we have data for two drugs on a two-valued scale, consisting of the numbers of patients who responded and did not respond to each of two drugs. We construct a contingency table with four cells, as shown in Figure 14.4. In that table, a represents the number of patients who were given drug D_1 and showed improvement, b, the number who did not improve, and c and d, the corresponding counts for drug D_2. We add the rows and columns and obtain the grand total, and place these sums in the margins of the table as shown. If we were using a response scale with more than two points, more columns would be added to the table, and if the factor possessed more than two levels, there would be more than two rows. In this book, we restrict ourselves to 2×2 tables like that of Figure 14.4.

To fix ideas, let's examine the contingency table of Figure 14.4 in more detail. If we were using specific trial data, the symbols a through d would be replaced with the numbers of patients in each cell. The sum $(a + b)$, at the right in the first row, would be replaced with the total number of patients on drug 1, whether or not they improved, and $(c + d)$ would be replaced with the total on drug 2. The sum of the first column (all patients who improved, regardless of which drug they were given) would appear where $(a + c)$

Drug	Improvement		Total
	Yes	No	
D_1	a	b	(a + b)
D_2	c	d	(c + d)
	(a + c)	(b + d)	N

Figure 14.4 Contingency table schematic using rows for treatment counts and columns for responses.

appears in the table, and would denote the total number of patients showing improvement. Similarly, the total number who did not improve would be placed where $(b + d)$ now appears. Finally, the total number of patients would appear where N now appears. Note that N can be obtained by adding *either* the two row or the two column totals. Such a table is often called a "two-by-two" table. The expression "two by two," or "2×2," means that two classifications are used for each cell, in this case, two drugs (the independent variable identified with the rows) and the two-valued (binomial) improvement scale (the response, identified with the columns).

If there were more than two drugs or more than two degrees of improvement, the table would have more rows, more columns, or both, but a 2×2 table as well as one with more rows, columns, or both would nevertheless both be called "two-way" tables, because they would possess only two dimensions, rows and columns. Three-way arrangements are possible (and not uncommon) in which the levels of a third variable are represented by the rows or columns in a set of additional tables, with one such table for each level of that variable. The structure would then have three dimensions: rows, columns, and tables.

14.7.3   Short Scales

In clinical studies, contingency tables are often used when the response scales are short. However, we should mention here that although there will be times when you must use very short response scales such as the binomial or three- or four-point scoring scales, you should try to avoid them. Of course, if you do so, you or your statistician will then not need the corresponding contingency table analyses described here. The reason for this warning is that a measurement using a limited scale, such as a binomial or trinomial, does not convey as much information as a continuous variable, and when you estimate sample size, you will find that you will require more patients for such data—often many more—than when the data are analyzable with parametric or rank tests. On the other hand, if such short-scale variables are minor components of a study, and your principal response or responses are analyzable with more powerful techniques, there is probably no harm in using one. Of course, you should remember that the addition of a response means that you should have increased the sample size to provide for the additional multiplicity, so you should plan for more responses only if you are convinced that they are necessary. On the other hand, at times (e.g., for testing adverse effects data), you will find contingency tables to be very useful. But even then, you should remember that if you sample sizes turn out to be just adequate for more powerful tests, you are unlikely to find significance with contingency table analyses of short-scale data, because they always require substantially greater sample sizes. If you wish to be conservative, as you should be in most clinical work, especially when dealing with safety data, one solution is to increase the value of alpha, such as 0.10 instead of 0.05, when testing adverse effects.

14.7.4 Responses

As noted, when we describe or exemplify contingency tables for clinical data here, they will hereafter be the kind in which a factor and a response are clearly identifiable. For consistency, we will show the factor in the rows and the response in the columns. The kinds of response variables for which contingency table analyses are commonly used in clinical work can be divided into four groups: nominal (in which the counts can be classified only into nonnumerical categories), binomial (two-valued), multinomial (multiple-valued), and normal. The response scales can be represented in words (cured, not cured) or they may take the form of integers or other symbols. For example, binomial data can be classified by sets of 0's or 1's (or any pair of integers), representing yes or no, plus or minus, improved or not improved, etc. Examples of multinomial scales are the common evaluation of a patient's condition as mild, moderate, or severe, which can be expressed as ordered integers such as 1, 2, and 3, etc. Sometimes a response has a normal distribution. In such a case, the column labels may be a number of ranges within the limits of the observations, or, sometimes, all the observations themselves.

14.7.5 Varieties of Contingency Tables

The short-form equation for the necessary calculations for a 2×2 table with independent cells, which appears later in this section as Equation (14.18), applies *only* to 2×2 tables. Larger tables and tables with more than two dimensions use different and more general methods of analysis, which are not described here. Your statistician will be familiar with the calculations. If you are interested, a number of the books listed in the Bibliography under "Clinical Trial and Medical Statistics" and "General Statistics," and some under "Nonparametric and Discrete Data Analysis" give the procedures, most of which are fairly simple. A particularly good reference is Fleiss [41]. You should note that most of these methods, as well as the chi-squared analysis described later in this chapter, are normal approximations.

There are still other kinds of tables and analyses. In addition to the larger two-dimensional tables just mentioned, which are analogous to 2×2 tables but have more rows and/or columns, there are others. For example, when the categories in a response scale can be arranged in ascending or descending order, there are contingency table tests that can utilize this information, conferring an increase in statistical power. An example is a scale such as mild, moderate, and severe. Additional dimensions can be used; for example, there might be *sets* of two-way tables (resulting in three dimensions rather than two), as already mentioned. Still another technique is described in a large body of application and theoretical information about the use of contingency tables for **log-linear** analysis, in which multifactor contingency tables are analyzed in a manner analogous to the use of the analysis of variance. If you are interested, see Agresti (14), Bishop, Fienberg, and Holland (15), Cox (16), Fienburg [40], Fleiss [41], Freeman [42], or Upton (17).

14.7.6 Example 14.8: Two-Way Table, Binomial Response

Contingency tables are usually used to analyze data classified in two ways (one response and one factor, or two responses) or more (more than two factors or responses). In clinical work, the analyses are almost always univariate (one response at a time) but one or more factors. As always, we use the word "factor" to mean an independent variable, and "response" for a dependent variable (a "measurement" variable, such as a judgment scale). In this example, we use a two-way table with two rows and two columns, in which the rows represent two treatments (i.e., one factor with two levels) and the columns, the levels of one response.

Suppose you have completed a trial comparing a placebo and a drug (D_1 and D_2, respectively), and that you had planned to investigate whether or not the use of the drug is associated with a gastrointestinal (GI) effect such as nausea. This can be tested appropriately with a contingency table analysis. The data for the table are first arranged in the form of frequencies or "counts" belonging to each category of the response scale. For example, you might have classified your patients during a trial into those having nausea and those reporting none. You should also have classified them according to whether they were assigned to D_1 or D_2. You would count the number of different *patients* (*not* the number of occurrences within patients) in each of these cases, and place the counts in the table, also showing totals for the rows, columns, and the overall count. Your two-way contingency table would then resemble that of Table 14.11.

Table 14.11 is designed to answer the question, "In the two populations represented by the D_1 and D_2 groups, is the *proportion* of patients reporting nausea greater for D_1 than for D_2?" (or D_2 than D_1?), or "Is there any

Table 14.11. Two-Way Contingency Table: Nominal Data, Binomial Response (Example 14.8)

Drug Used	Nausea		Totals
	No	Yes	
1	10	15	25
2	20	10	30
Totals	30	25	55

significant difference between the proportions of patients with nausea for the two drugs? You should usually run a two-tailed test, as the latter question implies, because, as you are aware, in a blind test, it is quite possible that patients on placebo ("drug" D_1) can experience substantial GI effects. You note that in the first row of Table 14.11, the proportion of patients exhibiting nausea for D_1 is 10/25, or 0.400, whereas in the second row, for D_2, the proportion is higher, 20/30, or 0.667. Before the significance test is done, therefore, the initial impression might be that there is a greater proportion of nausea in the *population* of patients taking the drug than in the placebo population. A significance test will provide an answer to the question, "Does this observed difference in proportions reflect a real population difference (i.e., is there a population difference between the drug and placebo, or is the sample difference an effect of chance)? Remember that there will still be a small probability alpha of finding significance even if there is no population difference.

There are several ways to analyze this kind of table. We will demonstrate the most convenient one only.[21] This method does not demonstrate the underlying rationale of the method as well as other procedures, but it is simple to use. You can obtain more complete information in the references cited.

Calculate the total value of chi-squared for the table (this is really the corrected sum of the chi-squared values for each of the four cells) using Equation (14.18):

$$\chi^2 = \frac{N(|ad - bc| - 0.5N)^2}{(a + b)(c + d)(a + c)(b + d)} \qquad (14.18)$$

The symbol χ^2 is correctly read "chi squared." The letters a, b, c, and d refer to the counts of patients in the four cells of Table 14.11, reading from left to right and starting at the first row (drug 1). N is the total count for the table, shown in the lower right-hand corner.

In this example, as shown in Table 14.11, the marginal totals are

$$(a + b) = 25$$
$$(c + d) = 30$$
$$(a + c) = 30$$
$$(b + d) = 25$$
$$N = 55$$

---

[21] This procedure includes provision for a continuity correction. It should be noted that even with the correction, this analysis and other chi-squared procedures appling to contingency table data are normal approximations.

Using the cell counts and these totals, we employ Equation (14.18) to calculate chi squared for the table:

$$\chi^2 = \frac{N(|ad - bc| - 0.5N)^2}{(a + b)(c + d)(a + c)(b + d)}$$

$$= \frac{55[|(10 \times 10) - (15 \times 20)| - (0.5 \times 55)]^2}{(10 + 15)(20 + 10)(10 + 20)(15 + 10)}$$

$$= 2.910$$

We must now compare this estimated chi-squared value (2.910) with a standard value from the chi-squared table in the Appendix (Table A.2). The two-way contingency table has one degree of freedom, because, *given the marginal totals*, the table can be reconstructed if the count in any *one* of the four cells is given and the other three are missing (try it). The table in the Appendix shows chi-squared values for 1 to 5 df, over a range of probability values. Using the Appendix table, we therefore look up the value of chi squared for 1 df and a probability of 0.05 (we assume that we specified 0.05 for alpha). We find the tabulated value to be 3.841. We compare this value with the calculated chi squared. Because the calculated value is less than this, the conclusion is that we cannot show a difference between the two treatments in terms of the sample distributions of GI symptoms observed. If the calculated value of chi squared had been greater than 3.841 but less than 5.024, the tabular value of chi squared for $p = 0.025$, we would have concluded that there was a significant difference between treatments, with a probability lying between 0.05 and 0.025.

A Caution

The contingency table test described here is an approximate test; the chi-squared procedure is an approximation to the normal. Small sample sizes, and particularly small cell sizes, can give very approximate results. Snedecor and Cochran [38] caution against using the chi-squared analysis for small contingency tables. This rule is that if the total sample size (N) is less than 20 *or* if any *expected* value is less than 5 when N lies between 20 and 40, the test should not be used. We call this Cochran's rule. In such cases, they recommend, instead, the use of Fisher's exact test. Although we have not described that test here, it is described in many references; see Snedecor and Cochran [38], Maxwell [44], and others. For small tables, it is quite simple to use, and is also included with many statistical computer packages.

To apply this rule, the *expected value* of the count in each cell is needed. The expected value for a cell in Table 14.11 is the value it would have, *given the marginal totals shown*, if the null hypothesis were true. Expected values for each cell are calculated as follows: Multiply the total for the column containing that cell by the total of its row, and divide by N. For example, in

Table 14.11, the expected value for cell "*a*" (containing a count of 10) is $(30 \times 25)/55 = 13.6$. By similar calculations, the expected values in cells *b*, *c*, and *d* are 11.4, 16.4, and 13.6, respectively. As a check on your calculations, the expected values should give the same row, column, and grand totals as the original data. Note that Table 14.11 does not violate Cochran's rule, so that Equation (14.18) was used legitimately.

14.8 MULTIPLE COMPARISONS

14.8.1 Definitions and Descriptions

When there is more than one treatment comparison to be made among the data for a given trial, you will almost always need to use an **experimentwise error rate**, rather than a **testwise error rate**. To review, an experimentwise error rate is an alpha error applying to each of an entire group of comparisons, considered together, whereas a testwise rate applies only to each single test, taken by itself. The latter is rarely used, and when it is, it is frequently interpreted incorrectly.

To employ an experimentwise error rate, you must use a multiple-comparisons procedure. If, for example, an ordinary *t* test is used instead to make several treatment comparisons from the same set of data, the actual alpha value applying to the tests taken as a group will be larger than your specified value, and you will therefore be likely to declare significance when there is none. In this connection, it is well to keep in mind that in any given single-factor design having more than two treatments, there are *always* more possible comparisons than treatments. When there are three treatments, there are three possible **pairwise comparisons**. When there are four treatments, there are six, and so on. But in addition to the pairwise comparisons, there are other, more complex contrasts that are sometimes of interest, such as the mean of treatments 1 and 2 versus that of treatment 3, etc. The usual case in which an ordinary *t* test can be used correctly in such as event exists when only a single comparison out of the several possible is to be made, and that one has been specified before examining any data. Note that an experimentwise error rate requires a multiple-comparisons test, and thus is almost invariably what is needed when you are testing several contrasts from a single trial.

In this section, we examine only one multiple-comparisons test in detail, although some others are mentioned. These tests are usually used to avoid the problems of multiplicity when more than one comparison must be made among a group of treatment data during the statistical analysis of a trial, as just discussed. However, they can also be used to control multiplicity introduced in other ways.

A multiple-comparisons test is a hypothesis (significance) test like the *t* tests or rank tests. When multiplicity is introduced by the use of more than one comparison of treatment means or combinations of means, the t test and its analogues are subject to experimentwise error rates that are too small. That is, in the long run, the number of tests giving significance when the null hypothesis is really true will actually be greater than the proportion specified by the alpha level used. Putting it another way, if you have specified an alpha level of 0.05 and multiple comparisons are made, the specified alpha will not hold true, and the true alpha level will be higher than that found—often seriously higher. In a series of such tests, you will thus claim more cases of significance than there really are.

For example, if you use an alpha specification of 0.05 and the null hypothesis is true, you will expect to claim significance falsely approximately five times in every hundred experiments of the same kind, that is, you will have a probability of 0.05 of falsely claiming significance in *each* test. But if there is multiplicity created by making more than one comparison within a single clinical trial, by using a test procedure like the t test, which is not intended for use in that way, this probability will be higher. How much higher it becomes increases rapidly with the number of comparisons you make.

The use of a good multiple-comparisons test avoids this problem completely.

14.8.2   Preparation during Planning

Most multiple comparisons tests will be run by the statistician. However, we discuss them briefly here because you should prepare for their use during planning.

If there are to be multiple hypothesis tests, the sample size estimated during planning should be greater than it would be if only a single test were to be done. The reason is that the values of alpha, beta, delta, and the sample size are all interdependent. If the sample size estimate is not increased, but several comparisons are nevertheless made, by using a multiple-comparisons test, the alpha level for each comparison will have been maintained as planned, but the beta level or the value of delta, or both, will have been increased beyond those specified.

14.8.3   Kinds of Multiple-Comparisons Tests

The Bonferroni Inequality
This procedure was described and recommended in Chapter 5. It is a simple and appropriate method for providing for the multiplicity introduced when you need to carry out more than one comparison using a t test or the equivalent.

If you are using a sample size table, such as Tables A.3 or A.4 in the Appendix, you need the specified values of alpha, beta, and delta, as well as an estimated value of sigma, to make your estimate. If, for example, you are planning a single-factor design with four treatments, there will be six possible pairwise comparisons. By calling the treatments *A*, *B*, *C*, and *D*, these will be *A* vs. *B*, *A* vs. *C*, *A* vs. *D*, *B* vs. *C*, *B* vs. *D*, and *C* vs. *D*. If you wish to test each of these contrasts with *t* tests using the Bonferroni procedure, *but maintain your specified values of beta and delta as well as alpha*, you can, but you must increase the sample size to do so. In the case of a parallel design, this is done by entering Table A.3 using a value of alpha calculated *by dividing your specified alpha (e.g., 0.05) by the number of comparisons you wish to make*. In this case, to make all six of these comparisons, the calculated alpha will be 0.05/6, or about 0.008. You could therefore enter Table A.3 using an alpha level of 0.01, the nearest tabular value to 0.008. This will produce a sample size slightly smaller than that strictly necessary. However, the Bonferroni method is somewhat conservative, so that your sample size will probably be adequate.

As pointed out before, you can use Bonferroni or any other suitable multiple-comparisons test without this compensation of the sample size, but you will be penalized by a distortion of beta, delta, or both.

Other Multiple-Comparisons Procedures

There are many multiple-comparisons procedures in addition to Bonferroni, but Bonferroni is simple to use and makes the adjustment of the sample size easy; it is recommended strongly, in spite of its conservatism. We list several others here, and you can find descriptions of their use in several of the books listed in the Bibliography. Four of the best known, which we recommend, are the following:

1. **Fisher's Protected LSD** (or the the variation described by Carmer and Swanson, which we call the **Fisher/Carmer and Swanson Protected *t* Test**) (8) or Bernhardson (9).
2. **Tukey's Honestly Significant Difference (HSD) Test** [33, 38].[22]
3. **Dunnett's Test** (18).
4. **Scheffé's Test** (3).

Other tests exist, but these four, and the Bonferroni, will be satisfactory for any multiple-comparisons problem you may encounter. There are others that are equally satisfactory, as well as some others that are the opposite of conservative.

The Fisher/Carmer and Swanson test allows the use of a series of *t* tests following an analysis of variance, but only if the analysis of variance has shown significance. In addition to Carmer and Swanson (8), Bernhardson (9) later published a paper that describes a similar study. Tukey's [33, 38] test is straightforward and simple, and is used as an LSD. Dunnett's (18) test is

---

[22]This test is described in Snedecor and Cochran [38], but it is called the *Q Method* there. The test is ascribed to Tukey in several sources, including Dixon and Massey [33].

designed for the particular situation in which several comparisons are to be made with a control or standard, but not *all* the possible pairwise comparisons are to be made. Finally, Scheffé's test allows *any* number of comparisons *of any kind* to be made, not only the pairwise comparisons, for example, but such combinations as means of treatments *A* and *B* vs. that of *C*, and the like. *None of these tests except the Fisher/Carmer and Swanson should be preceded by an analysis of variance.* If an ANOVA has been run beforehand and a significant result is obtained, and a multiple-comparisons test other than the *t* test of the Carmer/Swanson procedure is then used, the test may show significance at the originally specified alpha level *less often* than alpha percent of the time.

14.9   STATISTICAL PROCEDURES NOT DESCRIBED

Because of the emphasis upon planning and design in this book, all but a few statistical procedures have been omitted. These include many of those that are very commonly used, such as the analysis of variance (ANOVA). However, the biostatistician in your organization will be familiar with most or all of them. If you are interested in obtaining further information, descriptions and examples of those mentioned in what follows are available in many of the books listed in the Bibliography.

The more common techniques of statistical analyses that have been omitted from this book include the analysis of variance, the analysis of covariance, regression analysis, correlation, multivariate analysis, and survival analysis. There is a great deal of literature on these topics, as well as upon many others less relevant to the analysis of clinical trial data. Some of this can be found in books listed in the Bibliography. There is a landmark paper concerned with survival analysis, published in two parts in the *British Journal of Cancer* in 1976 and 1977 by Peto et al. (19). All of the authors are widely known in statistics, and the techniques described have applications far beyond those of mortality studies. Both papers were written for practitioners and researchers who are not experienced in statistics or experimental design, and are easy reading. We recommend them very highly.

14.10   SUMMARY OF THE CHAPTER

14.10.1   Error Estimation

The chapter begins with a discussion of the estimation of error. This sets the stage for subsequent discussions of hypothesis testing. Hypothesis testing or an equivalent, to compare new materials, standards, and/or placebos, has become a sine qua non in clinical trial work. For one thing, it is needed for any work intended for submission to the FDA when seeking regulatory approval for a "new drug." This section is devoted to the calculation of variance and standard deviation, and a discussion of their subspecies. Such calculations and related ones constitute the foundations of the procedures that you or your statistician will use in the analyses of your data.

14.10.2 Hypothesis Tests

The following sections of the chapter are restricted to the description of some common forms of several elementary statistical hypothesis tests and related procedures. These are the t tests, rank tests, and contingency table tests. Those described are designed for testing data from one-factor designs only. They are intended to convey sufficient understanding of statistical analysis to facilitate effective and correct selection of experimental designs during planning, as well as to pave the way for the treatment of essential sample size estimation procedures in the following and final chapter of this book. No effort was made to describe all the available varieties of any of these three test categories in this chapter.

All the topics in this book are confined to so-called **univariate** statistical methods, in which *only one response* (dependent variable) at a time is used in a given analytical procedure. Univariate methods include analyses of data with more than one *independent* variable (factor), although we have limited ourselves to one factor in this chapter.

The hypothesis tests described in this section include the independent groups t test, the dependent t test, and two related entities, the LSD (least significant difference) and confidence intervals. Following this, two common rank tests, the Wilcoxon procedures, which are the rank test equivalents of the two t tests, are described. Finally, the simplest member of the contingency table tests, using so-called 2-by-2 tables, is described. Such tables are useful in analyzing dichotomous data. Extensions, with more rows and/or columns, can be used for designs with more than two levels of a single factor, more than one factor, and response scales with more than two points.

14.10.3 Multiple Comparisons

A short review of the use of the Bonferroni inequality for performing multiple comparisons, using experimentwise error rates and estimating sample size while preserving specified values of beta and delta as well as alpha, was given. Other common multiple-comparisons tests were listed but not described.

14.10.4 Omitted Procedures

It was pointed out that because this book gives emphasis to trial planning and experimental design, only a few elementary methods of data analysis have been described. It was necessary that these be included to provide enough understanding of hypothesis testing and related analyses to make possible informed selection of experimental designs when planning a trial. Other statistical procedures were mentioned and referenced, but not described. It is expected that, with few exceptions, the statistician will perform the analyses.

14.11   APPENDIX: RESIDUALS, NORMALITY, AND VARIANCE TESTS

14.11.1   Calculation of Residuals

Nature and Advantage of Residuals
The use of residuals calculated from your data rather than the use of the data themselves is convenient in testing assumptions. In a one-factor design, the residuals are the quantities that remain after removing the estimated mean from each datum. They are estimates of the errors in the population. If there were no errors in a population of responses from a single treatment, the residuals would all be zero, and the "distribution" would comprise a mean, mu, with a standard deviation and variance of zero.[23] There is an important advantage to the use of residuals rather than original data when studying the distribution of error. Unlike the original data, if the variances of the original treatment groups are not greatly different, the residuals from two or more groups can be combined into one sample representing a single distribution of errors with a mean of zero. This allows the easy use of all of the data, providing more powerful tests of the assumptions.

Normality and Variance Tests Using Residuals
We describe and recommend Michael's test for nonnormality (20) with Nelson's modifications (21) to examine residuals derived from the data of Example 14.2, Table 14.3. We will also test the data for heteroscedasticity, but for that, we will begin with the two groups of data themselves, using Levene's test, also mentioned in the last chapter. This test also uses residuals, but they are handled differently, and are calculated integrally with the test.

Further Examination of Residuals
As suggested earlier, in addition to calculating residuals for the foregoing purposes, it is a good idea to ask the statistician to examine them in other ways, such as by plotting them against their fitted values. In a one-way (single-factor) design, the fitted values are the treatment means. The plot should show a set of points for each treatment group, with no trends related to treatments. In addition, other graphical tests of the residuals are often a good idea. They can be plotted against the order in which the patients were

---

[23]Of course, errors are *always* present in data from the real world.

examined and treated, which will show any trends that might suggest nonrandom influences. For example, if, in a single-center trial, some of the patients were treated and examined in different weeks, or in different locations, or by different investigators (although none of these events may occur in a well-conducted trial), plots of the residuals against weeks, locations, and/or investigators will often disclose anomalies. If the clouds of points surrounding each mean, week, location, or investigator appear at different levels, suggesting influences of these unplanned factors, you should investigate the conduct of the trial further.

The Residuals

For a single-factor design, the calculation is very simple, because the only influence expected to be imposed upon each datum is the effect of one of the treatments, if any. In a more complex design, such as a two- or three-factor trial with possible interactions, there would be several treatment and interaction effects representing fitted values to be removed, but the principle is the same.

As an illustration, we use the data from Example 14.2, Table 14.3. Table 14.A1 illustrates the results of the calculation for this example. The sum of squares of the residuals is found at the bottom of the table. The column headings illustrate the calculations. Because the sum of the residuals is theoretically zero, and is nearly zero in this example, the simple sum of squares of the residuals themselves—that is, the first term in Equation 14.5, for example—is adequate as a basis for a variance calculation. The data are shown in the first column, the group means in the second, the residuals in the third, and their squares in the last. If the variances were exactly the same in both groups, the two sample distributions would be the same except for the two means. The means will be different if the treatments have different effects upon the response. Once any effect of the appropriate mean is removed from each individual datum, if there is no evidence of unequal variances in the two groups of residuals as measured by a test such as the Levene test, the residuals from both groups can be combined into one single set of individual error estimates, shorn of nonrandom influences.

The squares of the residuals given in column 4 of Table 14.A1 (and their sum of squares shown at the bottom of the table) demonstrate that the latter is equal to the total sum of squares of deviations from the mean. This fact can be used as a check of your calculations. That is, if you add the two group SS values at the bottom of Table 14.3, you should get the same or almost the same result as the sum of squares of the deviations shown at the bottom of Table 14.A1 (117.5000 + 68.2143 = 185.71). Any difference will be a result of rounding errors. If agreement is not close, there is probably an error in the calculations. Also note the sum of the residuals column. In the population, the sum of the residuals (and therefore also the mean) is zero. Because of rounding errors, however, the calculations are unlikely to yield exactly zero. In the present case, we have -0.01 when the sum is rounded to two places.

Table 14.A1. Calculation of Residuals and Their Squares (Example 14.2)

Data (y_{ij})	Treatment Means $(\bar{T}_i)$	Residuals $(y_{ij} - \bar{T}_i)$	Residuals Squared (z^2)
49.5	48.00	1.5	2.2500
48.0	48.00	0.0	0.0000
52.5	48.00	4.5	20.2500
46.5	48.00	−1.5	2.2500
52.0	48.00	4.0	16.0000
48.5	48.00	0.5	0.2500
40.0	48.00	−8.0	64.0000
50.5	48.00	2.5	6.2500
46.0	48.00	−2.0	4.0000
46.5	48.00	−1.5	2.2500
47.5	44.93	2.57	6.6049
48.5	44.93	3.57	12.7449
40.5	44.93	−4.43	19.6249
43.5	44.93	−1.43	2.0449
49.0	44.93	4.07	16.5649
43.5	44.93	−1.43	2.0449
42.0	44.93	−2.93	8.5849
Sum		−0.01	
N		17	17
Sum of Squares			185.71

The mean, of course, although not shown in the table, is very small: −0.01/17, or 0.00 (−0.0006 to four places). This is the reason that it was not necessary to subtract it from each individual residual before squaring and summing, as would be done with any original data when calculating a sum of squares of deviations from the mean.

14.11.2 Michael's Probability Plot

Michael's Stabilized Probability Plot[24] was used to test the residuals for nonnormality. The method is useful for testing the **good of fit** of data to any of a number of different distributions, but we present it here as a normality test. It is a relatively new procedure, and, when used to construct a normal

---

[24]This procedure is described in the Michael and Nelson papers, which are referenced in Chapter 12 and above, repeated here for your convenience. See references (20) and (21) at the end of this chapter. Nelson's paper (21) gives a very clear description of the procedure, and includes a BASIC program for performing it. If you use the program, you may need to edit it a bit for your particular machine. We thank the American Society for Quality Control and Dr. Lloyd Nelson for permission to use Figure 14A.1, to display the output of the BASIC program in Table 14.A2, and to include the program itself in the Appendix to this book.

probability plot, represents a significant advance over the conventional graphical methods; the variances of the points in the plot are approximately equal, making a graphical significance test possible at a glance.

The traditional normal probability plot is a graph of a cumulative distribution of sample data plotted against a cumulative normal distribution. If the plot is a straight line, it indicates that the sample distribution is derived from a normal population. However, this method does not include a procedure for testing whether any deviation from linearity implies significant nonnormality. On the other hand, Michael's plot shows at a glance, at any selected alpha level, whether normality may be assumed. The method is more powerful than many other goodness-of-fit tests, such as the old Pearson chi-squared test. In fact, Michael states that, with a Monte Carlo study, he found that his procedure is nearly as powerful as the Shapiro-Wilks, the current favorite. It is also much easier to use than that test, requiring no tables if done as described here.

The analysis of residuals using Michael's method is complete in itself. The normal probability plot is optional, although you should find it very useful, especially for presentations and reports to management personnel who are not familiar with statistical procedures.

The "stabilization" in Michael's test involves the use of an arc sine function to adjust the variance of the data and the points of the normal distribution. This transformation allows the use of a uniformly spaced plotting scale rather than a normal probability scale. A simple diagonal line drawn from point $(0,0)$ to $(1,1)$ is used to represent the normal reference distribution. In his paper, Nelson uses the symbols X' and Y' to represent the transformed scales. See the Michael (20) and Nelson (21) papers.

The BASIC program given in Nelson's paper is reprinted with permission in the Appendix to this book. We have made some minor modifications to make it conform to MS DOS 3.x.[25] The output is a four-column table giving the residuals, the two values comprising each point of the transformed scale (X' and Y') and their absolute differences $|X' - Y'|$, sorted by order of magnitude of the residuals.[26] To do the test, you can run the BASIC program

---

[25]Since this was originally written, MS-DOS 5.0 and 6.0 have appeared. The BASIC interpreter accompanying those operating systems is completely compatible with the GW-BASIC used in Nelson's program, as reprinted and slightly modified in the Appendix. Note that this software and program, with perhaps minor changes, are designed to operate with any IBM or IBM-compatible desktop computer system using a DOS operating system, version 2.0 or later, including the original PC, PC/XT, PC/AT, PS-2 (MCA), or systems compatible with them. This form of BASIC, rather than one of the newer and more efficient versions such as Microsoft's QUICK BASIC[TM], was used because of its wide availability. The software and program are incompatible with the Apple hardware and operating system, however.

[26]You need not know the mathematical basis for Michael's procedure to use it successfully. If you are interested, however, the values X' are arc sine functions of the rank order numbers of the observations, and the Y' values are arc sine functions of the cumulative normal distribution. The critical values for the maximum absolute difference between these two among the N pairs of values are given in a table in Michael's paper, but are printed out by Nelson's BASIC program, so that no further reference materials are needed.

Table 14.A2. Output of BASIC Program for Michael's Test for Nonnormality (Example 14.2)

Residual	X'	Y'	$|X' - Y'|$
− 8.00	0.110	0.056	0.054
− 4.43	0.192	0.194	0.002
− 2.93	0.251	0.285	0.034
− 2.00	0.300	0.350	0.050
− 1.50	0.344	0.386	0.042
− 1.50	0.385	0.386	0.001
− 1.43	0.424	0.391	0.033
− 1.43	0.462	0.391	0.071
0.00	0.500	0.500	0.000
0.50	0.538	0.538	0.000
1.50	0.576	0.614	0.038
2.50	0.615	0.686	0.071
2.57	0.656	0.690	0.034
3.57	0.700	0.756	0.056
4.00	0.749	0.782	0.033
4.07	0.808	0.786	0.022
4.50	0.890	0.810	0.080

Alpha Value	Critical Absolute Difference
0.050	0.124
0.010	0.146

and compare the *largest* of these differences with the appropriate critical value given in the printout for your chosen alpha level. If you wish to use a value of alpha other than one of those given in Michael's paper (0.01, 0.05, 0.10, and above), you can extrapolate in his table.

Using the data of Example 14.2, the output of the Nelson program is shown in Table 14.A2. The table is slightly modified relative to that produced by the program. The residuals of this example are contained in the data statements of the program (statements 210 and 220), and the number of data are given in statement 240. When using the program for other data, the appropriate values are substituted in these statements. The values X' are the arc sine functions of the rank order numbers of the observations, and the Y' values are arc sine functions of the cumulative normal distribution.

In this example, an alpha level of 0.05 was specified before doing the test. The largest difference between X' and Y' is 0.080, which appears at the bottom of column 4 in Table 14.A2. Because this does not exceed the critical value of 0.124 for alpha = 0.05 shown at the bottom of the table, we conclude that lack of normality has not been shown. To understand this, remember that the test is used here in the "simplistic" version of the hypothesis test described in Chapter 12. That is, if the maximum absolute difference *exceeds* the critical value given, the null hypothesis would be rejected and the distribution being tested would be declared to be nonnormal. If the null hypothesis cannot be rejected, as in this example, we merely conclude that nonnormality has not been shown. Of course, because you have an estimated value of sigma (calculated from the data) and alpha, which you should have prespecified, it is permissible to postcalculate delta with some assumed "what-if" value of beta, or beta with a "what-if" value of delta (the latter would perhaps be more suitable here).

The conclusion of nonsignificance above is supported visually in Figure 14.A1, which is Michael's stabilized probability plot for the data of this example. This figure includes (a) a plot of the sample points X' and Y' from the BASIC program, as listed in the second and third column of Table 14.5; (b) a straight line extending from the lower left-hand corner of the figure, point $(0, 0)$, to the upper right-hand corner, point $(1, 1)$, which represents the stabilized cumulative normal distribution used for comparison with the sample points; and (c) two lines parallel to the normal line, one above and one below it, which represent the $(1 - \alpha)\%$ upper and lower confidence limits for the plotted points. The lines are straight and equidistant from the central line because of the use of the arc sine transformation. In the present case, we used a value of 0.05 for alpha, so that the two lines define a 95% confidence interval for individual points about the central line. The two lines

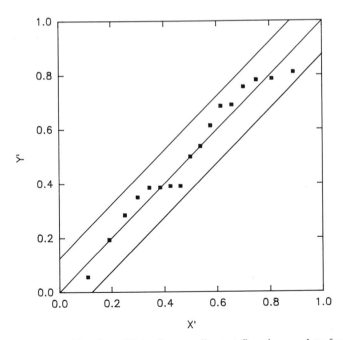

Figure 14.A1 Plot resulting from Michael's normality test (based upon data from Example 14.2).

Table 14.A3. Calculation of Absolute Deviations from the Group Means for Levene's Test (Example 14.2)

	Data		Absolute Deviations	
	T_1	T_2	$|T_1 - \bar{T}_1|$	$|T_2 - \bar{T}_2|$
	49.5	47.5	1.5	2.57
	48.0	48.5	0.0	3.57
	52.5	40.5	4.5	4.43
	46.5	43.5	1.5	1.43
	52.0	49.0	4.0	4.07
	48.5	43.5	0.5	1.43
	40.0	42.0	8.0	2.93
	50.5		2.5	
	46.0		2.0	
	46.5		1.5	
Sum	480.0	314.5	26.0	20.43
N	10	7	10	7
Mean	48.00	44.93	2.60	2.92

are plotted at vertical distances of $0.124Y'$ units above and below the normal line. A different value of alpha could have been used. For example, had we wished to use 99% limits, we would have located the two lines at $0.146Y'$ units above and below the normal line. If the plotted points shown formed a normal distribution exactly and without error, they would lie exactly upon the diagonal line representing the standard normal distribution, plotted in the middle of the graph.

14.11.3   Comparison of Variances (Levene's Test)

We now test whether it can be concluded that the variances of the two treatment populations represented by the samples of 7 and 10 data in Table 14.3 are different. To do this, we use Levene's test at an alpha level of 0.05.[27] This test uses the deviations of the observations from their means, so that the basic raw materials are identical to the residuals used in Michael's test, Table 14.4, except that they are taken as absolute values and are kept separated by their two groups of origin. They are shown in Table 14.A3.

Levene's test of the data in Table 14.A3 was done as follows: The absolute deviations from each group mean were calculated, as shown in the table. The means of the deviations were then taken. The two means in this case are 2.60

---

[27]It has been suggested that tests of the assumptions be made at alpha values higher than those customarily used in the final tests. Thus, if you use an alpha value of 0.05 in your regular hypothesis tests, you might use 0.10 in the tests of the assumptions. We have not done this here, but you may wish to do so to make your final hypothesis tests more reliable.

and 2.92, as shown at the bottom of the table.[28] The test relies upon a hypothesis test that will indicate whether these mean absolute deviations are sufficiently different to justify a claim, with a probability of error of alpha, that the distributions represented by the samples have different variances. You will recall that, in this example, we know that the population variances are the same, because the data were originally taken from a single distribution and then given different means. We therefore do not expect to find significance.

The kind of hypothesis test to be used in doing Levene's test can be anything suitable. Snedecor and Cochran [38] use an analysis of variance, relying upon its robustness if the data are not normally distributed. This might be used whenever the number of groups exceeds 2.[29] In the case of just two groups, however, an independent t test is completely equivalent to an analysis of variance, so that either could be used.

Alternatively, it might be preferable to use a test that does not depend upon the assumption of normality. For example, we could use Wilcoxon's Rank Sum test for two groups. Wilcoxon's Rank Sum test is described and exemplified in this chapter, and is the one that was used here.[30]

The procedure for the Levene test is described in Snedecor and Cochran [38]. If you wish, you can apply that procedure to the data of this example, for practice. In this case, no evidence of heterogeneity of variance was found. Instead of an analysis of variance, the Wilcoxon Rank Sum test, using a normal approximation procedure, was used as the hypothesis test for the Levene procedure, and yielded a probability value of 0.56, very far from the prespecified alpha value of 0.05. As a matter of interest, a t test was done on the same data to see how close the result would be to this. The probability was not determined as exactly, but lay between 0.50 and 0.75. Thus, there was good agreement between the two procedures.

14.12 LITERATURE REFERENCES

(1) Tukey, J. W., *Biometrics*, 5, 232 (1949).

(2) Satterthwaite, F. E., *Biometric Bulletin*, 2, 110 (1946).

(3) Scheffé, Henry, *The Analysis of Variance*, John Wiley, New York, 1959.

(4) Anscombe, F. J., and John W. Tukey, *Technometrics*, 5, 141–160 (1963).

---

[28]Levene's test is suitable for checking the variances among any number of treatment groups, not just two as in this example. For example, if, instead of a simple t test, we were running a multiple-comparisons test, we could use Levene's test to compare the variances among the data from several treatments with each other.

[29]The analysis of variance procedure is not described in this book. There are many variations, and numbers of them are described in many of the statistics books listed in the Bibliography.

[30]The use of rank tests in the Levene procedure was conceived by J. M. Becktel of the V.A. Research Hospital at Hines, Illinois.

(5) Daniel, Cuthbert, and Fred S. Wood, *Fitting Equations to Data*, John Wiley, New York, 1971.

(6) Searle, Shayle R., *The American Statistician*, 42, 211 (1988).

(7) Wooding, W. M., *Journal of Quality Technology*, 1, 175–188 (1969).

(8) Carmer, S. G., and M. R. Swanson, *Journal of the American Statistical Association*, 68, 66–74 (1973).

(9) Bernhardson, Clemens S., *Biometrics*, 31, 229–232 (1975).

(10) Edgington, Eugene S., *Randomization Tests*, Marcel Dekker, New York, 1980.

(11) Page, E., *Applied Statistics*, 26, No. 1, 75–76 (1977).

(12) Tiemstra, Peter J., *Journal of Quality Technology*, 3, No. 3, 149–156 (1981).

(13) Lien, David A., *The BASIC Handbook*, 3d ed., Compusoft Publishing, San Diego, 1986.

(14) Agresti, Alan, *Categorical Data Analysis*, John Wiley, New York, 1990.

(15) Bishop, Yvonne M. M., Stephen E. Fienberg, and Paul W. Holland, *Discrete Multivariate Analysis: Theory and Practice*, The MIT Press, Cambridge, Mass., 1975.

(16) Cox, D. R., *The Analysis of Binary Data*, Chapman and Hall, London, 1970.

(17) Upton, Graham J. G., *The Analysis of Cross-Classified Data*, John Wiley, New York, 1978.

(18) Dunnett, Charles W., *Journal of the American Statistical Association*, 50, 1096–1121 (1955).

(19) Peto, R., M. C. Pike, et al., *British Journal of Cancer*, 34 585–612 (1976), and ibid., 35, 1–39 (1977).

(20) Michael, John R., *Biometrika*, 70, 11–17 (1983).

(21) Nelson, Lloyd S., *Journal of Quality Technology*, 21, 213–215 (1989).

PART V

Details of Sample Size Estimation

CHAPTER 15

Sample Size Estimation

15.1 INTRODUCTION

15.1.1 About Sample Size Estimates

There are few procedures in clinical trial planning that are more important in the design of an effective study than the estimation of sample size. This is not an original observation, but so many clinical studies are planned and run without using *any* statistical sample size estimation that it cannot be emphasized too much. For example, a survey of 71 published clinical trials in which significance was not found was published in 1978 by Freiman et al. (1) in *The New England Journal of Medicine*. Among the 71 papers, the authors found "an almost total lack" of mention of the alpha and beta risks and little indication that there was any realization of the effects of the small sample sizes used upon the power of the tests. In many of the trials described, the beta risks calculated a posteriori by the authors of this survey, assuming common values of delta and alpha, were too large to provide reasonable expectations of significance. It might be supposed that in more recent work this situation has changed, but the current literature indicates little improvement.

Thus, obtaining a good estimate of the sample size for a clinical study goes a long way toward ensuring that the inconvenience to the patients undergoing a trial, as well as your and your company's time and expense, will be justified. To run a clinical trial without a prior sample size estimate is to ignore a major source of potential failure of your project.

15.1.2 Neyman-Pearson Esimates

In Chapter 5, we introduced the notions of sample size estimation and power using the Neyman-Pearson ideas, so that you would possess sufficient knowledge of them to allow you to deal adequately with subsequent topics up to this point. However, the development in that chapter was limited to a brief exposition of principles and an example using a *t* test. This chapter expands broadly upon the earlier material in order to provide you with the tools you need to estimate sample size for most of the common experimental designs you will probably be using in your work. It is intended to stand alone, without necessitating reference to Chapter 5.

You will recall that we have recommended that you should not carry out your statistical analyses yourself, or at least not without help from a statistician. However, this need not be true of much of your sample size estimation. For the simpler designs, the estimation of sample size, like the selection of an experimental design, can and probably should be done by you during your planning stage, rather than by the statistician. Of course, as a precaution, you probably should show your work to the statistician before putting your results into practice.

A number of the concepts and procedures introduced in this chapter also use terms and ideas that were presented in some detail in Chapters 13 and 14 (Part IV), as well as with the information about experimental designs in Part III. You may wish to review those chapters before reading this one.

In this chapter, we emphasize the Neyman-Pearson ideas of statistical hypothesis testing (2, 3, 4). The first step is to specify the smallest difference between treatments (delta) that you wish your study to detect, on the average.[1] You will also need to specify the usual alpha risk. In addition, you must specify another probability value, the beta risk, so that you can control your risk of *not* finding significance when a treatment difference as large as that specified really does exist in the population. Finally, you will need as good an estimate as possible of the standard deviation that you expect the data to show. Unless you have data from previous studies done under the same conditions as your projected trial, the most practical way to obtain that estimate is from a well-run pilot trail. Once you have specified alpha, beta, and delta and obtained an estimate of sigma, for the simpler designs, you will then be able to obtain your sample size estimates by merely using one of the tables in the Appendix to this book. Approximation formulas are also given for some cases so that you can use them instead of the tables if you wish.

Although we have not described the use of the analysis of variance (ANOVA) for the data analysis of one-factor trials with more than two levels, nor for multifactor studies, we do include information about the estimation of sample size for the former, as you will frequently need to design such studies. We do not describe the sample size estimation for the multifactor designs, which require multifactor analyses of variance for their analysis, except for randomized blocks designs. Your statistician will be familiar with

---

[1]Once in a while, you may be interested in contrasts other than the simple comparison of one or more pairs of treatment means, such as combinations of two or more means vs. another mean or similar combination. However, the procedures you would use in such cases are very similar. We speak of comparing means here because that is by far the most common use of hypothesis tests in clinical trial work.

the appropriate procedures in these cases, however. If you are interested, you can obtain information about some methods useful for sample size estimation in these cases through a special application of the Bratcher et al. tables described later (5), from Dallal [66], from Borenstein and Cohen's program [67], from [Cohen [27], or from Wheeler (6).

15.1.3 Multiplicity

A method for allowing for the multiplicity brought about by the use of multiple comparisons was shown earlier. This consisted of increasing the sample size estimate during planning, then, during the analysis of the data, compensating for the multiplicity by the use of the Bonferroni procedure. Other types of multiplicity, such as the use of interim tests, multiple responses, and the like, can also be allowed for beforehand by the use of Bonferroni during planning. Further discussion of these ideas needed to be postponed until after the chapters on design and analysis.

15.1.4 Literature

The literature of statistics teems with references to sample size estimation, so much so that it would be almost impossible to present an exhaustive list of citations. But most of the *applications* literature confines itself to estimating sample size for rather simple designs, and much of the rest is not suitable for a book at the introductory level. However, an important exception is the excellent treatment by Bratcher et al. (5). Their procedure is intended for the estimation of sample size for one-way studies having more than two treatments, but is is also extendable, as an approximation, to certain two-way designs (randomized blocks). A portion of these tables is reprinted in the Appendix, with permission. Another notable exception is Jacob Cohen's [27] book.

Although Cohen's book has been issued in two editions, the first in 1969 and the second in 1988, it is not well known in the pharmaceutical industry, possibly because of its title. It is certainly as useful in medicine as in the behavioral sciences. To my knowledge, there is one other professional book stressing applications that is in print (Kraemer and Thiemann [28]), but it does not cover as broad a field as Cohen. There has been at least one further volume (Mace), but it is now out of print. On the other hand, the periodical literature is copious, as the sample in the References section for this chapter may suggest.

There is a companion to Cohen's book, a computer program suitable for the IBM PC, PC/XT, PC/AT, PS/2, (TM) and compatibles, including the 80286, 80386, and 80486 and Pentium (TM) series. This is Borenstein and Cohen [67]. However, it will be helpful for you to become familiar with Cohen's book before using the program. The book will require a bit of study, but the material you are now reading, together with the preceding two chapters on data analysis (Part IV), should provide adequate preparation. If you are able to find time to study this material and Cohen's concept of *effect size*, you should have no trouble using the program for the designs analyzed in the preceding two chapters. The program and Cohen's book goes further than we do here, covering multifactor designs, multiple regression and correlation as well as the one-way analyses described here. Of course, for many of your designs, your can use the equations in this chapter and/or the tables in the Appendix.

We have abstained from frequent references to software, but the foregoing as well as one more program must be mentioned because, although there are some others available, this and the Borenstein/Cohen package appear exceptional in their approach, breadth, and ease of use. This second program is called DESIGN, was written by Gerard E. Dallal, and is available as a supplementary module to the SYSTAT package listed in the Bibliography [66]. It is written at a somewhat more advanced level than the Borenstein-Cohen program, but it is useful and well-done.

These two small-computer software packages for calculating sample size and power have been available for some time. However, by the time this book appears, there may be others to choose from.

15.1.5   Limitations of the Coverage in This Chapter

In this chapter, sample size and power are treated as thoroughly as I feel to be necessary for our purposes, and for a majority of your applications. Most of the elementary introductory material was adequately covered in Chapter 5. An appreciation of experimental design and analysis is a necessary prerequisite for the effective use of sample size estimation, and design and analysis have been covered as fully as needed for the aims of this book in Parts III and IV (Chapters 8 through 14). Some points are repeated here for emphasis and to provide a more integrated exposition in one place. But as for many other issues in this volume, we must be concerned with no more than a limited study of the most useful procedures. You are encouraged to gain further information through the references given here, to others they may lead to, and discussions with a biostatistician.

15.1.6   A Caution

A weak point in many studies is the lack of specific planning of which and how many comparisons among treatments are to be made. Sometimes this point is not mentioned at all in the protocol, and when it is, it is often decided upon without consideration of the multiplicity introduced by multiple testing. To estimate sample size for your studies, regardless of who performs the actual estimates, you must lay out, *ahead of time*, which and how many comparisons are to be made, which of your responses are most important if there are more than one, and your specifications of alpha, beta, and delta. These things can only be decided adequately by you, as the person responsible or sharing responsibility for the study. An important point to remember is that, except for sequential studies (which you will rarely, if ever, need), you cannot legitimately adjust your sample sizes during a trial; they must be decided a priori.

15.2 SPECIFYING RISKS AND DELTA

15.2.1 The Null and Alternate Hypotheses

When you plan a significance test, you imply the formulation of null and alternate hypotheses to clarify your objective. We will not do that here for every example, but you will find it a useful exercise. The following is an example for a **two-tailed test**:

$$H_0: \mu_1 - \mu_2 = 0 \tag{15.1}$$

$$H_1: |\mu_1 - \mu_2| = \delta \tag{15.2}$$

In the test of the null hypothesis of Equation (15.1), the investigator wishes to "test for significance" to determine whether to reject that hypothesis. The procedure is the following:

1. Assume that you are planning a parallel trial to compare two drugs. Two groups of patients are selected randomly, and one of the drugs is assigned to all the patients in each group. During the planning, you *specify* values of **delta, alpha, and beta**, and *obtain an estimate* of **sigma**, the last preferably by running a pilot trial. These four quantities have been been explained previously but are briefly reviewed here for your convenience. All four are needed if you are to use the most appropriate hypothesis test available, and they are necessary for the preparation of sample size estimates.

2. **Delta** is the minimum population difference that you wish to be detectable when you use a hypothesis test to compare the data from the two samples. You consider this difference to represent the smallest difference of interest clinically.

3. **Alpha** is the probability of being wrong if the test leads you to claim significance (e.g., if you state that two treatment group averages are different by an amount delta, favoring one or the other treatment).

4. **Beta** is the probability of being wrong if the test leads you to claim that no difference of delta or greater exists between the two group means.

5. **Sigma** is the estimate of the experimental error or variation of each measurement, on the average.

6. After the trial has been run, the statistician tests H_0, the null hypothesis, using a **hypothesis test (significance test)** such as a t test or other suitable technique.

7. The statistician either accepts or rejects the null hypothesis, Equation (15.1), depending upon the outcome of the test.

8. Suppose the test results in the *acceptance* of the null hypothesis. In that case, the alternate hypothesis, Equation (15.2), is *rejected*. One or the other must be true, but not both. Because the null hypothesis has been accepted, the investigator concludes that a difference as great as delta does *not* exist between the two treatment population means. But there is a probability of beta that the alternate hypothesis is really true, and, thus, that the investigators' decision was incorrect.

9. If, instead, the null hypothesis is *rejected*, then the alternate hypothesis must be *accepted*. The investigator then concludes that a difference of delta, *in one or the other direction*, does exist. In this case, there is a probability of alpha that this conclusion is wrong.

A **one-tailed test** is one in which the investigator wishes to obtain significance if the mean of the population treated with, say, treatment 1 (μ_1), is delta units *less* than that for the other population, but cannot imagine that the opposite configuration could exist, or is not interested in it. The hypotheses for such a test are written as follows:

$$H_0: \mu_1 - \mu_2 = 0 \tag{15.1}$$

$$H_1: \mu_2 - \mu_1 = \delta \tag{15.3}$$

As you can see, the alternate hypothesis now refers to a difference in one direction only, because the absolute symbols are now absent from the alternate hypothesis, Equation (15.3) (note also that the null hypothesis is unchanged). The absence of the "absolute" symbols of Equation (15.2) is equivalent to stating that it is concerned only with the case in which μ_2 is *larger* than μ_1. If interest lay in the opposite situation, in which the magnitudes of the two values of mu were reversed, the opposite alternate hypothesis could be used instead, with μ_1 being the larger of the two means.

The **power** of the t test or other hypothesis test is one minus the value of beta, or $1 - \beta$. Thus, if you chose to specify beta as 0.10, the power would be 0.90. This means that if there really is a difference of delta between the two population means, you will find significance in 90 out of 100 such trials.

15.2.2   The Alpha and Beta Risks

Definition

Let us clarify the concepts of alpha and beta a bit more. As just pointed out, alpha and beta are probabilities specified a priori by the designer of a trial. They refer mainly to the samples you are testing, not to the populations.

Alpha is the probability that the difference between the observed means being tested could be as large as they are seen to be if there were really no population difference. Beta is the probability that there really is no difference of concern to you between the two populations, although you have concluded, based upon sample data, that such a difference exists. *The smaller the value of alpha, the more unlikely it is that you will falsely reject the null hypothesis.* This probability is almost always set to a low value. *The smaller the value of beta, the smaller the probability that you will incorrectly conclude that there is no difference between the two treatments by falsely accepting the null hypothesis.*

Using Alpha without Specifying Beta and Delta

If you or your statistician plan to use significance tests when your trial is completed, you *must* specify a value for alpha *before the data are available for inspection.* You may specify alpha but omit specifications for beta and delta if you wish, but this is not recommended; we have called this the "simplistic procedure" (see Chapter 13, Section 13.2.6). If you do specify alpha only, omitting beta and delta (e.g., to compare two treatment groups), your study will have the following disadvantages:

1. You will be unable to estimate the sample size needed. That is, except by a lucky chance, you will *not* be able to arrange for significance to be obtained *only* when a clinically significant difference between the treatments (population means) is detected. The magnitude of any detectable difference will depend upon the sample size that you happen to use. Your test may not be powerful enough to detect a difference as small as you wish, and you may be forced to conclude that no difference has been shown. Or, if the sample size is too large, you may conclude that there is an important difference when the population difference is really too small to be of interest or clinical importance.

2. If you do not obtain significance when the data are analyzed, you will be unable to *accept* the null hypothesis. It will be possible to state only that *the null hypothesis cannot be rejected*—quite a different conclusion. You will know only that significance has not been shown. You will not be even reasonably sure that there is *no* difference of a specified size. You will not know whether you would have found significance if the sample size had been larger.

3. You will not know the magnitude of the treatment difference (delta) that the test will detect until the test is over and the analysis has been done (so that the estimated standard deviation has been calculated). Even then it will not be possible to calculate delta except by specifying beta after the event (assuming that you correctly specified alpha when the test was planned). If you then find that the sample size used was too small to detect a delta value of the size you wished, you will need to repeat the trial.

When the simplistic procedure was discussed in Chapter 13, it was illustrated with Equations (13.1) and (13.2), the appropriate null and alternate hypotheses, respectively, for that procedure. If you now refer to them, you will see that they are different, and simpler in a way, than Equations (15.1), (15.2), and (15.3), which were just shown. However, it is an unnecessary gamble to use the simplistic procedure. It is almost always possible to greatly increase the probability of a successful trial by estimating your sample size using a value of sigma based upon the principal response and the values of alpha, beta, and delta that you wish to use. The potential loss of time and money with the use of the simplistic procedure nearly always justifies avoiding it.

There is one kind of situation, however, in which the simplistic procedure is frequently used, and for which we recommend it. When you must test for nonnormality or heteroscedasticity, or run other tests that are not comparisons of response means or other treatment contrasts of interest, you will often be forced to use the simplistic procedure. To obtain significance tests of the best obtainable power and to take delta and sigma into account with respect to a selected and important response, your must carry out your sample size calculations with that response in mind. You cannot reasonably plan your trial with sample sizes arranged, for example, according to the desired power of a normality or variance test. If you were to do otherwise, the resulting sample size would be unlikely to be appropriate for your major purpose. Similar considerations apply to the testing of adverse effects.

15.2.3 Specifying Beta and Delta (Neyman-Pearson Procedure)

The recommended procedure (Neyman-Pearson), which includes the specification of both beta and alpha risks, as well as a value for delta, should be used in all but the most casual clinical trials. Although this method will not guarantee success, it will greatly increase your proportion of effective trials, because, to use it, you must estimate and use the appropriate sample size. Further, you will then gain complete control of the power of your tests. You will be able to arrange things to obtain *any* degree of assurance (short of 100%) of detecting *any* magnitude of treatment difference or other effect that you desire. If you do not specify beta and delta, these things are impossible. Of course, there is a catch—two, in fact. The first is not a major drawback. When you plan tests based upon continuous distributions such as the normal, you need estimates of sigma that are as reliable as possible. Frequently, you may have previous data obtained with the same kind of responses that can be used for these estimates. If not, you should use a pilot trial (see what follows).

15.2.4 Sample Size When Specifying Alpha, Beta, and Delta

The second catch is related to the magnitude of the sample size you are willing or able to use. If everything goes well, after you specify selected values of alpha, beta, and delta, you will obtain a sample size estimate that is not excessively large or difficult to achieve. But you may find it to be much larger, or smaller, than is desirable, affordable, or even possible. If it is smaller than you expected, first check your work. If that is satisfactory, you may still feel that the calculated value is too small to be a good representative sample of the patient population. If so, you may have no choice but to increase it.

If the sample size is much larger than provided for in the budget or in the time allowed, again be sure that you check the calculations. A mistake can be expensive. Even a computer procedure should be rechecked. The program used may or may not be bug-free, but remember that many errors are made in manually entering data. If you find the calculations to be correct, you need to rethink your specifications. Is the delta value that you specified smaller than you really need? Did you select a smaller delta then necessary "just to be sure"? If so, you have unnecessarily increased the sample size. Everything else being equal, the smaller delta becomes, the greater the sample size you must use. If you decide that you can safely increase delta, do so and then recalculate the sample size. If the sample size is still too great and you feel that you cannot increase delta further, the next step is to think about the value of sigma. The smaller sigma is, the smaller the sample size can be. Therefore, you should be sure that you have specified the most precise experimental procedure, response, and statistical analysis possible, as each of these factors can affect the value of sigma, and therefore of the sample size. Note, however, that the response you use in the pilot trial, if it is the principal response, should be the least precise among those planned, so that if there is a clinically important difference, it will be detectable at a power you specify.

The next step in trying to reduce the sample size is to examine the alpha and beta probabilities. Increasing the value of either alpha or beta will reduce the sample size estimate. The probability is high, however, that you will be unable to do very much with alpha. The greatest probability that you should generally use for this is 0.050, if for no other reason than that it is unlikely that the FDA will find a larger value acceptable. In fact, in your own and your organization's interests as well, especially if your trial will be long and/or costly, you may wish to decrease alpha to 0.025, 0.010, or even a smaller probability, thus improving your chance of being right if and when you find it possible to claim significance. Here, you must balance the likelihood of finding a clinically important difference (the power; see the next paragraph), with its associated eventual advantages in the form of patient benefits and a successful product, against the costs, both ethical and economic, of increasing the sample size. Of course, you must also try to avoid being in error by concluding that there is a difference when there really is not, thus causing you to continue with an expensive loser. There is little further advice that we can offer regarding the level of alpha.

You may wish to consider increasing the value of beta. Think of the additive inverse of beta, $1 - \beta$, which is the power that you have specified for the eventual hypothesis test. The power is the probability of *detecting* a treatment difference or effect equal to the magnitude that you have specified as delta, if such an effect exists (beta is the probability of *not* detecting such an effect). Increasing the value of beta, while holding alpha and delta constant, will allow use of a smaller sample size (of course, at the cost of decreasing your chances of finding an important treatment effect). If you do increase the value of beta, you should perhaps only rarely go beyond 0.200. A common and often reasonable value is 0.100 or less.

As you can see, the magnitudes of five quantities are interdependent: alpha, beta, delta, the sample size, and sigma. *Increasing* alpha, beta, *or* delta (and remembering that sigma is an inherent property of the type of response and general precision of the trial), while holding the other two constant, will *decrease* the required sample size. Sigma can be reduced only if or when more precise experimental procedures or conditions, or a more precise response measurement, can be found. If you can find a way to reduce sigma, the sample size will be smaller, assuming that alpha, beta, and delta remain the same. For more discussion of the estimation of sigma, see Section 15.4, which follows.

If you have specified values of alpha and beta and do not wish to change them further, your only remaining resource for reducing the sample size beyond reducing sigma by changing your experiment conditions is to increase delta. You may not wish to do so, but at this point you will have no further choice beyond abandoning the project.

15.3   MULTIPLICITY

If there will be multiplicity in a study that you are planning, this must be taken into account when estimating the sample size. Suppose that you wish to run a trial using two treatments, and that you will have two different responses, but wish to use an overall alpha value of 0.050. To compensate for the multiplicity brought about by making two comparisons (testing more than one response using the same patients in the same trial), you decide to use the Bonferroni inequality described earlier. As a reminder, this is done as follows: You make two *t* tests, one using each response, but, although you will claim a difference at the 0.050 level if significance is found, you do each test at the 0.025 level (i.e., 0.050 divided by the number of comparisons to be made).[2]

---

[2]When using Bonferroni in this manner, you will frequently find that you must interpolate in the *t* table to find the appropriate standard value of *t*. Linear interpolation is an adequate approximation for this purpose. If you use Table A.1 in the Appendix, you will find that *t* is given for 0.02 and for 0.05, but not for any values between these two. Therefore, in this example, you would need to interpolate between 0.050 and 0.020 to obtain the value of *t* for 0.025. In this case, 0.025 lies one-sixth of the distance from 0.020 and 0.050. To get *t* for 0.025, therefore, you would add one-sixth of the difference between *t* for 0.050 and *t* for 0.020 to the value of *t* for 0.020. That is, $t_{0.025} = 2.764 - (2.764 - 2.228)/6 = 2.675$.

If you plan to use 0.025 in the test, you should also use it for alpha when estimating the sample size. The reasoning is the following: If you do two *t* tests at the 0.050 level using the same groups of patients, the *true* overall alpha risk is really *greater* than 0.050, because it is 0.050 for *each* of the two tests. You would then wrongly reject the null hypothesis *not* five times out of every 100 such trials, but at a higher frequency. To compensate for this, you can do each test at a new level of alpha that will be *roughly* equivalent to the use of 0.050 for one *t* test (the Bonferroni procedure is conservative). But when you use a smaller alpha value in this way, the power of the test will be lower than you intended unless you compensate during planning by recalculating to obtain a larger value of *n*. That is, reducing alpha without changing any other variable can increase beta and reduce the power. You can obtain the appropriate value of *n*, the sample size estimate, by using the Bonferroni-derived value (0.025 in this case) instead of 0.050 for alpha. This sample size will preserve the levels of beta and delta that you specified.

The same reasoning—and remedies—can be applied when sources of multiplicity other than multiple responses are present, such as the repetition of hypothesis testing because of interim testing or multiple comparisons among more than one pair of treatments.

15.4 ESTIMATING SIGMA FROM A PILOT TRIAL

This subject needs further discussion. If you have data at hand that has been obtained fairly recently, under conditions very similar to those that you expect for the present trial, you can use them to obtain an estimated value of sigma. However, a pilot trial is almost always preferable, for a number of reasons. Some of these reasons are that you will be doing the pilot trial with a specific major study in mind, and it will (or should) resemble that study closely; it will (or should) use the same or some of the same facilities and investigators; patients will (or should) come from the same source as the study you are planning; and the pilot will be done shortly before the study begins so that the experimental conditions should be similar. The experimental design (structure) need not be identical to the trial you are planning, if the same response is used under similar conditions.

The value of sigma needed will usually be the standard deviation of individual items from their mean (see Chapter 14). If the data are part of a multifactor experiment, the standard deviation must be that corresponding to the error of single cells in the design, so that it will be free of the influence of any of the controlled factors. The biostatistician will be able to calculate this by obtaining the error mean square from an analysis of variance (ANOVA) of the pilot trial data for the principal response. The error mean square is the square of the needed standard deviation. This will not work with fractional designs such as latin squares or other types of incomplete designs, however.

Once you make your choice and run the pilot study, you will be more or less committed. If you were then to schedule another measurement method, less precise than the principal response, your sample size, based upon the original principal response, would be too small for the new one, not to mention the additional multiplicity introduced by adding another response.

15.4.1 Choosing the Principal Response

It is usually easy to judge which of several measurements to select as a principal response. Of course, the one you choose should be the one you believe to be the most important. Keeping that in mind, there are several other things to consider: (a) Binomial or short-scale multinomial measurements, analyzed by the appropriate statistical methods, are not very powerful, often requiring many more patients than responses that are normally or near normally distributed, or at least have a continuous distribution. (b) Most judgment scales, although they are usually longer and therefore more powerful than the foregoing, are often used as integer scales and therefore yield less information per measurement than continuous scales, such as measurements of blood pressure to the nearest 2 millimeters or so. (c) It is likely, among judgment scales, that the one having the least possible points will be the least precise. Therefore, if your projected most important responses include some such scales, you should make one of them the principal response to ensure that the sample size obtained will be large enough.

Taking these considerations and the multiplicity introduced by the use of more than one response into account, you can see that you should select as few and as precise responses as possible if it is important to minimize your sample size (as it almost always is). Measuring everything in sight may sound like a method of exercising appropriate precautions, and, regrettably, many trials use numbers of responses without compensating by increasing the sample size appropriately. And if you do attempt to compensate for the multiplicity in such a trial, you will often find that the sample size needed will be impractically large. The moral is that using more responses than are absolutely required "just to make sure" ensures only trouble.

Your pilot study need not possess the same degree of complexity of design as your trial. The important features are as follows: (a) You need not use more than one kind of response measurement, the one you plan to use as the principal response in the main trial. (b) If possible, the pilot should be run by the same investigator or investigators who will run the trial itself. (c) The size of the pilot should be reasonable, although you need not plan for significance tests, of course. The larger the pilot, the more precisely you will be able to estimate sigma.

A pilot trial can sometimes be run using a single treatment, and sometimes none at all, if you can be sure that assigning a treatment or treatments to the sample(s) of patients will not change the variances of the response data. However, the safest procedure is to use the treatments planned for your main study in order to obtain responses at the same or nearly the same level as you expect later. As to the size of the pilot trial, numbers like four to eight patients or subjects are not enough to give even reasonably reliable estimates of sigma. Such small numbers are also less likely to represent the gamut of potential patient characteristics in the population. Remember that in a pilot trial, you will be interested in the precision with which you can estimate sigma; it is not one for which you need a significance test. The aim is to get an adequately precise estimate of sigma using a *representative* sample of the target population. Although the procedure is not covered in this book, it is a simple matter to calculate a confidence interval about sigma (see Snedecor and Cochran [38], Dixon and Massey [33], or other texts).

In the planning of industrial trials, even when adequate estimates of sigma are not available, pilot trials are not infrequently omitted, because time is usually short. But this is a shortsighted policy, exchanging a much improved probability of success in a trial for the exigencies of the moment. A brief contemplation of the cost and consequences of a failed trial, which is common enough with the greatest care, should carry adequate conviction. We therefore strongly urge that you run a pilot trial whenever no other reasonably precise estimate of sigma is available.

15.5 ESTIMATING SAMPLE SIZE FOR *t* TESTS

15.5.1 Introduction

In this section, we will consider two kinds of *t* test—the **independent** and the **dependent**. An independent *t* test is one that uses two independent patient groups. Each patient in a given group receives one of the two treatments. In other words, the design for an independent *t* test is a parallel arrangement. A dependent *t* test is one that uses a single group of patients, with each patient receiving both treatments in random order. The design is thus a randomized-blocks arrangement, with patients as the blocks, and with each block consisting of two plots (for a review of this kind of design, see Chapters 12, 13, and 14).

In Chapter 5, the only sample size estimation procedure demonstrated was a brief example using an independent *t* test, referencing tables of sample sizes in the Appendix (Tables A.3a through A.3d). In this section, we examine a more thorough example for use with an independent *t* test, and a second for the dependent or "one-sample" test. There are two sets of tables in the Appendix that are easy to use in obtaining the estimated sample sizes for these tests. They are derived, with some condensation and rearrangement, from Davies [14]. They are approximate to a slight degree, but are at least as accurate as necessary, because the estimate of sigma itself, upon which they are based, will always have uncertainty about it. Beyond that, unless sigma is known exactly, a really accurate estimate requires an iterative solution. Such a procedure is described by Neyman et al. (2, 3), and discussed later by Owen (7). The method described here, using both alpha and beta risks, was firstdescribed by Neyman and Pearson (4) and is the modern basis of hypothesis testing. The tables in the Appendix, as well as the equations that follow, will agree fairly closely with published exact values; see Neyman et al. (2, 3, 4), Owen (7), and Hodges and Lehman (8), as well as with other published approximations; for instance, see Croarkin (9), Dupont and Plummer (10), Wheeler (6), Bowman and Kastenbaum (11), Wheeler (12), Feigl (13), Fleiss et al. (14), and Ury and Fleiss (15).[3]

Approximate sample sizes can also be obtained by the use of equations. These serve the same purposes as the tables, and are about equally precise. They appear in much of the literature, including Dixon and Massey [33], Fleiss [8], and Snedecor and Cochran [38]. We give them here because some of you will find them more convenient than the tables, and they are more instructive. Like the latter, there is one equation for the independent and one for the dependent case. Both are simple to use. If you are interested in exact calculations, see the foregoing papers. The approximate equations that follow give results very close to those in the Appendix tables, and in many cases they are identical.

Certain sample size equations have been shown by Kupper and Hafner (16) to give estimates of n that are too low. The two given here, however, are satisfactory.

15.5.2   Example 15.1: Sample Size for an Independent t Test

In this example, the "data" were obtained from a computer-generated pair of samples taken from two normal distributions having two different known values of the mean but the same sigma. We will estimate the sample size for the trial, using *specified* values of alpha, beta, and delta, and the "estimate" of sigma for that distribution. We will assume that the two normal distributions comprise diastolic blood pressures of populations of patients given the two treatments to be compared. Hereafter, we assume that the data are real data and describe the example accordingly.

A sample of patients is drawn from a population of patients with mild hypertension. Half of them are treated with the test drug, while the other half receives a currently marketed drug. The size of the two groups will be estimated as described in what follows to conform to our specifications of alpha, beta, and delta. We then compare the two samples using a t test. Later examples in this chapter, with one exception, will not be as elaborate as this one. In this example, we are more thorough in order to display the

---

[3]There are so many papers on the topic of sample size that it is not practical to list them all; the references cited here and listed at the end of this chapter are a selected sample of the periodical literature; the Bibliography references a number of recommended textbooks and professional books.

process of carrying through an actual study, using the estimated sample size. Of course, we will have an advantage not usual in actual trials because we will know the parameters of the two patient populations exactly, will not need a pilot trial, and will thus be able to see how closely these typical samples might come to the population values.

Specifying Risks and Delta

A sponsor wishes to run an early phase trial of a new mild antihypertensive agent, D_1, against a current treatment, D_2. The population to be sampled will consist of patients classified as mild primary hypertensives. A pilot trial was not thought necessary, in view of the common belief that 7 mm is the approximate standard deviation to be expected for both systolic and diastolic measurements for most patients.[4] In this example, although both systolic and diastolic pressures will be assumed to be recorded (to the nearest millimeter, if possible), we will illustrate the use of diastolic values only. The *t* test will be two-tailed. The null and alternate hypotheses will be those given by Equations (15.1) and (15.2), shown in Section 15.2.1. Note that the alternate hypothesis is two-tailed.

The following specifications were set up:

$$\text{alpha } (\alpha) = 0.05$$
$$\text{beta } (\beta) = 0.10$$
$$\text{delta } (\delta) = 7 \text{ mm}$$

Sample Size Using the Table

Based upon the foregoing values of sigma and delta, delta/sigma (δ/σ) becomes 1.00.

Using Table A.3c in the Appendix (for comparison of the means of two independent groups with a *t* test, with alpha = 0.05), for beta = 0.10, we find, in the row labeled delta/sigma = 1, a sample size of 23 patients per treatment.

Sample Size Using the Equation

To obtain the sample size for a trial corresponding to this example, you may choose to use the table as just described, or an equation. Equation (15.4), which follows, as well as that for the dependent case, Equation (15.7), appears in several of the books cited in the Bibliography, including Snedecor and Cochran [38], Colton [20], and Dixon and Massey [33]. However, we have modified both equations slightly by the addition of a term (*c*; see what follows), based upon Cochran's procedure as described in Snedecor and

---

[4]We are currently investigating this belief. I have been unable to find a reference that suggests its origin. It is possible that the distributions of blood-pressure data are not normal, and that the standard deviation for systolic and diastolic pressure data differ. Of course, in this example, we *know* the population values of both sigma and the means, and the distributions are normal.

Cochran [38], and mentioned earlier. The examples to be shown for both this and the dependent t test are cases in which sigma is known because the data have been computer-generated. However, we are assuming that it is unknown, as is the usual situation in planning a trial. Equation (15.4) estimates the sample size *per group* for tests of two independent groups, then, as follows:

$$n = \frac{2(Z_\alpha - Z_\beta)^2 S_{y_i}^2}{\delta^2} + c \qquad (15.4)$$

In this example, alpha, beta, and delta have the values given before. The term $S_{y_i}^2$ is the variance of individual items, the square of the value of sigma mentioned before. The values of Z_α and Z_β can be obtained from the abbreviated table of Z, Table A.5, in the Appendix, or from any published normal area table. In this example, the first of these is the value of the abscissa (Z) of the standardized normal distribution corresponding to the alpha value (i.e., the sum of two tail areas) selected before, two tailed in this example, and having units that are the numbers of standard deviations above or below the mean of the distribution. The second, Z_β, is *always a one-tailed* value of Z. Unless beta is 0.500 (not 0.050) or larger, this value must be made negative to represent the *lower* tail value. In Table A.5, the one-tailed values of Z are shown as positive, because they are labeled upper-tail values. The lower-tail values of Z are always negative if beta is less than 0.500.

The value of c, the second term in Equation 15.4, is based upon the suggestion in Snedecor and Cochran [38] mentioned earlier. If alpha is 0.050, c has a value of 1. If alpha is 0.010, 2 is used for c. Although c values for smaller alpha probabilities are not mentioned, we use 3 for c if alpha is 0.001. This has given satisfactory results here, perhaps a bit conservative, in cases in which that value of alpha is needed.

By using Equation (15.4), the sample size was calculated as follows:

$$n = \frac{2(Z_\alpha - Z_\beta)^2 S_{y_i}^2}{\delta^2} + c \qquad (15.4)$$

$$= \frac{2(1.96 + 1.281)^2 (7)^2}{(7)^2} + 1$$

$$= 22.01$$

$$\approx 23$$

We follow the conservative custom of using the next greater value of n if the equation yields a number with *any* decimal part. This is the reason that the value of 22.01 was changed to 23 patients per treatment for the final result. You will note that this agrees with the value obtained from the table. In using this equation, note that because Z_β in the numerator is negative but is preceded by a $(-)$ sign in the equation, its contribution becomes positive.

The Trial and Results

The two normal distributions that were generated and sampled had the following parameters:

	Group 1 (to receive D_1)	Group 2 (to receive D_2)
Mean	97	90
Sigma	7	7

A sample of 23 was drawn from each of these two populations. The samples did not and could not be expected to reflect the foregoing values exactly, because of sampling variation. The sample data are shown in Table 15.1, labeled Treatment 1 and Treatment 2, and simulate the two treatment groups.

Table 15.1. Data for Example 15.1

Treatment 1 (D_1)	Treatment 2 (D_2)
87	90
97	85
98	87
89	91
100	91
98	84
93	84
92	93
103	101
92	87
94	76
91	86
98	88
94	90
95	111
98	85
96	101
93	88
91	87
107	86
102	87
102	84
92	97

Table 15.2. Results of Analysis of Data (Example 15.1)

Statistic	T_1	T_2	Difference
$\bar{y}$ (mean)	95.7	89.5	6.2
S_{y_i} (standard deviation)	4.901	7.286	
$S_{y_i}^2$ (variance)	24.02	53.09	
n (sample size)	23	23	
t (calculated t) value		3.396	
df (degrees of freedom)		44	

A t test for independent groups was performed on the data of Table 15.1. The means of the two groups, their standard deviations, variances, and other relevant statistics are shown in Table 15.2. The population variances could not be shown to be significantly different, although the observed difference was moderately large, and of course there was no nonnormality for either group.

As Table 15.2 shows, the t value found was 3.396, and that required to reject the null hypothesis (see Appendix table under the 0.05 column and 44 df) was less than 2.021. The null hypothesis of equal means was accordingly rejected and the alternate hypothesis accepted and it was concluded that the difference between the two group means *in the populations* was compatible with the postulated delta value of 7. This conclusion could perhaps be illustrated more concretely by calculating confidence limits about the observed difference of 6.2, which would be found to include 7.

Note the results shown in Table 15.2. You will recall that the standard deviation in the population was 7, and the difference between the means was also 7. The sample standard deviations were 4.9 and 7.3, with a pooled value of 6.2. It happened that the difference between the sample means was also 6.2. This represents reasonable agreement with the population values for small samples.

15.5.3 t Test of Differences (Dependent t Test)

Introduction
The estimation of the sample size needed for testing whether the mean of a population of differences is equal to zero is given in the following example. This test is a version of the so-called **one-sample** or **dependent** t test. If you have occasion to use this kind of t test for a different purpose, such as the comparison of a mean of a single set of data with a standard or known value other than zero, the same sample size table and equation will nevertheless apply. However, the difference test is by far the most common application.

This kind of t test is appropriate when the data come from a changeover study in which each patient receives two treatments in random order (see Chapter 12). You will recognize that pattern as a particular variety of the

randomized blocks design, in which the patients form the blocks.[5] If the population of differences forms a normal or nearly normal distribution, a *t* **test of differences** is appropriate. This is done using the set of individual differences between the two response values provided by each block (patient). In such a test, the null hypothesis states that the mean of the group of differences is zero; see Equations (15.5) and (15.6) which follow.

Another very common method of analysis is a two-way ANOVA for randomized blocks, which will give the same results. ANOVA calculations are not described in this book, but if you are interested, the ANOVA for randomized blocks is described in Box et. al. [32], Chapter 7; Fleiss [8], pages 125–129; Neter et al. [37], Chapters 27 and 28; and Snedecor and Cochran [38], Chapter 14. Note that it is not correct to analyze the two sets of responses obtained from each patient as if they were independent, that is, the independent *t* test and an ANOVA for two treatments are not the correct kinds of analysis for this design. The reason is that the design is not a one-way design; it possesses two factors, both of which must be accounted for (treatments and patients).

As you do when designing a trial to be analyzed using the independent *t* test, you should prespecify values for alpha, beta, and delta, and obtain an estimate of sigma. The null and alternate hypotheses for the *t* test now refer to the mean of the distribution of *this single set of individual differences* obtained from the pairs of observations for each patient. The null hypothesis is that the mean of the population of such differences is zero. The alternate hypothesis might state that this mean has a value *greater or less than* zero, or it might state that it is equal to some specified value. The latter reflects the situation that obtains if we specify both alpha and beta, along with a value of delta (minimum mean difference of interest). In this case, if the test were two-tailed, the hypotheses would be written as shown by Equations (15.5) and (15.6) that follow. The vertical bars in Equation (15.6) signify that absolute values are to be taken, so that the hypothesis is two-tailed, that is, if the mean of the differences is not zero, but delta, they show that its sign is immaterial.

$$H_0: \mu = 0 \qquad\qquad (15.5)$$

$$H_1: |\mu| = \delta \qquad\qquad (15.6)$$

In a one-tailed test, a mean of the population of differences would be considered of interest only if it existed in a specified direction.

Tables A.4a through A.4d in the Appendix give sample sizes for the two-tailed dependent *t* test. They are used in the same way as described for the independent *t* test tables, Tables A.3a through A.3d. An approximation equation that gives values that are very nearly exact can also be used. The

---

[5]This design is frequently called a *repeated measures* design among workers in the behavioral sciences, but that term is rarely used elsewhere.

remarks given in Section 15.5.1 and in Section 15.5.2 under the heading "Sample Size Using Equation" apply here as well. The equation for this case, Equation (15.7), follows:

$$n = \frac{(Z_\alpha - Z_\beta)^2 S_{D_i}^2}{\delta^2} + c \tag{15.7}$$

This equation is the same as Equation (15.4) for independent groups except for the omission of the constant, 2, in the numerator, and the use of a different variety of variance, $S_{D_i}^2$. In the equation, n represents the number of *differences*, that is, the number of patients, because we are considering a paired design. The values of Z are obtained as before, from any table of normal areas or from the condensed table in the Appendix. Alpha, beta, and delta are specified during planning according to the monitor's or sponsor's preference and needs. The variance should be obtained from a pilot study or other data, and converted by calculation to the variance of an individual difference, as shown in what follows.

In this equation, c becomes 2 if alpha is 0.050 and 3 if it is 0.010. These values are given in Snedecor and Cochran [38], as were two of those for Equation (15.4).

In Equation (15.7), you must be sure to use the appropriate variance in the numerator. In the independent groups case, because the comparison is between means of individual data, the correct variance for use in the sample size equation, Equation (15.4), was that for individual measurements—the square of the pooled standard deviation of single items. In the present case, for estimating the sample size needed to test a mean difference, Equation (15.7) also requires a variance of single items; this time, however, it is the variance of individual *differences*. Therefore, the pilot trial should be designed so that you can obtain a set of such differences, and this statistic is the one that must be estimated from them and used in getting the sample size. We identify this variance here as $S_{D_i}^2$. The first step in its calculation is illustrated in Chapter 14, Section 14.2.4, Example 14.1, which yields the variance of individual items for a single set of data, $y_1, \ldots, y_n$. See Equations (14.2), (14.5), and (14.6) in that section. In the present case, the data will be differences, but the calculations are the same.

For the t test itself, the statistic required is *not* the same; it is the standard error of the **mean difference**. This is calculated from the data (the set of differences to be tested) in the same way as that in the case of independent groups, except that no comparison of variances or pooling is needed because there is only one group. The appropriate calculations were illustrated in Chapter 14, Section 14.3.9, Example 14.4, and are represented in Equations (14.12) and (14.13) in that section. We use the symbol $S_{\bar{D}}$ for the standard error of a mean difference.

You should be careful to avoid confusion between the variances in the sample size equations and the standard deviations used as denominators in the corresponding t tests. Also, you should carefully note that although both the independent and dependent t tests are concerned with means, they are otherwise very different. The independent test is meant to compare two means estimated from samples of two independent populations of patients, each having a different treatment and each patient having been assigned to only one of the two. The error in such a test is derived from the *patient-to-patient* variation. The dependent test, when it is a difference test, uses a sample of patients, each of whom has received *both* treatments and for which the data are the set of individual *differences* between the two treatments. The appropriate denominator for the independent t test, which compares two means, is the standard error of a difference between two means, so that the error is derived from the *within-patients* variations.[6] On the other hand, the error for the difference test, which compares a single mean difference with zero, is the standard error of a mean difference. Both of these are quite distinct quantities. In addition, they must not be confused with the similar quantities used in the sample size equations, which are *variances* (squares of standard deviations) in both cases, and refer to individual measurements, in the independent case, or *individual* differences between measurements in the other. The dependent t test is illustrated in Example 15.2, which follows.

Example 15.2: Sample Size for the Dependent t Test

A skin irritation test was planned, to be performed by a dermatologist. The object of the test was to evaluate the irritation potential of a new product (T_2) for application to the skin, comparing it with a standard irritant, a mild soap solution (T_1). The test was to use a paired arrangement, placing twenty 1-centimeter-square patches upon the back of each subject. Ten of the patches were to use the soap solution, and the other ten the test product. The 20 patches were to be arranged symmetrically in four columns of five upon the back of each subject, and the identity of the treatment for each patch was to be randomized individually for each subject to eliminate any bias caused by position. This randomization was done ahead of time by the sponsor, and a schedule for removing the patches in pairs was supplied to the dermatologist, who was not to be aware of the identity of the treatment positions.

The intervals for removal of the patches were to be 4, 6, 8, 10, 12, 16, 24, 32, 40, and 48 hours, chosen on the basis of previous experience. Thus, the response was to be an elapsed time with a possible maximum of 10 integer values—in effect, a 10-point scale. Based upon previous experience, all involved were sure that the maximum period of 48 hours was great enough.

At each of these 10 intervals, two specified patches, selected upon the basis of a schedule given to the dermatologist, were to be removed. The

---

[6]An analysis of variance for randomized blocks can be used instead of the t test for differences. When this is done, both sources of variation, patient to patient and between patients, are explicitly considered.

measurement was to be the time required for the new treatment and the standard to show the first perceptible erythema relative to the surrounding skin. If any erythema was noted under either patch, the time of observation was to be recorded.

If any irritation was observed at such a point, the dermatologist was then to open a sealed envelope supplied by the sponsor, listing the patches to be permanently removed from that subject's back at that time, that is, those having the treatment that had just shown irritation. For example, if treatment T_1 was used under patches 1, 2, 3, 4, 6, 8, 12, 18, 19, and 20, and the first one of these removed on schedule, as just described, showed faint erythema, all of the other nine in that set were to be removed. No readings were to be taken on the skin areas thus revealed; the area evaluated at the time would have already been randomly specified and observed. The remaining nine patches, having the other treatment, were to be left on the subject's back until irritation was noted under one of them, at which time the time would be recorded and the remaining patches removed. Of course, this scheme would break the blinding, but it would ensure that there was no effect of position to confound the analysis. Alternative arrangements, such as locating the treatments one on each side of the back, would not have eliminated the necessity of removing half of the patches once one treatment showed irritation, and might have introduced a position bias. The final data were thus to be one of the earlier time intervals for each subject and each treatment.

It was not expected that either treatment would remain on the subjects' backs for the entire interval without irritation, but, if so, that fact was to be recorded. For the statistical analysis, differences were taken between the two responses for each subject. If, in spite of this, any subject had not shown irritation after 48 hours, that subject's data were not to be used in the efficacy analysis, although they would be included in the final report. As it happened, this did not occur.

It was believed that a t test, in view of its robustness, would be suitable for this trial. However, it was possible that the scale would not be linear; if not, it could not be normal. In addition, the restriction of the measurements to integers guaranteed nonnormality of a different kind. Therefore, instead of merely depending upon the robustness of the t test, it was planned to supplement the analysis with a Wilcoxon Signed Ranks test, and to use these results if the two tests differed substantially. Of course, the rank test alone could have been used, but the sponsor was interested in noting whether there was any substantial difference between the two procedures. The slightly greater sample size required for the Wilcoxon test was not considered important; it was expected to increase the probability of not finding significance to a small degree if the data were normal, but would be more appropriate than the t test if they were not.

The sponsor decided upon the use of a "clinically significant" delta value of 3 hours. Here, delta was the skin contact time in hours by which the treatment could be either poorer or better than the standard before significance would be shown. In other words, a two-tailed test was to be done.

Previous data had yielded a standard deviation of 4.8 hours for individual differences. If irritation did not appear for the new treatment (T_2) until after a significantly longer period than that for the standard (T_1), the sponsor would then wish to run additional efficacy trials of the new product. If the treatment gave significantly greater irritation (shorter mean time) than the standard, or if there was no significance, indicating that the difference between the new product and the soap solution was less than delta, further work with the new product was to be discontinued.[7] Both alpha and beta were set at 0.050. By using these values of sigma, alpha, beta, and delta, Equation (15.7) was used to find the sample size, with the following results:

$$n = \frac{\left(Z_\alpha - Z_\beta\right)^2 S_{D_i}^2}{\delta^2} + 2 \qquad (15.7)$$

$$= \frac{(1.96 + 1.645)^2 (4.8)^2}{3^2} + 2$$

$$= 35.27$$

$$\approx 36$$

As you see, 36 pairs of data (36 subjects) were needed. A comparison of this result with a value obtained from Table A.4c in the Appendix will show the same result. To use that table, find the subtable headed alpha (two-tailed) = 0.05, then the column for beta = 0.05. Delta over sigma is 3/4.8, or 0.625. If you therefore interpolate between the two rows for delta/sigma = 0.60 and that for 0.65, you will find a sample size of 36. Because of the need for interpolation, if you are using a pocket calculator, you may find the use of the equation equally fast.

15.5.4   Use of t Test Equations

We emphasize again that Equation (15.4) and (15.7), and Tables A.3 and A.4, give approximate results, although they should be as accurate as needed for any practical work. Another important point is to be certain of the meaning of n in each case. In Equation (15.4) and Table A.3, the sample size for an *independent* t test, n represents the number of *patients per treatment*, and if you are using equal sample sizes, this must be doubled to get the total

---

[7]You might suppose that a one-tailed test might be appropriate here, because the sponsor was not interested in further development of the new product unless it was significantly superior (longer time required to cause irritation) than the standard. Because of other considerations not relevant to the purposes of this example, however, there was also interest in whether there would be a significant failure of the test product.

number of patients, because there will always be two treatments.[8] On the other hand, in Equation (15.7) and Table A.4, the value of n represents the number of *pairs of data* when you are using a difference test. Putting it another way, to be absolutely sure that there will be no error in estimating the sample size: The value of n you find for either test, using the equations or the tables, *always* represents the number of patients needed for one treatment group.

15.6 SAMPLE SIZE FOR RANK TESTS

15.6.1 Introduction

A large variety of rank tests is described in the literature. Convenient references are Conover [39], Hollander and Wolfe [43], Siegel [45], and Wilcoxon and Wilcox [46]. The best known are two of these, which we discuss here; they are Wilcoxon's Rank Sum and Signed Ranks tests. There is voluminous literature on both of them. They were first described by Wilcoxon (17) in 1945, but the above references are perhaps the most easily available, especially the first two.[9] They were exemplified in Chapter 14, Section 14.4.

15.6.2 Sample Size for Rank Tests under Normality

To obtain the estimated sample size when you contemplate running one of Wilcoxon's rank tests, a convenient approximation that is often adequate is to use the equations or tables recommended before for use with the t test—Equations (15.3) and (15.7) or Tables A.3 or A.4. Woolson [10] indicates that the use of the sample size equations is reasonable if the underlying distribution is normal. As mentioned earlier, in that case, these two tests possess an "asymptotic relative efficiency" of about 95.5% (3/pi), compared to the t tests. Therefore, it could be recommended that the calculated sample size or that obtained from the tables be multiplied by the inverse of this factor to obtain a better sample size estimate. However, if the distribution were exactly normal, this would account for an increase of only 4.7%, or about five patients more for every hundred initially estimated. In using this procedure, it should be remembered that the equations are approximations, and also that a further, perhaps small, degree of approximation is added because the ranks do not form a continuous distribution. Because of this, it may be reasonable to suppose that, like the use of the normal approximation for the significance test, the avoidance of the use of very small sample sizes is advisable.

---

[8]This equation and table, as well as those for the dependent case, are for use in planning trials with two treatments only except under special circumstances.
[9]A test that gives results identical to Wilcoxon's Rank Sum test, called the Mann-Whitney test (18) was published 2 years after Wilcoxon's paper, in 1947.

15.6.3 Nonnormal Distributions

If the parent distribution is not normal, the appropriate sample size may be either greater or smaller than that obtained with the equations. Thus, if you find that the distribution is reasonably normal, you can use either the rank tests or the *t* test. If it is not normal, the rank tests are of course appropriate,[10] but the method of estimating sample size just suggested will no longer be suitable.

In recent years, more attention than in the past has been paid to developing more precise methods for estimating sample size for the Wilcoxon rank tests, especially when the distribution sampled is not normal, but also in the normal case. The most recent paper at the present writing appears to be one by Hamilton and Collings (19). For additional information, see also the other papers cited there. The authors describe an approximation method for estimating sample sizes for rank tests, with an example using Wilcoxon's Rank Sum test. The method is compared to two others described in the literature. Although normality is not required, the distribution is assumed to be continuous. Hence, because ranks are discrete, this is one source of approximation. This paper is one of only a few that have dealt with this topic. However, it is considerably more advanced than the level of this book, and hence is not described or exemplified here.

To conclude this topic, therefore, when the original data are known to be substantially nonnormal, there does not yet appear to be a fully satisfactory method for estimating sample size for rank tests. Our suggestion for routine work, therefore, is to assume normality if the departure is not great, and to use the *t* test tables or equations.

15.6.4 The Wilcoxon Rank Tests

Only the Wilcoxon Rank Sum test will be exemplified here, although we discuss both that and the Signed Ranks test. The Rank Sum test is intended for use with any pair of independent groups; it is the rank test analogue of the independent groups *t* test, and is subject to the same assumptions with the exception of that of normality. The Signed Ranks test is intended to be used with single groups, as for difference tests. It is the rank test analogue of the dependent (paired) *t* test. However, this test is not only free of the assumption of normality, but also of that of homogeneity of variances, because only one set of data (the differences) is used. A reference to a publication by Wilcoxon and Wilcox, although not the first edition, is given in the Bibliography [46]. As we indicated earlier, these two famous tests were first described by Frank Wilcoxon in 1945 (17), and are also discussed in

---

[10]An exception occurs when there is a known nonnormal distribution such as the binomial, for example, for which there is a specified sample size estimation procedure. Usually, in such cases, however, as for the binomial, neither the rank tests nor the *t* tests are the most appropriate ones. See Section 15.8.

Hollander and Wolfe [43] in the Bibliography, as well as in some of the general statistics tests and other references and professional books cited there.

15.6.5 Ties

In doing the rank tests, if you encounter more than about 10% ties among the data to be ranked, it is best to make a correction (see Hollander and Wolfe [43]). If there are fewer than 10% ties, a correction will do no harm but is probably not necessary. In the Signed Ranks test, in addition to correcting for ties, any differences equal to zero (when the two data for a given patient are the same in a difference test) must be dropped from the set of differences. The sample size value and degrees of freedom used are then revised accordingly.

15.6.6 Example 15.3: Sample Size for Wilcoxon Rank Sum Test

Introduction

Example 15.3 will show the comparison of two equal-sized groups of independent data with known means and equal variances, to demonstrate the Rank Sum test. We will use Equation (15.4) to estimate the sample size. The results will show that the final calculated sample size was adequate. The original data (before ranking them) were not truly normal, because they were integers. We will not show data for the Signed Ranks test, but it can be handled similarly, except for the use of the dependent sample size table or formula.

Description of Trial

The trial was early Phase II, with the object of comparing two antibiotics for use against middle ear infections. T_1 was an antibiotic commonly used for this purpose, and T_2 was a new product that had shown promise in early Phase I trials. In a manner similar to that of Example 15.1, to simulate the data, samples from two normal distributions with known parameters were drawn and then rounded to integers. The distributions had means of 17 and 11 days, and standard deviations of 4 days. Samples of equal sizes were taken from each. The samples were then compared by means of a Wilcoxon Rank Sum test.

Data Collection

The response was the number of days, to the nearest day, required for the infection to disappear, in the judgment of an otolaryngologist/investigator. In such cases, there can be some patients who do not respond to the antibiotic treatment, or who show an allergic reaction. Such patients, of course, must be dropped from the trial and receive alternate treatment(s). If the work is to be reported to the FDA, the records of these patients should be submitted nevertheless. It would thus be wise for you to try to estimate the number of dropouts and allow for them beforehand. For simplicity, however, we are assuming that there were none in this case.

The specifications were

$$\text{alpha} = 0.01$$
$$\text{beta} = 0.10$$
$$\text{delta} = 6 \text{ days}$$

When the two distributions were generated, a sigma value of 4 days was used. Because delta was specified to be 6 days, the means of the two distributions were $T_1 = 17$ days and $T_2 = 11$ days, delta days apart, and delta/sigma, for use in the sample size table, became 6/4, or 1.5.

Estimating Sample Size

By using Equation (15.4), the sample size suitable for an independent t test using the previous specifications and parameters was calculated as follows (c was equal to 2 in this case, because alpha was 0.01). The values of Z were obtained from Appendix Table A.5:

$$n = \frac{2(Z_\alpha - Z_\beta)^2 S^2}{\delta^2} + c \qquad (15.4)$$

$$= \frac{2(2.575 + 1.282)^2(4)^2}{(6)^2} + 2$$

$$= 15.2235$$

$$\approx 16$$

To use the table for independent groups instead of the equation, first find Appendix Table A.3a (for alpha = 0.01). Then find the row labeled with 1.5 for delta/sigma. Find the column headed with 0.10 for beta, and follow it down to the row labeled 1.5. You will find a value of 15 for the sample size per group. Because the equation was slightly more conservative than the table in this case, to be safe, we will use 16 patients per group.

The data, created as just described, are shown in Table 15.3.

Results of Data Analysis

Because the Rank Sum test is sensitive to heteroscedasticity, although not to nonnormality, the variances of the two groups of data were calculated and found to be 16.00 and 13.27, respectively. A comparison of these at the 0.05 significance level disclosed no significant difference. There was thus no reason, based upon the assumptions underlying the rank test, that might prevent its use.

The rank test (see Chapter 14 for method) showed the two treatment medians[11] to be sharply and significantly different, with the median days for

---

[11] In this case, the medians were very close to the averages, because the distributions, except for the rounding to integers, were known to be normal. This will never be the case in your work with

Table 15.3. Data for Wilcoxon Rank Sum Test (Example 15.3)

T_1	T_2
12	16
17	12
22	18
12	10
17	11
23	7
17	8
24	4
19	10
23	10
23	12
12	10
19	12
20	16
19	7
18	9

the old treatment (T_1) being 18.6 days and that for the new (T_2), 10.8. The probability of the observed difference under the null hypothesis, using the normal approximation, was 0.00003.[12] As a matter of curiosity, the pooled standard deviation based upon the original samples was 3.71. You will recall that the distributions had standard deviations of 4 and means of 17 and 11, so there was good agreement between these and the medians and standard deviation.

A t test was not run. Even though its robustness would probably have made it suitable for these data, the fact that they were patently nonnormal (they were integers) could have created some doubt. On the other hand, the sample variances were tested using Levene's test and were not significantly different. The rank test was therefore unquestionably applicable. Of course, the use of the sample size table and equation was approximate, because of the nonnormality.

---

data from actual trials, however. You will never be certain that your data are taken from a normal distribution. Therefore, you should remember that the Rank Sum test compares medians, not averages, and that these are not the same when the distribution is not symmetrical. If a distribution is skewed in either direction, the median more accurately estimates the most frequent value than does the arithmetic mean ("average").

[12] Woolson [10] indicates that the normal approximation is reasonable if the sample size is at least 10 for the smaller of the two groups in the Rank Sum test, and at least 20 for the Signed Rank test.

15.6.7   Signed Ranks Test

The sample size for this test can be estimated using the dependent table or equation for the t test, if the data are expected to be derived from an approximately normal parent distribution. The procedure for running this test was illustrated in Chapter 14, and will not be repeated here.

15.7   SAMPLE SIZE FOR ONE-WAY ANALYSIS OF VARIANCE (ANOVA)

15.7.1   Introduction

When there are more than two levels of a single factor (such as a trial comparing three different drugs), a very common kind of statistical analysis of the data is the analysis of variance (ANOVA). This method has not been described in this book, but the biostatistician will be very familiar with it, and will use it often. Therefore, the method for estimating sample size for it is given here. Aside from the discussion of randomized blocks that follows, we do not consider the estimation of sample size in detail for multifactor designs. Although the appropriate procedures are quite complex, again, your statistician should be well versed in their use.

If an analysis of variance is used to process data from a trial having one factor at more than two levels, if the comparison of more than one of the several treatment means is desired, and if the ANOVA shows significance, the analysis will not yet be complete. Following a finding of significance, it is necessary to determine *which* of the comparisons is responsible for that outcome. In such cases, many analysts commonly follow up the ANOVA with a multiple-comparisons procedure such as the Bonferroni or the Tukey HSD test (see Chapter 14). However, this procedure is too conservative, that is, it will fail to detect some contrasts that, nevertheless, should be detectable at the alpha level specified. Fortunately, there are two procedures that will operate at the specified alpha level: (a) Use the multiple-comparisons procedure *without* preceding it with an ANOVA or (b) use the ANOVA, following it, if significance was found, with a procedure we call the Fisher/Carmer and Swanson method (20). Its use is extremely simple. Carmer and Swanson showed that in such a case, the correct test is the ordinary t test, even though that test is not normally meant for use in making more than one comparison from a group.

Aside from the randomized-blocks design, the single-factor design with two levels is the most complex design for which analyses are described in this book. You should rely upon the biostatistician for the sample size estimation and analysis of most single-factor designs using more than two treatments, and for most *multifactor designs*. Nevertheless, the *design* of such studies is not difficult, and it was believed important in the design chapters to include multifactor factorials, because you will be likely to use studies with such designs, and you should be closely involved in selecting them. If you are interested in going further with multifactor sample size estimation, two excellent sources of help are Cohen's book [27] and the Borenstein-Cohen sample size program referred to earlier [67]. The Dallal program is also available, but is somewhat more difficult for nonstatistical professionals [66]. Methods suitable for practically all the designs you will need can be found in these references. However, there is one simple approximate procedure that is suitable in the case of a randomized blocks (two-factor) design. That is the use of the Bratcher et al. tables.

15.7.2   Use of the Bratcher et al. Tables

In Fleiss [8], basic procedures for the *exact* calculation of sample size in the multiple-treatments case (one-way ANOVA, more than two treatments) are described, but, as the author points out, they are not simple. This approach is beyond the level of this book, but some may find Fleiss's text of considerable interest. However, for some designs in this group, there are convenient tables available in the literature, including those given by Cohen [27]. The procedures in Cohen's book were designed for scientists and other technical people who must use statistics in the practice of their professions, but who are not statisticians. They nevertheless require some study.

The Borenstein-Cohen program [67] can be used for the present application (multiple treatments in a one-way design), but the Bratcher et al. paper mentioned in the introduction to this chapter (5) and discussed in what follows will probably be easier and faster, because an adaptation of their tables is given in the Appendix to this book (Tables A.6a through A.6c). Furthermore, they have the advantage of also being usable in the case of common randomized-blocks designs, when two factors only are used (the blocks and a treatment factor).

The Bratcher tables (5) are excellent, and encompass probably the easiest sample size estimation method available for use when designing a trial with a single factor (one-way), with three or more treatment levels.[13] These tables are based upon approximations, but the authors state that the beta values (actually, $1 - \beta$ in their paper) possess five-place accuracy in most cases, and three-place accuracy at worst.[14] As indicated, they are designed principally

---

[13]These tables also include sample sizes for two-treatment one-factor ANOVAs, but the tables designed for the *t* test in the independent case apply here, and you will probably find them more convenient to use. You will recognize that the *dependent* case (i.e., a "paired" test with more than two treatments given to each subject, or other type of block) is a randomized-blocks design. This is a two-factor design (blocks and treatments), and is therefore not discussed in detail in this section on estimating sample size for ANOVA. It is mentioned briefly in what follows because the authors of the Bratcher paper show that their table may be used for obtaining approximate sample sizes for randomized-blocks designs (two factors, blocks and one other, only), as well as for its primary purpose (one-way multiple-treatment designs).

[14]The authors state that in most cases, approximations to the noncentral F distribution were used; see page 158 in their paper. When cell sizes were very large, a less exact procedure, giving three-place accuracy, was employed.

for use with completely randomized one-way designs. However, as shown on pages 160 and 164 of the paper and in the authors' Table 5, the use of the tables for a two-way design when the design is randomized blocks gives quite accurate and generally conservative results, using n, the values in the body of the tables, to mean the number of *blocks*, rather than the number of patients per treatment.[15]

These tables are recommended for use when designing studies to be analyzed by one-way ANOVAs, and for two-way randomized-blocks analyses. The first few times you use them for the latter purpose, you may wish to compare your results with those you can obtain using the Borenstein-Cohen program [67], until you are satisfied that, for your studies, the Bratcher tables are satisfactory for this two-way design. As in the last chapter, however, we restrict our examples here to the one-way designs.

We now show an example of the use of the Bratcher tables for a single-factor three-treatment design that is to be analyzed either by the use of a multiple-comparisons test directly, or by using an ANOVA, followed, *if F is significant*, by protected t tests of the three pairwise contrasts. The Bratcher tables, as well as those of Cohen and the Borenstein-Cohen program, take the number of comparisons planned into account, so that there is no need to compensate for the multiplicity introduced by the use of more than one comparison by further increasing the sample size. Of course, any additional multiplicity brought about by other sources, such as interim analyses, multiple responses, or the like, if they exist, should be compensated for. Also, you should bear in mind that if you decide to make more comparisons than originally planned for when estimating the sample size, and you use some appropriate multiple-comparisons procedure (*not* preceded by an ANOVA), you will have a correct analysis but, because the sample size will be smaller than is needed for the intended power, you will run a risk of not detecting important contrasts.[16]

---

[15]The authors emphasize the beta risk, or rather the power $(1 - \beta)$, as would be normal in research and exploratory work. Because much of your work will relate to submissions to the FDA to support petitions for NDAs, for which you may often already feel sure that efficacy exists, your emphasis will more likely be on the alpha risk. The statements relating to randomized blocks in the Bratcher paper are based upon calculations using alpha values of 0.10 and 0.30, larger than most of those likely to be used in clinical studies (0.05 or less). However, the "bottom line" is that the tables themselves will probably be satisfactory for this purpose, considering how approximate the estimation of sigma may be. You can compare sample sizes obtained from these tables with Cohen's tables or the Borenstein/Cohen program for the randomized-blocks case.

[16]Some writers have suggested that multiple comparisons decided upon before a trial is run need not compensate for multiplicity, although if such a decision is made a posteriori, there should be compensation. My attitude is that this is difficult to explain, and, indeed, it is not borne out by the work of Carmer and Swanson (20) or by similar work published by Bernhardson (21). In both of these papers, multiple comparisons were fully intended a priori, and were used, yet their work clearly showed that the use of uncompensated multiple comparisons resulted in distorted experimentwise error frequencies.

15.7.3   Example 15.4: One-Way Design, More Than Two Levels

Description of Trial

A dietician wishes to compare three reducing diets. Each diet will use a different combination of menus. Moderate weight loss for the average patient is the objective. The diet producing the greatest *loss* in 3 months, up to a specified maximum, will be considered the most desirable. The subjects will first come to a hospital clinic for a fitness examination and initial (baseline) weighing. Each will return twice more for weighing during the following 2 weeks, to establish a reliable baseline, and will be given their menus during the last of these visits.

During the trial, the subjects will come to the clinic to be weighed every 2 weeks to assure that their health continues satisfactory and to check compliance. To improve the precision of the data, averages of the three baseline weights will be taken for each subject, and the means of the last two weights taken during the trial will be calculated and subtracted from these baseline means. These differences will be used as the data for analysis. Because intermediate results will be available, the dietician plans to examine those data for characteristics of the weight function during the trial, but they will not play a part in the final data analysis.

Specifications, Statistics, and Sample Sizes

The values of the specifications selected will be alpha, 0.010, and beta, 0.100. The dietician is interested in differences in weight loss of as small as 2 kg during the 3-month period, so delta will be specified to be 2 kg. A previous study has yielded a pooled standard deviation of 1.60 kg, and this value is to be used in the sample size estimation.

Among the Bratcher tables, Tables A.6a through A.6c in the Appendix, find the subtable for an alpha of 0.01. Delta sigma is 2/1.60, or 1.25, so in the first column, we find 1.25, which labels the five rows designated in the second column. In the second column, find the row label, 3 (three levels of the treatment variable). In the fourth column (for beta = 0.10), third row, you will find a value of 24, the number we are seeking. The dietician will therefore randomly assign each diet to 24 subjects.

Examining the Results of the Trial

As a rough test of this result, we synthesized a set of 24 data from three known normal distributions, differing only in their means. We assigned a mean weight loss of 5 kg to the distribution representing diet 1, 6 kg to that for diet 2, and 3 kg to that for diet 3. We specified sigma values of 1.75 for all three distributions, just slightly higher than our estimate. We then took a random sample of 24 from each of the three distributions and analyzed them as if they were data from an actual experiment. If we find that diets 1 and 2, to which we assigned 5- and 6-kg mean weight losses, are each significantly different than diet 3 (3 kg), but that they do not differ significantly between

Table 15.4. Weight Losses (kg) After 3 Months with Three Diets (Example 15.4)

Diet 1	Diet 2	Diet 3
5.4	7.9	0.7
6.1	6.3	2.2
8.3	7.9	3.7
4.5	4.2	6.0
3.6	3.8	4.7
4.2	5.5	1.5
6.4	6.4	1.4
1.8	7.9	1.8
7.2	2.5	4.8
2.1	6.3	4.2
4.7	4.1	6.1
7.1	7.6	2.7
4.1	4.6	6.0
4.4	7.5	5.1
5.4	5.4	2.2
6.9	6.4	3.5
4.0	3.7	2.2
3.3	6.8	5.5
4.2	7.7	2.3
3.9	5.5	3.8
5.5	6.0	3.3
7.0	4.8	3.0
4.5	5.1	3.6
2.9	4.0	3.7

themselves, we will have an indication that our system is working, at least for this one experiment, chosen randomly from any number of repetitions of the trial that we might perform.[17] Of course, it is obvious that a truly reliable test can only be made in a reasonable time by carrying out a Monte Carlo study (running a large number of such "synthetic" trials and noting the average conformance to our conditions).

---

[17] In the next section, we will go further, actually drawing data representing 100 clinical trials from the postulated distributions. We will then count the frequency that failures to find significance occurs. This should be approximately equal to a proportion beta of the total number of trials, because, like the present case, we will build in treatment differences large enough to show significance in most cases. We could have tested alpha in an analogous manner (in that case, the two distributions would have the same mean, and the null hypothesis would therefore be true). Such a "Monte Carlo" procedure is less time-consuming on a small computer when the responses are binomial, as in the next section, than when they are continuous, as they are in this example.

Table 15.5. Means and Standard Deviations (Example 15.4)

Diet	Mean	Std. Dev.
Diet 1		
Population	5	1.6000
Sample of 24	4.896	1.6732
Diet 2		
Population	6	1.6000
Sample of 24	5.746	1.5662
Diet 3		
Population	3	1.6000
Sample of 24	3.500	1.5632

The data obtained are given in Table 15.4. The weight losses of the individual patients were taken to the nearest 0.1 kg.

Since the data were obtained from a single distribution known to be normal, we did not check the group variances or their normality. An ANOVA was done to determine whether there were any significant contrasts among the three groups.

Although we have not described the ANOVA procedure in this book, we show the results in order to complete this example. In an ANOVA, the statistic of interest in determining significance is called F. In this case, the F value was 12.029 at 2/69 df, representing the degrees of freedom for the three treatments ($= 2$) and that for error ($= 69$). These F and df values correspond to a probability of $\ll 0.001$ and indicate that there were one or more significant contrasts in the data. Table 15.5 shows the means and standard deviations—those originally specified for each of the populations generated, and those found in the three samples of 24, representing the results of the trial. Because the ANOVA gave significance, protected t tests were done and, along with other numbers, their results are shown in Table 15.6, considering the three paired comparisons only.

As can be seen in Table 15.6, the results agreed well with those intended when the populations were established. The difference between diets 1 and 2 was not significant. Note that in this case, the population difference was less than delta (the difference between the two population means was 1.0). That between diets 1 and 3 was found significant, but the probability was not much smaller than alpha (alpha was 0.010; the p value found was about 0.005). This was reasonable, because, as shown in Table 15.6, delta was 2.00 for the populations, and these two population means differed by just that amount (cf. Table 15.5), so that this comparison was borderline. Finally, the difference between diets 2 and 3 was found highly significant, which again was to be expected, because the population difference was 3, as compared to the delta value of 2.

Table 15.6. Results of Analyses (Protected t Tests): Pairwise Comparisons of Diets (Example 15.4)

Statistic	Pairwise Comparisons of Diets		
	Diet 1 − Diet 2	Diet 1 − Diet 3	Diet 2 − Diet 3
Difference	−0.85	1.40	2.25
t Found, 46 df	−1.817	2.986	4.972
Probability	0.076	0.005	< 0.00001
Signif. Level	Not significant	Significant	Significant

Note: Specifications set a priori:

$$\alpha = 0.010$$
$$\beta = 0.100$$
$$\delta = 2.000$$

15.8   SAMPLE SIZE FOR DESIGNS WITH TWO OR MORE FACTORS

As indicated, the *analyses* and *sample size estimation* of designs with more than one factor (with the exception of some material on simple randomized-blocks designs) are not covered in this book. Of course, we have described the preparation of such designs. When there is more than one factor, the statistician will be able to carry out sample size estimations and analyze the data. We suggest Cohen's book [27] or the Dallal [66] or Borenstein and Cohen programs [67] as sources of tables and methods for the estimates.

15.9   CONTINGENCY TABLE TESTS USING BINOMIAL RESPONSES

15.9.1   Introduction

We present an illustration of sample size estimation for binomial response studies for the most common case only. That case is the approximate analysis of data using 2×2 tables (1 df), in which we wish to examine two *independent* treatment groups to compare the proportions of **successes** for the two treatments. A *success* is one of the two possible outcomes in a **Bernoulli trial**. As defined in Kotz and Johnson [57], a Bernoulli trial is an observation, usually one of a series, with the following characteristics: (a) The result is binomial (it must be either a success or a failure). (b) Each trial is independent of the others. (c) The probability of success is the same in each. An example of one Bernoulli trial is a coin toss. Another is a single independent observation of a patient's condition, in which the data will indicate only whether he or she is improved or not. Note that the word "trial" is used differently here than the usual usage in this book.

Binomial data from a group of Bernoulli trials for two treatments might be analyzed conveniently using either chi-squared contingency table tests or

Fisher Exact tests,[18] but we limit ourselves here to the 2×2 chi-squared tests, as described in Chapter 14. The sample size procedure described in the example that follows (use of a table) is suitable for this method of analysis. You can also use a normal approximation (with a Z value).[19] In addition to the sample size estimation and data analysis methods for independent groups described here, equivalent methods for dependent (paired) data also exist. If you have occasion to use them, you will find descriptions of both exact and approximate methods of analysis in Siegel [45] or Conover (McNemar Test) [39], and in Colton (analysis and sample size estimation [20]).

15.9.2   Example 15.5: Sample Size for Binomial Responses

Outline of the Trial

Let's assume that you are planning a trial in which two antihistamines, an established treatment and a new drug, are to be compared for the relief of certain allergies. You are interested in comparing the proportion of patients whose symptoms are relieved and who are assigned to the new product, with the corresponding proportion for the other product. Putting it more simply, you wish to compare the relative proportions of *successes* for the two drugs. The measurement scale will have two points, "substantial" vs. "average to poor" effectiveness, in which a response of "substantial" is to be counted as a success and "average to poor" as a failure. The established drug has been shown to give success in 40% of patients examined, on the average. If the new drug is superior to the old by at least 20 percentage points, your management has indicated that a major clinical trial series will be mounted.

Hypotheses

Interest is in a one-tailed test, because there will be no further testing of the new drug if it is not superior to the old. We thus have the following null and alternate hypotheses:

$$H_0: \pi_2 - \pi_1 = 0 \tag{15.8}$$

$$H_1: \pi_2 - \pi_1 = \delta \tag{15.9}$$

In the foregoing hypotheses, π_i (pi sub i) stands for the parameter of distribution i ($i = 1$ or 2), which is the known or postulated fraction (proportion) of successes (probability of success) in that binomial population. A binomial distribution possesses only one parameter—pi; the standard deviation of the distribution is a function of pi. Note that we use fractions here (percentages divided by 100) rather than percentages per se. The value of the symbol δ (delta), of course, denotes the difference between the two popula-

---

[18]This test is discussed briefly in Section 15.9.3, but is not described in this book.
[19]The value of Z is related to chi squared at 1 df. For example, if you square a two-tailed Z value for the probability 0.05 (which is 1.96), you obtain 3.84, which is the value of chi squared for 1 df.

tion parameters that is desired if significance is to be found, in units of the parameter. Note that the alternate hypothesis is one-tailed, and states that π_2 is greater than π_1. The null hypothesis is expressed as a difference with π_2 given first. It could have been written $\pi_2 = \pi_1$ or as $\pi_1 - \pi_2 = 0$ with the same meaning. It states that the two populations have the same proportion of successes (the same parameter); that they are equal.

Our test of the null hypothesis will result in its rejection or acceptance. If it is accepted, we will conclude that the drugs do not differ in effectiveness, with a probability beta of being wrong in that conclusion if, in fact, H_1 is really true. If it is rejected, we will conclude that there is a difference in effectiveness of delta (20 percentage points), in favor of π_2, with a probability alpha of being wrong.

Sample Size

We will use an alpha value of 0.050 and a beta of 0.100. In this test, the information corresponding to a value of delta in a normal statistics test is the specification that you will require superiority of the new drug of 20 percentage units, or a difference of 0.200 in proportions. Sample size equations for this test are given in several of the books listed in the bibliography—Colton [20], Dixon and Massey [33], and Snedecor and Cochran [38], and Fleiss [41] are examples. Although all of these are based upon approximations, the first three use more approximate procedures than Fleiss, although they indicate that there are more precise methods. And although other books contain tables based upon the sample size equations, Fleiss has given one of the best. We therefore have reprinted a condensed form of his table in the Appendix, with permission. It results in slightly greater sample sizes than the other methods because it allows for the use of the Yates continuity correction (see Chapter 14, Section 14.5.6, Example 14.18) in the calculation of chi squared or Z. We recommend its use for your independent 2×2 chi-squared table tests.

To use one of the group of modified Fleiss tables (Table A.7a to A.7r) in this example, proceed as follows: The values of P_1 and P_2 are statistics (sample values) that correspond to π_1 and π_2, respectively. Find the page for $P_1 = 0.40$. This is the proportion of successes we are assuming for a group of patients treated with the old treatment, T_1. In the table, the extreme left-hand column gives values of P_2, the proportion for the new treatment, T_2. Find the set of rows corresponding to the specification of the sponsor, $P_2 = 0.60$. There are four of these, for alpha values of 0.01, 0.02, 0.05, and 0.10. You will note that the table is labeled as a two-tailed table. Because this is a one-tailed test, the previously selected alpha value, 0.05, is multiplied by 2, giving 0.10. The row labeled 0.10 is now used to find the sample size. The columns of the table are labeled with values of beta. Choose the column headed by 0.10. Going down this column to its intersection with the row just described, we find a value of 115. We will therefore use 115 patients per treatment group in this trial.

Table 15.7. Contingency Table Comparison of Antihistamines (Example 15.5)

Drug Used	Successes	Failures	Totals
T_1	41	74	115
T_2	65	50	115
Totals	106	124	230

Note the fairly large sample size. If you do many binomial designs, you will find that although binomial trials are frequently easier to design, execute, and analyze than those using continuous-variable responses, they suffer from the serious disadvantage of requiring substantially larger groups of patients, which can be both an ethical and an economic problem. When you use a larger sample size than would be necessary with a different design, you are inconveniencing or perhaps endangering a larger number of patients than may otherwise be necessary. As to the economics, each binomial datum carries much less information—only one of two possible values, one or zero or an equivalent—so that you will need many more patients to supply the required total quantity of information. It is better to avoid the use of binomial responses when you can. Nevertheless, this example is given because avoidance may not be possible.

The Trial
As was done for previous examples, two distributions (in this case, binomial rather than normal) were generated, and a sample of 115 "patients" was drawn from each, representing the two treatment groups. The parameters specified were simply the two proportions, 0.40 and 0.60, here called π_1 and π_2. The results are shown in Table 15.7.

Table 15.7 is the contingency table containing the results of the drawings from the two distributions, and shows the *numbers* of successes and failures for each drug. The sample *proportions* of successes can be calculated for each by dividing the number of successes in each case by the appropriate row total. In this case, the proportions are $41/115 = 0.357$ for the old drug (T_1) and $65/115 = 0.565$ for the new (T_2), a difference of 0.209 in favor of T_2.

Table 15.7 was analyzed by the use of Equation (14.18) from Chapter 14. You will remember that this equation gives the continuity-corrected chi-squared value for the data in the table. In this case, we have

$$\chi^2 = \frac{N(|ad - bc| - 0.5N)^2}{(a + b)(c + d)(a + c)(b + d)} \qquad (14.18)$$

$$= \frac{230[|(41 \times 50) - (74 \times 65)| - 0.5 \times 230]^2}{115 \times 115 \times 106 \times 124}$$

$$= 9.2567$$

For the one-tailed test, the chi-squared value required for significance at an alpha value of 0.05 can be found in Snedecor and Cochran [38], for 1 df and is 2.71 (remember to use a value of 0.100 for alpha, because the table of chi squared is two-tailed, but you are doing a one-tailed test). Because the value just calculated exceeds this value, we reject the null hypothesis of equal proportions of successes in the two groups and accept the alternate hypothesis, which says that the difference between the two proportions in the population is (at least) 0.20. By inspection, we see that the difference is in favor of T_2.

A Small Monte Carlo Study

Let us see how we might determine whether the Fleiss table sample size of 115 that we used in Example 15.5 was reasonable. As promised in the footnote to Section 15.7.3, we use a Monte Carlo procedure for this. Many types of problems can be studied with this technique. It derives its name from Monte Carlo because of its use of probability to arrive at a result; it is an empirical method of investigating probabilistic phenomena.

In the present case, two binomial populations, one representing the old and one the new treatment, were generated. The parameter of the one representing the old treatment was 0.40, and that of the other was 0.60. One hundred pairs of data, representing 100 trials, were drawn from these, each pair derived from 115 hypothetical patients and giving the number of successes—the number of patients obtaining relief—for each. Of course, the number of failures in each simulated treatment group was 115 minus the number of successes. Thus, each of these 100 "trials" consisted of two "data" giving the number of successes for each of the two treatments out of totals of 115 patients on treatment 1 and 115 on treatment 2.

For each of the 100 sets of treatment groups (i.e., each simulated trial of 230 patients), a value of chi squared was calculated, just as was done in Example 15.5 (which actually was one of the 100 pairs, selected randomly). Finally, the number of times that this chi squared turned out to be too small to produce significance was counted. Because beta was set at 0.10, in 100 experiments, the expected number of such failures to produce significance between the treatments would be 10. In fact, the number of these nonsignificant results was 8. If several thousand simulated trials had been done, rather than 100, a number closer to 10 might have been obtained.

Finding eight nonsignificances in the 100 trials was gratifying close to theory, but, of course, it might have been an unusually good result. However, it certainly suggests that the sample size of 115 was reasonable. Note also that this exercise has demonstrated the nature of beta; as you know, beta is the probability of failing to find significance when the proportions of successes in the two populations really do differ by delta (i.e., when the alternate hypothesis is really true). Because we generated the two distributions, we know the real proportions. For the outcome, we expected beta to be 0.10, or 10% of all of the experiments; the value we found was 0.08, or 8%.

A similar study could be done to demonstrate the nature of alpha by generating sets of two distributions having *the same* proportion of successes, drawing a large number of samples from each, and noting the frequency with which significance was found. Because there really would then be no difference between such a pair of distributions, if alpha was 0.05, for example, we could expect to get a number of wrongly significant results in the neighborhood of 5% of the total number of experiments.

15.9.3 The Use of Normal Approximations vs. Exact Tests

As was pointed out in Chapter 14, the chi-squared test of a contingency table is a normal approximation applied to binomial data. And as mentioned there (Section 14.5), the degree of approximation becomes poorer as the sample size becomes smaller. The degree of approximation is also affected by the size of the expected values in the cells. Snedecor and Cochran [38] give the following rules: If the *total* sample size is less than 40 and the expected value in any cell is less than 5, do not use the chi-squared test.[20] If the sample size is less than 20, do not use it in any case. In either event, use the Fisher Exact test instead (see what follows). Another way to look at the use of a chi-squared test is to note that the degree of approximation will be reasonably satisfactory if the value of $n\pi(1 - \pi)$ is greater than 5. If it is not, use the Fisher test. Fisher's Exact test is valid with large samples also, but if you decide to use it with counts in the cells as large as those in Example 15.5, you will probably wish to choose a computer program or at least a programmable calculator, because the test will become very tedious. In the example given here, both of the previous criteria were satisfied; the sample size was greater than 40, and we used $n = 115$, $p_1 = 0.40$ and $p_2 = 0.60$, so that the previous expression for either p_1 or p_2 was $(115)(0.40)(0.60) = 27.6$. We were therefore safe in using the chi-squared test.

The Fisher Exact test is described in many texts, for example, a clearly presented example is given in Maxwell [44]. Another discussion appears in Snedecor and Cochran [38]. The test is easy and fast if you use a programmable calculator (and the cell sizes are small),[21] and is also available on several statistical computer packages. It has been criticized by Berkson (22), but it nevertheless appears to fill a useful niche and continues to be recommended in the applications literature, particularly when expected values are too small for a legitimate chi-squared test. The probability values given by this test have been compared with those for the chi-squared test demonstrated in Example 15.5 (see Maxwell [44]) (the Fisher test gives a one-tailed probability, which is multiplied by 2 for a two-tailed test). Agree-

---

[20]See Chapter 14, in the section referenced before, for the definition and calculation of expected values in a contingency table.

[21]If the numbers in the contingency table are large, care must be taken in programming to avoid overflow.

ment with the chi-squared test of the same table is very good down to quite small sample sizes.

15.10   SUMMARY OF THE CHAPTER

15.10.1   Nature of the Null and Alternate Hypotheses

Sample size estimation is closely related to hypothesis testing, as you have seen. Therefore, the formation of the null and alternate hypotheses are reviewed briefly. A hypothesis test is a test of whether or not to reject the null hypothesis. If that occurs, the alternative hypothesis must be accepted. Alpha, the probability of being wrong when claiming significance, must always be specified a priori when a hypothesis test is planned. A low probability such as 0.050 or 0.010, or even 0.001, is usually selected. If beta and delta have also been specified, and a reliable estimate of sigma is available, and if the null hypothesis cannot be rejected, it can be *accepted*. However, if beta and delta are not specified and H_0 cannot be rejected, one may correctly state only that significance has not been shown. The null hypothesis *cannot* then be accepted.

15.10.2   Risk Specifications, Sigma, and Hypothesis Testing

The first step in estimating sample size in the manner recommended here is to obtain specifications of alpha, beta, and delta. Alpha is defined in the previous paragraph. Beta is the probability of being wrong when claiming that the null hypothesis cannot be rejected. A beta probability lying between 0.05 and 0.20 is common. This process has been discussed thoroughly; the principal requirements for setting alpha and beta are to carefully consider the objectives of your trial. Delta has been equally thoroughly discussed, and its value is also dependent upon your objectives. It is defined as the smallest difference that you wish to detect between two treatments in a trial, using a given type of response, when a hypothesis test is eventually performed. If there are several treatments, it is the minimum detectable difference between *any* two treatments.

The *power* of a test is the additive inverse of beta. That is, if beta is equal to 0.100, then the power is $1 - 0.100$, or 0.900. A power of 0.900 can be interpreted as a statement that, if H_1 is true, there is a probability of 0.900 that the null hypothesis will be rejected.

There is a need for an estimate of sigma when a sample size estimate is to be prepared. Unless there is recent and relevant information about it, the use of a pilot trial is advocated in spite of the additional time and labor required. Guessing at your sample size, or estimating it with inadequate information, can be very costly.

Alpha and beta may be prespecified as having any possible values at all, short of one or zero, by the test planner, but the values mentioned earlier are those frequently used. The value of delta depends upon the nature of the response and the planner's idea of the magnitude of a clinically important difference between the means to be tested. The smaller you make alpha, beta, or delta, the larger the sample size must be. On the other hand, although you do not have any direct ability to specify sigma—it is a parameter of the distributions of treated patients from which the sample groups are drawn—the *smaller* the value of sigma (or its estimate from a pilot trial), the smaller the sample size will be found to be.[22]

15.10.3 Multiplicity

Problems of multiplicity that affect the validity of your sample size estimates or your hypothesis tests are considered again, and methods of avoiding them are discussed. Multiplicity problems arise when (a) a test designed to compare two means is used for more than two; (b) hypothesis tests are repeated for response measurements made at two or more different times, whether they are the same or different kinds of measurements; (c) tests are improperly done on repeated measurements of the same group of subjects in the same trial; (d) interim tests are done during a trial; and similar situations. Multiplicity may often be necessary, and it can be compensated for if you plan ahead. If you do not do so, your significance tests will possess actual alpha values that are substantially greater than those that you have specified.

15.10.4 Sample Size Estimation

Like most sample size estimation procedures, those given here give approximate, albeit quite accurate, results. Such procedures, using tables, equations, or both, are given for both independent and dependent *t* tests, two kinds of rank tests, one-way analysis of variance (when more than two treatments must be tested in a single trial), and 2 × 2 contingency table tests when there are two independent treatment groups and the response is binomial (dichotomous; yes/no, 0/1, etc.). Five examples are given to illustrate the use of

---

[22]The value of sigma can sometimes be reduced by improving the precision of the response measurement or choosing a different method with an inherently greater precision. As a crude example, if you read a sphygmomanometer only to the nearest 10 mm, or if you read it carelessly, your measurements will convey less information than if you read the scale to the nearest 5 mm or less. In such cases, sigma values estimated from sets of such measurements will be larger than if the readings had been done more precisely. Also for reasons of precision, when selecting a judgment scale, you should avoid a binomial or trinomial scale if possible. On the other hand, scales having five points or higher (*all of which are used in the data*) can often be satisfactorily analyzed, to a reasonable degree of approximation, with a parametric procedure. You should note that all points of a scale should be useful, however. If one or both extreme points are never used, the scale is really shorter than is implied.

these procedures. References to procedures for other designs are given. A short discussion of the use of normal approximations is presented, and a small Monte Carlo study to test roughly whether the binomial sample size used in the illustrative example was correct is given.

15.11 LITERATURE REFERENCES

(1) Freiman, Jennie A., Thomas C. Chalmers, Harry Smith, Jr., and Roy R. Kuebler, *New England Journal of Medicine*, 299, 690–694 (1978).

(2) Neyman, J., K. Iwaskiewicz, and S. Kolodziejczyk, *Journal of the Royal Statistical Society*, 2, 114 (1935).

(3) Neyman, J., and B. Tokarska, *Journal of the American Statistical Association*, 31, 318–326 (1936).

(4) Neyman, J., and E. S. Pearson, *Philosophical Transactions of the Royal Society of London*, *A*, 231, 289–337 (1933).

(5) Bratcher, T. L., M. A. Moran, and W. J. Zimmer, "Tables of Sample Sizes in the Analysis of Variance," *Journal of Quality Technology*, 2, 156–164 (1970).

(6) Wheeler, Robert E., *Technometrics*, 16, 193–201 (1974).

(7) Owen, D. B., *Journal of the American Statistical Association*, 60, 320–333 (1965).

(8) Hodges, J. L., and E. L. Lehmann, *The Annals of Mathematical Statistics*, 39, 1629–1637 (1968).

(9) Croarkin, Mary C., *Journal of Research—B*, National Bureau of Standards, 66B, 59–70 (1962).

(10) Dupont, William D., and Walter D. Plummer, Jr., *Controlled Clinical Trials*, 11, 116–128 (1990).

(11) Bowman, K. O., and M. A. Kastenbaum, *Technometrics*, 16, 349–352 (1974).

(12) Wheeler, Robert E., *Technometrics*, 17, 177–179 (1975).

(13) Feigl, Polly, *Biometrics*, 34, 111–122 (1978).

(14) Fleiss, Joseph L., Alex Tytun, and Hans K. Ury, *Biometrics*, 36, 343–346 (1980).

(15) Ury, Hans K., and Joseph L. Fleiss, *Biometrics*, 36, 347–351 (1980).

(16) Kupper, Lawrence L., and Kerry B. Hafner, *The American Statistician*, 43, 101–105 (1989).

(17) Wilcoxon, Frank, *Biometrics Bulletin*, 1, 80–83 (1945).

(18) Mann, H. B., and D. R. Whitney, *Annals of Mathematical Statistics*, 18, 50–60 (1947).

(19) Hamilton, Martin A., and Bruce Jay Collings, *Technometrics*, 3, 327–337 (1991).

(20) Carmer, S. G., and M. R. Swanson, *Journal of the American Statistical Association*, 68, 66–74 (1973).

(21) Bernhardson, Clemens, S., *Biometrics*, 31, 229–232 (1975).

(22) Berkson, Joseph, *Journal of Statistical Planning and Inference*, 2, 27–42 (1978).

Appendix

A.1 EXPLANATION AND DISCUSSION OF TABLES AND PROGRAMS

A.1.1 Remarks

In most cases, the explanations for the use of the tables in this section repeat similar descriptions given in the book. They are reiterated here for your convenience, to save your searching through the chapters for textual material, and to serve as refreshers if your use is only occasional or occurs some time after reading the book. In cases in which you are already familiar with their use, of course, there will be no need for further clarification.

The descriptive material for the programs does not appear in the text in any detail, and is included here as a guide if you wish to write similar programs of your own.

A.1.2 Tables

Table A.1 (Two-Tailed t Table)
This table is reprinted from Table 12 of Pearson and Hartley's tables, Volume I [51]. It is reproduced here with the kind permission of the BIometrika Trust at University College, London. The first column, labeled df, shows the degrees of freedom for error for your data. For example, if you have two groups to compare, one having 10 data and the other having 6, you would have a total error df of $(10 - 1) + (6 - 1)$, or 14. The remaining seven columns give t values, and are labeled with probability values in the top row. These correspond to the alpha values that you specify in your designs when planning your studies. The t values in the last row of the table, labeled with the symbol for infinity (∞), are equal to the two-tailed Z values for the normal distribution shown in Table A.5, as far as those go. This is so because the t distribution approaches the normal as a limit.

The t values in the table are critical values, to which you should compare any calculated t. When and if the calculated t *exceeds* the tabular value, you

472

can claim significance at the probability shown at the top of the column in which the critical t value is found. Note that the table is *two-tailed*. If you decide to run a one-tailed test, you can use the same table by dividing the probability values by 2. For example, for 15 df, the tabulated two-tailed t value for alpha = 0.05 is 2.131. The one-tailed value for the same alpha is 1.753, shown in the 0.1 column.

Note: The use of alpha values greater than 0.05 is emphatically **not** recommended for industrial clinical studies. The table includes a column for alpha = 0.1 because you may occasionally need it for one-tailed tests at alpha equals 0.05, as just discussed.

Table A.2 (Abbreviated Chi-Squared Table)

This table is also reprinted from Pearson and Harley, Volume I [51] (their Table 8). This, too, is used here with the generous permission of the Biometrika Trust at University College, London. Only a portion of the original is shown here. If you test 2×2 contingency tables as described in Chapter 14, you will use row 1 of this table. Other rows are needed when contingency tables larger than those with two rows and two column are to be analyzed. Tables of chi squared such as this one have numerous uses in addition to the analysis of contingency tables, many of which are described in the volumes in the Bibliography. The full table from Pearson and Hartley gives a much greater range of probability values and a range of 1 to 100 df.

See Chapter 14 for details of the use of this chi-squared table when you wish to analyze a 2×2 contingency table. For the analysis of contingency tables with more than two rows, columns or both, see, for example, Fienberg [40], Fleiss [41], Freeman [42], and Maxwell [44]. For any number of rows and columns in a contingency table, including a 2×2 table, you determine the correct degrees of freedom (df) as follows[1]:

1. Let R be the number of rows and C the number of columns in your table. Subtract 1 from R and 1 from C and multiply the results together. The result is the degrees of freedom for the table, and the number to use when you are choosing which row to use in Table A.2. In

---

[1]The foregoing procedure is pragmatic; it does not help to explain the meaning of degrees of freedom. The following procedure does not fully explain the concept, but it may help: If you look at the top row in any 2×2 contingency table, note that if you accept the row total as fixed, you can vary *either* of the two entries in the row, changing it to any value without altering the total. The other entry, however, must then assume a new specific value, and only that one value, without freedom to change. Circle the value you selected. Repeat this in the second row. You will see that neither of the two second row entries can be altered at all if the row totals are to remain constant. Because you have only one circled value in the table, we say that the table has 1 df. This procedure can be used with the columns rather than the rows, if desired. When a table has, say, three columns and two rows, you will find that you can circle *two* entries rather than one, so such a table will have 2 df. The procedure can be extended to tables of any size.

symbols,

$$df = (R - 1)(C - 1)$$

2. After you find the row in Table A.2 corresponding to the df of your contingency table, find the correct column. This is the one headed by a probability value equal to the alpha level you specified when planning your trial. The critical chi-squared value for comparison with your computed chi squared is found at the intersection of that row and column.

Table A.3 (Sample Sizes for the Two-Tailed Independent t Test)
These tables are adapted from a set that appear in Davies [14]. We refer to these and Table A.4 as the *Sillitto tables*, as they were prepared originally by George P. Sillitto, one of the authors of the Davies book. They are reproduced here with the permission of the Longman Group, UK Ltd., in Harlow, Essex, England. They are for use when planning a *t* test to compare two means, and for extended uses such as the Bonferroni or the Carmer and Swanson procedure mentioned in Chapters 5 and 14, in that case for comparing more than two means.

To enter the Sillitto tables and get an estimate of the number of patients **per treatment group** needed, in addition to obtaining an estimate of sigma (preferably from a pilot trial), you must also have specified delta (the smallest difference between means that you wish to detect with your *t* test), alpha (the significance level of the test you plan), and beta (the risk of falsely failing to find significance).

The Sillitto tables consist of four subtables, one for each of four alpha levels as shown just under their titles. The first step is to select the table corresponding to the alpha level that you need. Next, divide the specified delta value by the estimate of sigma and round the result to one or two decimal places (the tables use two places for delta/sigma up to 1.00, and one place thereafter). Locate this calculated value of delta/sigma in the leftmost column of the table.[2] This defines the row of the table you will use. Finally, find the column corresponding to the beta value you specified. The intersection of that row and column will give you the sample size estimate. You should use that number of patients for each treatment. Because this table is for use with parallel tests, each patient will receive only one treatment.

For small values of delta/sigma, you may find that there is no entry in the table for your calculated and selected values of delta/sigma and beta. This can occur if the intersection of your selected row and column lies in one of the blank spaces in the upper portion of one of the four tables. In such a case, the sample size necessary is greater than the largest number given in

---

[2]You may find that the value you calculated lies between two of the tabular values of delta/sigma. In this case, you must interpolate, as described in Chapter 15.

the table. You must then use the equation given in Chapter 15. One value in Table A.3d was incorrect, and has been corrected here.

Table A.4 (Sample Sizes for Dependent t Tests)
These tables are also from Davies [14], were also prepared originally by Sillitto, and are also reproduced by permission of the Longman Group, UK Ltd., of Harlow, Essex. There are four of these, as for Tables A.3. They are intended for use when you plan to test a single set of values, such as a set of differences, using the dependent *t* test. They are used in exactly the same way as just described for the A.3 tables.

Table A.5 (Abbreviated Table of Z Values)
These values are some of those often shown in graphs of the normal distribution, usually along the bottom axis. They can be used to define the lower or upper limits of tail areas of that distribution corresponding to various probabilities. The values in this table were calculated using a program that I wrote for an HP-42S pocket calculator, using definite integrals corresponding to the areas (probabilities) shown (the upper limits were taken as 5.0, which was far enough out on the tail of the distribution to give the required accuracy). The first column gives the probability, the second the one-tailed (upper tail) value of Z, and the third, the two-tailed value.

This table was designed to supply you with the most frequently needed values of Z for use in the equations given in Chapter 15 to calculate sample size.

We are suggesting several ways to obtain the Z values you will need if you use the *t* test sample size equations instead of Tables A.3 or A.4. The first and fastest is the use of Table A.5, if its values are within the range you need, as they usually will be. The next most rapid method is the use of published tables, if they are available to you. Tables of the normal distribution appear in almost any statistics text, as well as in every volume of statistical tables, but the two normal distribution tables in Colton [20] are among the easiest and simplest to use. Probably the next fastest procedure is to use Program AC.1 (see what follows) if you have a Hewlett-Packard 42S calculator. Finally, we suggest two desk computer programs. The first is one I wrote, described in what follows (BASIC Program AP.3). If you have a PC, and can spare the time to copy the program to your hard disk, the method is very rapid, and you can easily obtain estimates of either Z or P. It has the disadvantage of only fair accuracy for Z values, but for sample size estimates, this is usually satisfactory. The second is commercial application software, *Electronic Tables* [68], which will give any desired value of Z or P at almost any desired accuracy.

Table A.6 (Sample Sizes for One-Factor ANOVA)
This table, in reduced form, is reproduced here with the generous permission of the American Society for Quality Control of Milwaukee, and Dr. Lloyd S.

Nelson, Director of Statistical Methods at the Nashua Corporation in New Hampshire. It is a condensation of a most interesting and useful paper by Bratcher, Moran, and Zimmer that appeared in the *Journal of Quality Technology* when Dr. Nelson was Founding Editor of that publication.[3]

This set of tables can be used to obtain sample size estimates for any one-factor trial to be analyzed using an analysis of variance, for any number of levels of the factor from two to six. When there are only two levels, you may find Tables A.3a through A.3d more convenient, although either set of tables can be used. When there is only one factor, and it possesses only two levels, either a *t* test or an ANOVA may be used; they are completely equivalent.

The original tables published by Bratcher et al. gave sample sizes for 2 to 31 levels of the treatment factor in a one-factor design, but the adaptation presented here is limited to six for simplicity and because the use of more than six treatments in a one-way design is very rare in clinical trials. If you have a design for which you need to intercompare more than six treatments, you can use the original tables given by Bratcher et al. (see the reference footnote 3).

When you are planning a trial for which it is appropriate, the table is used as follows:

1. Obtain an estimate of sigma from a pilot trial or from previous similar data, as explained in Chapter 15 and earlier.

2. Obtain specifications for the values of alpha, beta, and delta, as also explained in Chapter 15.

3. You should note that in the condensed tables supplied here, the value of alpha is limited to 0.01, 0.05, and 0.10. These are the only values below 0.20 given in the original published tables, but they should serve most of your needs. The values for beta in the tables given here are those most commonly used in clinical trials; they are 0.05, 0.10, and 0.20. Again, if you need specifications outside this range, the original tables include a fourth beta value, 0.30. You should note that in those tables, these values are expressed as powers of the test, $1 - \beta$, rather than as beta risks.

4. Find the table for the alpha level you want, for example, 0.05 (Table A.6b). Divide the specified value of delta by the estimated sigma value, and round the result to two places. Find this value in the leftmost column of Table A.6b. If your value lies between two of the tabulated values, use linear interpolation as described in what follows.

5. If your rounded value of delta/sigma is equal to one of the values printed in the first column of the table, find the number of treatments

[3]"Tables of Sample Sizes in the Analysis of Variance," *Journal of Quality Technology*, 2, 156–164 (July 1970).

that you plan to use; this appears in the second column. This identifies the line of the table you need in the next and last step. In that line, find the column on the right-hand side of the table that is labeled with your specified beta value. In that column, find the sample size, or number of patients assigned to each treatment, that must be used.

6. For example, suppose that you have specified a value of delta of 2, in the units of the response to be used. Say that your estimated value of sigma is 1.330, so that delta/sigma would be 1.5038, or, rounded to two places, 1.50. Assume that you are planning to use three treatments (a test drug, a placebo, and a standard), and have specified alpha as 0.05 and beta as 0.10. To get the sample size, in Table A.6b, you find the lines for delta/sigma of 1.50 and then follow the line for three treatments across to the column headed by a beta value of 0.10. In the cell you have thus located, you will find the required sample size to be 13 patients per treatment, or 39 altogether.

7. There will be many cases in which you must interpolate, however, because your calculated value of delta/sigma will lie between two of the entires in the first column.[4] For example, suppose that your value of delta is 1.5 and sigma is 1.11. In such a case, you will obtain a value of 1.3514 for delta/sigma, or 1.35 when rounded to two places. This value lies 2/5 of the distance between 1.25 and 1.50.[5] The range of sample sizes over this interval in the table, for a beta value of 0.10 and three treatments, is 18 to 13, or 5. If you multiply 5 by 2/5 and subtract the result from 18, the first value in the range, you get 16 (you subtract rather than add because the values *decrease* as you proceed from 18 to 13). If this result had had any decimal digits following it, you would use the next higher value. This is the required number of patients per treatment. You would therefore use 48 patients for the three-treatment trial. Although this example is somewhat simplistic, it should illustrate the procedure satisfactorily.

Table A.7 (Sample Size for Two Independent Proportions).
These tables are a shortened version of Table A.3 in Fleiss [41]. They are reproduced with the permission of Wiley-Liss, a division of John Wiley & Sons, Inc., and are intended for the estimation of sample size for studies in which the responses are binomial—that is, in which the data consist of only two possible response values, yes or no, 0 or 1, not improved or improved, etc., as for Example 15.5, Chapter 15.

---

[4]If delta/sigma lies outside the range 1.00 to 3.00, you will need to change your specification of delta in order to use either these tables or the originals, because that is the range used in both.
[5]That is so because the distance between 1.35 and 1.25 is 0.10, and the total distance is 1.50 −1.25, or 0.25. Thus, the distance of the desired sample size from the beginning of the range is 0.10/0.25, or 2/5.

In Example 15.5, the proportion of successes ("substantial effectiveness") for each of two antihistamines is measured. To estimate the sample size for this trial, we used an alpha value of 0.05 and a beta of 0.10. The two drugs to be compared comprise a test drug and an established one used as a standard. The established drug has been shown previously to be successful in about 40% of the patients using it. This value, expressed as a proportion (0.40) is our estimate of P_1, the proportion of successes believed to exist for the standard drug. You have specified a delta value of 0.20, meaning that you will consider the test drug to be of interest if its proportion of successes, P_2, is 0.60 ($P_1 + 0.20$). Here is how to use Table A.7 in this case:

1. Find the subtable headed "$P_1 = 0.40$." This is Table A.7h. The table consists of two six-column segments. In the left-hand segment, column 1, find the four rows for $P_2 = 0.60$.

2. Table A.7 is a two-tailed table, but in this example, you wish to run a one-tailed test. That is, you will not be interested in a significant difference between the two products unless your test product is *superior* to the standard. To use Table A.7 as a one-tailed table, simply multiply your specified value of alpha by 2, and use the result in entering the table (remember, your actual alpha will still be 0.05).

3. The fourth row under the label $P_2 = 0.60$ is the alpha = 0.10 row. Follow this row across to the column labeled 0.10 for beta, where you will find 115 for the appropriate sample size to use for each of the two treatment groups.

A.1.3 BASIC Programs

Nelson's Program for Michael's Normality Test (Program AP.1)
This is a modification of a program by Dr. Lloyd S. Nelson (*Journal of Quality Technology*, 21, 213–215, 1989). It is described in some detail in the Appendix to Chapter 14 and an example is given. It is used here with the kind permission of the American Society for Quality Control of Milwaukee, and of Dr. Nelson. It is based upon a paper by John R. Michael [see reference (21), Chapter 14].

Wilcoxon's Rank Sum Test (Program AP.2)
This program was written by the author. It carries out the Wilcoxon Rank Sum test for two independent groups of data, usually representing two groups of patients assigned to two different treatments, such as two drugs. It uses a normal approximation to calculate a Z value and a fifth-order polynomial to approximate the normal distribution and obtain a probability, obviating the necessity of using a normal table. If the total number of data is 15 or 20 or more, and if the numbers of data in the two groups are not too

disparate, its resulting probabilities, although approximations, are quite accurate to two or three places.

Of course, you can obtain a still more accurate result if your sample sizes are within the commonly tabulated range (usually a maximum of 25 for each group). To do so, you can run the program, then, using the rank sum values obtained, refer to one of the Wilcoxon tables appearing in any of several of the references in the Bibliography. Such tables can be found in Hollander and Wolfe [43] and Snedecor and Cochran [38], among others. Or you can modify the program to print out the Z value (this is an approximation because the ranks are discontinuous) and then compare it with Z in any table of the normal distribution. Two very convenient normal tables, one one-tailed and the other two-tailed, are given in the Appendix to Colton [20].

Because the final probabilities given by this program are based upon normal approximations, it is most useful when you have a large sample size. Not only are there no conveniently available tables for such cases (greater than 25 data in one or both groups), but it is difficult and slow to rank two combined groups totaling 20 or 25 data without error. The program, of course, does this easily and very rapidly on any reasonably fast desktop micro. On my machine, the entire computation with the exception of the printout for an example using groups of 12 and 35 data given by Conover [39] pages 218–220, requires less than 1 second. The printing takes much longer —about 8 seconds on a laser printer.

Logistic Approximation to Normal Distribution (Program AP.3)

I wrote this BASIC program as a convenient and rapid method for obtaining either probabilities or Z values. It uses a logistic approximation rather than the methods used in the Wilcoxon program, and can be very useful. Its principal drawback, as mentioned in what follows, is that its degree of approximation extends only to about two decimal places for Z. See the last paragraph under the description of programs AC.1 and AC.2 in the next section for more information.

A.1.4 Hewlett-Packard Calculator Programs

Normal Probabilities (HP-42S Programs, Numbers AC.1 and AC.2)

I wrote these two programs to supply you with a convenient and rapid method of obtaining normal probability values, provided you have a Hewlett-Packard 42S (c) pocket scientific calculator.

Although the programs are written to give normal probabilities (areas under the standard normal curve between definite limits), it is quite easy to use them to obtain the corresponding Z values. The first of the two, NORMPR, is the main program, and the one you load and use to get a probability, given a value of Z. The second, AREA, is called and used as a subroutine by the first. Actually, the AREA program can be used alone. However, it is more convenient to use NORMPR.

The area obtained by NORMPR closely approximates that under the upper tail, and has a positive sign. The area is really a definite integral with limits consisting of the appropriate one-tailed Z value as the lower limit (LLIM) and a value of any constant greater than about 3 or 4 as the upper limit (ULIM). Of course, at the tail of a standard normal curve, the true upper limit is at infinity. However, *most* of the area under the curve is subtended when you reach an upper limit as small as 5, although I customarily use 10. You can use larger values, but you will see little difference in the probability values obtained if you do so and you are rounding them to, say, three places, and you will slow down the computation a bit. On the other hand, for safety, do not use values less than 5.

When starting the NORMPR program, you must enter upper and lower limits and an accuracy factor, called ACC. The calculator divides the total area into small segments, calculates the area of each, and adds them. ACC is the size of each such segment, expressed as a fraction of the total. A value of 0.001 is satisfactory for probabilities to three places. The value of the upper limit, if it is 20 or less, does not affect the speed of the calculation very much, nor does the accuracy factor. For example, with a value of ACC of 0.001, the calculation requires about 8 seconds; a value of 0.00001 requires about 16.

NORMPR is used as follows, after entering it into the calculator:

1. Start the program by pressing the orange function button on the HP-42S, and then the integral key ($\int$). A menu is displayed, showing any programs you may have stored in the calculator's memory.[6] The menu items replace the top-row key functions, as long as they are displayed. Press the key under NORM in the menu (the LOG key).[7]

2. A second menu is displayed by the program, showing LLIM, ULIM, ACC, and X above the first four of the top row of keys. Key in your upper limit, for example, key in 1.645, and then press the key directly below LLIM.

3. Repeat step 2 to enter the ULIM (say, 10) and the ACC (I use 0.001). Then press X, the last menu item.

4. A third menu appears. The last item, at the far right, is an integral sign. Press the key below it twice. In about 8 seconds, the probability, (0.0500) will appear (this example assumes that you have set the number of decimal places to four).

---

[6]The memory is nonvolatile, that is, data or programs stored in it do not disappear when the calculator is shut off, as long as the batteries are good.
[7]If there are more menu items that can be displayed in one row, there is provision for accessing additional rows.

5. To get a Z value using a known probability, try several Z values successively, "zeroing in" on Z (the one that yields the given probability). This can be done quite rapidly.

6. After you have made one calculation, you can make additional ones without restarting the program. Enter any new limits or ACC factors on the last menu, and then press the integral sign on that menu (on the display above the XEQ key) once. For example, if you wish to use the same upper limit and accuracy factor, just key in a new lower limit and press the integral sign key.

If you wish to program the calculator, there is a more convenient approximation procedure that was used in the BASIC program AP.3 described earlier. It will calculate approximations to either Z or the probability directly. Its major disadvantage is that it is accurate only to about two decimal places for Z (which, however, will often be adequate in sample size calculations). It uses a logistic approximation to the normal distribution. See the references to Page and to Tiemstra [references (11) and (12)] at the end of Chapter 14. Z, the abscissa value for the standard normal distribution at the point where measurement y occurs, is defined as $(y_i - \bar{y})/s_{y_i}$. To calculate Z when P is known, the equations for use in such a program are

$$u = \ln \left[P/(1 - P) \right]$$
$$v = -7u$$
$$w = 67/9$$
$$s = \sqrt{v^2 + w^3}$$
$$Z = (s - v)^{1/3} - (s + v)^{1/3}$$

and to calculate P, the tail area or probability at point Z when Z is known:

$$u = Z(3Z^2 + 67)/42$$
$$P = e^u/(e^u + 1)$$

A.2   TABLES AND PROGRAMS

The following tables are discussed in the foregoing sections.

Table A.1. Two-Tailed Probability Points for Student's *t* Distribution

| df | \multicolumn{7}{c}{Probability} | | | | | | |
	0.1	0.05	0.02	0.01	0.005	0.002	0.001
1	6.314	12.706	31.821	63.657	127.32	318.31	636.62
2	2.920	4.303	6.965	9.925	14.089	22.327	31.598
3	2.353	3.182	4.541	5.841	7.453	10.214	12.924
4	2.132	2.776	3.747	4.604	5.598	7.173	8.610
5	2.015	2.571	3.365	4.032	4.773	5.893	6.869
6	1.943	2.447	3.143	3.707	4.317	5.208	5.959
7	1.895	2.365	2.998	3.499	4.029	4.785	5.408
8	1.860	2.306	2.896	3.355	3.833	4.501	5.041
9	1.833	2.262	2.821	3.250	3.690	4.297	4.781
10	1.812	2.228	2.764	3.169	3.581	4.144	4.587
11	1.796	2.201	2.718	3.106	3.497	4.025	4.437
12	1.782	2.179	2.681	3.055	3.428	3.930	4.318
13	1.771	2.160	2.650	3.012	3.372	3.852	4.221
14	1.761	2.145	2.624	2.977	3.326	3.787	4.140
15	1.753	2.131	2.602	2.947	3.286	3.733	4.073
16	1.746	2.120	2.583	2.921	3.252	3.686	4.015
17	1.740	2.110	2.567	2.898	3.222	3.646	3.965
18	1.734	2.101	2.552	2.878	3.197	3.610	3.922
19	1.729	2.093	2.539	2.861	3.174	3.579	3.883
20	1.725	2.086	2.528	2.845	3.153	3.552	3.850
21	1.721	2.080	2.518	2.831	3.135	3.527	3.819
22	1.717	2.074	2.508	2.819	3.119	3.505	3.792
23	1.714	2.069	2.500	2.807	3.104	3.485	3.767
24	1.711	2.064	2.492	2.797	3.091	3.467	3.745
25	1.708	2.060	2.485	2.787	3.078	3.450	3.725
26	1.706	2.056	2.479	2.779	3.067	3.435	3.707
27	1.703	2.052	2.473	2.771	3.057	3.421	3.690
28	1.701	2.048	2.467	2.763	3.047	3.408	3.674
29	1.699	2.045	2.462	2.756	3.038	3.396	3.659
30	1.697	2.042	2.457	2.750	3.030	3.385	3.646
40	1.684	2.02	2.423	2.704	2.971	3.307	3.551
60	1.671	2.000	2.390	2.660	2.915	3.232	3.460
120	1.658	1.980	2.358	2.617	2.860	3.160	3.373
∞	1.645	1.960	2.326	2.576	2.807	3.090	3.291

Table A.2. Abbreviated Chi-Squared Table

df	Probability				
	0.001	0.005	0.010	0.025	0.050
1	10.828	7.879	6.635	5.024	3.841
2	13.816	10.597	9.210	7.378	5.991
3	16.266	12.838	11.345	9.348	7.815
4	18.467	14.860	13.277	11.143	9.488
5	20.515	16.750	15.086	12.833	11.071

Source: From E. S. Pearson and H. O. Hartley, *Biometrika Tables for Statisticians*, *Volume I*, Third Edition (1966), corrections, 1976. Published by the Biometrika Trust. Reprinted with permission of the Biometrika Trustees, London, England.

Table A.3a. Sample Sizes (Numbers of Observations per Group) for a Two-Tailed Independent _t_ Test for the Comparison of Two Means[1] (Alpha = 0.01)

Delta/Sigma	Beta = 0.01	Beta = 0.05	Beta = 0.10	Beta = 0.20
0.05				
0.10				
0.15				
0.20				
0.25				
0.30				
0.35				
0.40				
0.45				118
0.50				96
0.55			101	79
0.60		101	85	67
0.65		87	73	57
0.70	100	75	63	50
0.75	88	66	55	44
0.80	77	58	49	39
0.85	69	51	43	35
0.90	62	46	39	31
0.95	55	42	35	28
1.00	50	38	32	26
1.1	42	32	27	22
1.2	36	27	23	18
1.3	31	23	20	16
1.4	27	20	17	14
1.5	24	18	15	13
1.6	21	16	14	11
1.7	19	15	13	10
1.8	17	13	11	10
1.9	16	12	11	9
2.0	14	11	10	8
2.1	13	10	9	8
2.2	12	10	8	7
2.3	11	9	8	7
2.4	11	9	8	6
2.5	10	8	7	6
3.0	8	6	6	5
3.5	6	5	5	4
4.0	6	5	4	4

[1]Divide alpha by 2 for a one-tailed test.

Source: Tables A.3a through A.3d reprinted from Owen L. Davies, _The Design and Analysis of Industrial Experiments_, Second Edition (1956), Longman House, Essex, England, with permission of the copyright owner, Longman Group UK, Limited, Harlow, Essex, England.

Table A.3b. Sample Sizes (Numbers of Observations per Group) for a Two-Tailed Independent t Test for the Comparison of Two Means[1] (Alpha = 0.02)

Delta/Sigma	Beta = 0.01	Beta = 0.05	Beta = 0.10	Beta = 0.20
0.05				
0.10				
0.15				
0.20				
0.25				
0.30				
0.35				
0.40				
0.45				101
0.50			106	82
0.55		106	88	68
0.60		90	74	58
0.65	104	77	64	49
0.70	90	66	55	43
0.75	79	58	48	38
0.80	70	51	43	33
0.85	62	46	38	30
0.90	55	41	34	27
0.95	50	37	31	24
1.00	45	33	28	22
1.1	38	28	23	19
1.2	32	24	20	16
1.3	28	21	17	14
1.4	24	18	15	12
1.5	21	16	14	11
1.6	19	14	12	10
1.7	17	13	11	9
1.8	15	12	10	8
1.9	14	11	9	8
2.0	13	10	9	7
2.1	12	9	8	7
2.2	11	9	7	6
2.3	10	8	7	6
2.4	10	8	7	6
2.5	9	7	6	5
3.0	7	6	5	4
3.5	6	5	4	4
4.0	5	4	4	3

[1]Divide alpha by 2 for a one-tailed test.

Table A.3c. Sample Sizes (Numbers of Observations per Group) for a Two-Tailed
Independent t Test for the Comparison of Two Means[1] (Alpha = 0.05)

Delta/Sigma	Beta = 0.01	Beta = 0.05	Beta = 0.10	Beta = 0.20
0.05				
0.10				
0.15				
0.20				
0.25				
0.30				
0.35				
0.40				100
0.45			105	79
0.50		106	86	64
0.55		87	71	53
0.60	104	74	60	45
0.65	88	63	51	39
0.70	76	55	44	34
0.75	67	48	39	29
0.80	59	42	34	26
0.85	52	37	31	23
0.90	47	34	27	21
0.95	42	30	25	19
1.00	38	27	23	17
1.1	32	23	19	14
1.2	27	20	16	12
1.3	23	17	14	11
1.4	20	15	12	10
1.5	18	13	11	9
1.6	16	12	10	8
1.7	14	11	9	7
1.8	13	10	8	6
1.9	12	9	7	6
2.0	11	8	7	6
2.1	10	8	6	5
2.2	9	7	6	5
2.3	9	7	6	5
2.4	8	6	5	4
2.5	8	6	5	4
3.0	6	5	4	4
3.5	5	4	4	3
4.0	4	4	3	

[1]Divide alpha by 2 for a one-tailed test.

Table A.3d. Sample Sizes (Numbers of Observations per Group) for a Two-Tailed Independent t Test for the Comparison of Two Means[1] (Alpha = 0.10)

Delta/Sigma	Beta = 0.01	Beta = 0.05	Beta = 0.10	Beta = 0.20
0.05				
0.10				
0.15				
0.20				
0.25				
0.30				102
0.35				
0.40			108	78
0.45		108	86	62
0.50		88	70	51
0.55	112	73	58	42
0.60	89	61	49	36
0.65	76	52	42	30
0.70	66	45	36	26
0.75	57	40	32	23
0.80	50	35	28	21
0.85	45	31	25	18
0.90	40	28	22	16
0.95	36	25	20	15
1.00	33	23	18	14
1.1	27	19	15	12
1.2	23	16	13	10
1.3	20	14	11	9
1.4	17	12	10	8
1.5	15	11	9	7
1.6	14	10	8	6
1.7	12	9	7	6
1.8	11	8	7	5
1.9	10	7	6	5
2.0	9	7	6	4
2.1	8	6	5	4
2.2	8	6	5	4
2.3	7	5	5	4
2.4	7	5	4	4
2.5	6	5	4	3
3.0	5	4	3	
3.5	4	3		
4.0	4			

[1]Divide alpha by 2 for a one-tailed test.

Table A.4a. Sample Sizes (Numbers of Items) for a Two-Tailed Dependent _t_ Test of a Single Mean vs. a Standard Value (Such as a Test of Differences)[1] (Alpha = 0.01)

Delta/Sigma	Beta = 0.01	Beta = 0.05	Beta = 0.10	Beta = 0.20
0.05				
0.10				
0.15				
0.20				
0.25				
0.30				134
0.35			125	99
0.40		115	97	77
0.45		92	77	62
0.50	100	75	63	51
0.55	83	63	53	42
0.60	71	53	45	36
0.65	61	46	39	31
0.70	53	40	34	28
0.75	47	36	30	25
0.80	41	32	27	22
0.85	37	29	24	20
0.90	34	26	22	18
0.95	31	24	20	17
1.00	28	22	19	16
1.1	24	19	16	14
1.2	21	16	14	12
1.3	18	15	13	11
1.4	16	13	12	10
1.5	15	12	11	9
1.6	13	11	10	8
1.7	12	10	9	8
1.8	12	10	9	8
1.9	11	9	8	7
2.0	10	8	8	7
2.1	10	8	7	7
2.2	9	8	7	6
2.3	9	7	7	6
2.4	8	7	7	6
2.5	8	7	6	6
3.0	7	6	6	5
3.5	6	5	5	
4.0	6			

[1]Divide alpha by 2 for a one-tailed test.

Source: Tables A.4a through A.4d reprinted from Owen L. Davies, _The Design and Analysis of Industrial Experiments_, Second Edition (1956), Longman House, Essex, England, with permission of the copyright owner, Longman Group UK, Limited, Harlow, Essex, England.

Table A.4b. Sample Sizes (Numbers of Items) for a Two-Tailed Dependent t Test of a Single Mean vs. a Standard Value (Such as a Test of Differences)[1] (Alpha = 0.02)

Delta/Sigma	Beta = 0.01	Beta = 0.05	Beta = 0.10	Beta = 0.20
0.05				
0.10				
0.15				
0.20				
0.25				
0.30				115
0.35			109	85
0.40		101	85	66
0.45	110	81	68	53
0.50	90	66	55	43
0.55	75	55	46	36
0.60	63	47	39	31
0.65	55	41	34	27
0.70	47	35	30	24
0.75	42	31	27	21
0.80	37	28	24	19
0.85	33	25	21	17
0.90	29	23	19	16
0.95	27	21	18	14
1.00	25	19	16	13
1.1	21	16	14	12
1.2	18	14	12	10
1.3	16	13	11	9
1.4	14	11	10	9
1.5	13	10	9	8
1.6	12	10	9	7
1.7	11	9	8	7
1.8	10	8	7	7
1.9	10	8	7	6
2.0	9	7	7	6
2.1	8	7	6	6
2.2	8	7	6	5
2.3	8	6	6	
2.4	7	6	6	
2.5	7	6	6	
3.0	6	5	5	
3.5	5			
4.0				

[1]Divide alpha by 2 for a one-tailed test.

Table A.4c. Sample Sizes (Numbers of Items) for a Two-Tailed Dependent *t* Test of a Single Mean vs. a Standard Value (Such as a Test of Differences)[1] (Alpha = 0.05)

Delta/Sigma	Beta = 0.01	Beta = 0.05	Beta = 0.10	Beta = 0.20
0.05				
0.10				
0.15				
0.20				
0.25				128
0.30			119	90
0.35		109	88	67
0.40	117	84	68	51
0.45	93	67	54	41
0.50	76	54	44	34
0.55	63	45	37	28
0.60	53	38	32	24
0.65	46	33	27	21
0.70	40	29	24	19
0.75	35	26	21	16
0.80	31	22	19	15
0.85	28	21	17	13
0.90	25	19	16	12
0.95	23	17	14	11
1.00	21	16	13	10
1.1	18	13	11	9
1.2	15	12	10	8
1.3	14	10	9	7
1.4	12	9	8	7
1.5	11	8	7	6
1.6	10	8	7	6
1.7	9	7	6	5
1.8	8	7	6	
1.9	8	6	6	
2.0	7	6	5	
2.1	7	6		
2.2	7	6		
2.3	6	5		
2.4	6			
2.5	6			
3.0	5			
3.5				
4.0				

[1]Divide alpha by 2 for a one-tailed test.

Table A.4d. Sample Sizes (Numbers of Items) for a Two-Tailed Dependent _t_ Test of a Single Mean vs. a Standard Value (Such as a Test of Differences)[1] (Alpha = 0.10)

Delta/Sigma	Beta = 0.01	Beta = 0.05	Beta = 0.10	Beta = 0.20
0.05				
0.10				
0.15				
0.20				
0.25			139	101
0.30		122	97	71
0.35		90	72	52
0.40	101	70	55	40
0.45	80	55	44	33
0.50	65	45	36	27
0.55	54	38	30	22
0.60	46	32	26	19
0.65	39	28	22	17
0.70	34	24	19	15
0.75	30	21	17	13
0.80	27	19	15	12
0.85	24	17	14	11
0.90	21	15	13	10
0.95	19	14	11	9
1.00	18	13	11	8
1.1	15	11	9	7
1.2	13	10	8	6
1.3	11	8	7	6
1.4	10	8	7	5
1.5	9	7	6	
1.6	8	6	6	
1.7	8	6	5	
1.8	7	6		
1.9	7	5		
2.0	6			
2.1	6			
2.2	6			
2.3	5			
2.4				
2.5				
3.0				
3.5				
4.0				

[1]Divide alpha by 2 for a one-tailed test.

Table A.5. Abbreviated Table of Z Values (Normal Distribution)

Probability	Z Value	
	Upper Tail	Two Tail
0.005	2.576	2.807
0.010	2.326	2.576
0.025	1.960	2.241
0.050	1.645	1.960
0.100	1.281	1.645
0.200	0.842	1.281

Table A.6a. Sample Size per Treatment Group for Specified Alpha and Beta Risks in One-Factor Univariate ANOVA (Alpha = 0.01)

Delta over Sigma	Number of Levels of the Factor	Beta		
		0.05	0.10	0.20
1.00	2	38	32	26
	3	43	37	30
	4	47	40	33
	5	51	43	35
	6	53	46	38
1.25	2	25	21	17
	3	29	24	20
	4	31	27	22
	5	33	28	23
	6	35	30	25
1.50	2	18	15	13
	3	20	18	14
	4	22	19	16
	5	23	20	17
	6	25	21	18
1.75	2	14	12	10
	3	16	13	11
	4	17	15	12
	5	18	15	13
	6	19	16	13
2.00	2	11	10	8
	3	12	11	9
	4	13	12	10
	5	14	12	10
	6	15	13	11
2.50	2	8	7	6
	3	9	8	7
	4	9	8	7
	5	10	9	7
	6	10	9	8
3.00	2	6	6	5
	3	7	6	5
	4	7	6	5
	5	7	7	6
	6	8	7	6

Source: Tables A.6a through A.6c from T. L. Bratcher, M. A. Moran and W. J. Zimmer, "Tables of Sample Sizes in the Analysis of Variance," *Journal of Quality Technology*, 2, No. 3, 159–163 (July 1970). Reprinted with the permission of The American Society for Quality Control.

**Table A.6b. Sample Size per Treatment Group for Specified Alpha and
Beta Risks on One-Factor Univariate ANOVA (Alpha = 0.05)**

Delta over Sigma	Number of Levels of the Factor	Beta 0.05	Beta 0.10	Beta 0.20
1.00	2	27	23	17
	3	32	27	21
	4	36	30	23
	5	39	32	25
	6	41	34	27
1.25	2	18	15	12
	3	21	18	14
	4	23	20	15
	5	25	21	17
	6	27	23	18
1.50	2	13	11	9
	3	15	13	10
	4	17	14	11
	5	18	15	12
	6	19	16	13
1.75	2	10	8	7
	3	12	10	8
	4	13	11	9
	5	14	12	9
	6	14	12	10
2.00	2	8	7	6
	3	9	8	6
	4	10	9	7
	5	11	9	7
	6	11	10	8
2.50	2	6	5	4
	3	7	6	5
	4	7	6	5
	5	7	6	5
	6	8	7	6
3.00	2	5	4	4
	3	5	5	4
	4	5	5	4
	5	6	5	4
	6	6	5	4

Table A.6c. Sample Size per Treatment Group for Specified Alpha and Beta Risks in One-Factor Univariate ANOVA (Alpha = 0.10)

Delta over Sigma	Number of Levels of the Factor	Beta 0.05	Beta 0.10	Beta 0.20
1.00	2	23	18	14
	3	27	22	17
	4	30	25	19
	5	33	27	21
	6	35	29	22
1.25	2	15	12	9
	3	18	15	11
	4	20	16	13
	5	22	18	14
	6	23	19	15
1.50	2	11	9	7
	3	13	11	8
	4	14	12	9
	5	15	13	10
	6	16	14	11
1.75	2	8	7	5
	3	10	8	6
	4	11	9	7
	5	12	10	8
	6	12	10	8
2.00	2	7	6	4
	3	8	7	5
	4	9	7	6
	5	9	8	6
	6	10	8	7
2.50	2	5	4	3
	3	6	5	4
	4	6	5	4
	5	6	5	4
	6	7	6	5
3.00	2	4	3	3
	3	4	4	3
	4	5	4	3
	5	5	4	4
	6	5	4	4

Table A.7a. Binomial Sample Size for Each of Two Independent Proportions, Two-Tailed Test ($P_1 = 0.05$)

P_2	Alpha	Beta 0.01	0.05	0.10	0.20	P_2	Alpha	Beta 0.01	0.05	0.10	0.20
0.10	0.01	1368	1025	863	686	0.55	0.01	38	30	26	22
	0.02	1235	911	760	595		0.02	35	27	23	19
	0.05	1054	758	621	474		0.05	30	23	19	16
	0.10	910	637	513	381		0.10	26	19	16	13
0.15	0.01	447	337	285	228	0.60	0.01	32	26	22	19
	0.02	404	300	252	199		0.02	29	23	20	17
	0.05	345	251	207	160		0.05	25	19	16	14
	0.10	299	212	172	130		0.10	22	16	14	11
0.20	0.01	241	183	155	125	0.65	0.01	28	22	19	16
	0.02	218	163	137	109		0.02	25	20	17	14
	0.05	187	136	113	88		0.05	21	16	14	12
	0.10	162	115	94	72		0.10	18	14	12	10
0.25	0.01	157	120	102	83	0.70	0.01	23	19	17	14
	0.02	142	107	90	72		0.02	21	17	15	13
	0.05	122	90	75	58		0.05	18	14	12	10
	0.10	106	76	62	48		0.10	16	12	10	9
0.30	0.01	113	87	74	60	0.75	0.01	20	16	15	13
	0.02	102	77	66	53		0.02	18	15	13	11
	0.05	88	65	54	43		0.05	15	12	11	9
	0.10	76	55	45	35		0.10	13	10	9	7
0.35	0.01	86	66	57	46	0.80	0.01	17	14	13	11
	0.02	78	59	50	41		0.02	15	13	11	10
	0.05	67	50	42	33		0.05	13	10	9	8
	0.10	58	42	35	27		0.10	11	9	8	7
0.40	0.01	68	53	45	37	0.85	0.01	15	12	11	10
	0.02	62	47	40	33		0.02	13	11	10	8
	0.05	53	39	33	27		0.05	11	9	8	7
	0.10	46	34	28	22		0.10	9	8	7	6
0.45	0.01	55	43	37	31	0.90	0.01	12	10	9	8
	0.02	50	38	33	27		0.02	11	9	8	7
	0.05	43	32	27	22		0.05	9	8	7	6
	0.10	37	27	23	18		0.10	8	6	6	5
0.50	0.01	46	36	31	26	0.95	0.01	10	9	8	7
	0.02	41	32	27	23		0.02	9	8	7	7
	0.05	35	27	23	18		0.05	8	6	6	5
	0.10	31	23	19	15		0.10	6	5	5	4

Source: Tables A.7a through A.7r adapted from Joseph L. Fleiss, *Statistical Methods for Rates and Proportions*, Second Edition, copyright © 1981 by John Wiley & Sons, Inc. Reprinted by permission of Wiley-Liss, a division of John Wiley & Sons, Inc.

Table A.7b. Binomial Sample Size for Each of Two Independent Proportions, Two-Tailed Test ($P_1 = 0.10$)

P_2	Alpha	Beta				P_2	Alpha	Beta			
		0.01	0.05	0.10	0.20			0.01	0.05	0.10	0.20
0.15	0.01	2137	1595	1340	1060	0.60	0.01	42	33	28	24
	0.02	1928	1416	1176	916		0.02	38	29	25	21
	0.05	1642	1174	957	725		0.05	32	24	21	17
	0.10	1415	984	787	579		0.10	28	21	17	14
0.20	0.01	627	471	397	316	0.65	0.01	35	27	24	20
	0.02	566	419	349	274		0.02	31	24	21	18
	0.05	483	348	286	219		0.05	27	20	18	14
	0.10	417	293	236	176		0.10	23	17	15	12
0.25	0.01	316	238	202	162	0.70	0.01	29	23	20	17
	0.02	285	212	178	140		0.02	26	21	18	15
	0.05	244	177	146	113		0.05	22	17	15	12
	0.10	211	149	121	91		0.10	19	15	13	10
0.30	0.01	196	149	126	102	0.75	0.01	25	20	17	15
	0.02	178	133	112	89		0.02	22	18	15	13
	0.05	152	111	92	71		0.05	19	15	13	11
	0.10	131	94	76	58		0.10	16	13	11	9
0.35	0.01	136	104	88	72	0.80	0.01	21	17	15	13
	0.02	123	93	78	62		0.02	19	15	13	11
	0.05	105	77	64	50		0.05	16	13	11	9
	0.10	91	65	54	41		0.10	14	11	9	8
0.40	0.01	101	77	66	54	0.85	0.01	18	14	13	11
	0.02	91	69	58	47		0.02	16	13	11	10
	0.05	78	58	48	38		0.05	13	11	9	8
	0.10	68	49	40	31		0.10	11	9	8	7
0.45	0.01	78	60	51	42	0.90	0.01	15	12	11	10
	0.02	71	54	46	37		0.02	13	11	10	9
	0.05	60	45	38	30		0.05	11	9	8	7
	0.10	52	38	31	24		0.10	10	8	7	6
0.50	0.01	62	48	41	34	0.95	0.01	12	10	9	8
	0.02	56	43	37	30		0.02	11	9	8	7
	0.05	48	36	30	24		0.05	9	8	7	6
	0.10	42	30	25	20		0.10	8	6	6	5
0.55	0.01	51	39	34	28						
	0.02	46	35	30	25						
	0.05	39	29	25	20						
	0.10	34	25	21	16						

Table A.7c. Binomial Sample Size for Each of Two Independent Proportions, Two-Tailed Test ($P_1 = 0.15$)

P_2	Alpha	Beta 0.01	0.05	0.10	0.20	P_2	Alpha	Beta 0.01	0.05	0.10	0.20
0.20	0.01	2810	2094	1756	1388	0.60	0.01	54	42	36	30
	0.02	2534	1858	1541	1198		0.02	49	37	32	26
	0.05	2157	1538	1252	945		0.05	42	31	26	21
	0.10	1856	1287	1027	753		0.10	36	27	22	17
0.25	0.01	783	586	494	392	0.65	0.01	44	34	30	25
	0.02	707	521	434	340		0.02	40	31	26	22
	0.05	603	433	354	270		0.05	34	26	22	18
	0.10	520	363	292	216		0.10	29	22	18	15
0.30	0.01	380	286	241	193	0.70	0.01	36	29	25	21
	0.02	343	254	213	167		0.02	33	26	22	18
	0.05	293	212	174	134		0.05	28	21	18	15
	0.10	253	178	144	108		0.10	24	18	15	12
0.35	0.01	229	173	147	118	0.75	0.01	30	24	21	18
	0.02	207	154	130	102		0.02	27	21	19	16
	0.05	177	129	106	82		0.05	23	18	15	13
	0.10	153	109	88	67		0.10	20	15	13	10
0.40	0.01	155	118	100	81	0.80	0.01	25	20	18	15
	0.02	140	105	89	70		0.02	23	18	16	13
	0.05	120	88	73	57		0.05	19	15	13	11
	0.10	104	74	60	46		0.10	17	13	11	9
0.45	0.01	113	86	73	60	0.85	0.01	21	17	15	13
	0.02	102	77	65	52		0.02	19	15	13	11
	0.05	87	64	53	42		0.05	16	13	11	9
	0.10	75	54	44	34		0.10	14	11	9	8
0.50	0.01	86	66	56	46	0.90	0.01	18	14	13	11
	0.02	78	59	50	40		0.02	16	13	11	10
	0.05	66	49	41	32		0.05	13	11	9	8
	0.10	57	42	34	26		0.10	11	9	8	7
0.55	0.01	67	52	45	37	0.95	0.01	15	12	11	10
	0.02	61	46	39	32		0.02	13	11	10	8
	0.05	52	39	33	26		0.05	11	9	8	7
	0.10	45	33	27	21		0.10	9	8	7	6

Table A.7d. Binomial Sample Size for Each of Two Independent Proportions, Two-Tailed Test ($P_1 = 0.20$)

P_2	Alpha	Beta				P_2	Alpha	Beta			
		0.01	0.05	0.10	0.20			0.01	0.05	0.10	0.20
0.25	0.01	3386	2522	2114	1668	0.65	0.01	56	44	38	31
	0.02	3053	2236	1853	1438		0.02	51	39	33	27
	0.05	2597	1850	1504	1134		0.05	44	33	27	22
	0.10	2235	1547	1233	901		0.10	38	28	23	18
0.30	0.01	915	685	576	456	0.70	0.01	46	36	31	25
	0.02	826	608	506	395		0.02	41	32	27	22
	0.05	704	504	412	313		0.05	35	26	22	18
	0.10	607	423	339	250		0.10	30	22	19	15
0.35	0.01	433	325	274	219	0.75	0.01	37	29	25	21
	0.02	391	289	242	190		0.02	34	26	23	19
	0.05	334	240	197	151		0.05	29	22	19	15
	0.10	288	202	163	122		0.10	25	18	16	12
0.40	0.01	256	193	164	131	0.80	0.01	31	24	21	18
	0.02	232	172	144	114		0.02	28	22	19	16
	0.05	198	143	118	91		0.05	23	18	16	13
	0.10	171	121	98	74		0.10	20	15	13	11
0.45	0.01	171	129	110	88	0.85	0.01	25	20	18	15
	0.02	154	115	97	77		0.02	23	18	16	13
	0.05	132	96	79	62		0.05	19	15	13	11
	0.10	114	81	66	50		0.10	17	13	11	9
0.50	0.01	122	93	79	64	0.90	0.01	21	17	15	13
	0.02	110	83	70	56		0.02	19	15	13	11
	0.05	94	69	57	45		0.05	16	13	11	9
	0.10	82	58	48	37		0.10	14	11	9	8
0.55	0.01	92	70	60	49	0.95	0.01	17	14	13	11
	0.02	83	63	53	43		0.02	15	13	11	10
	0.05	71	52	44	34		0.05	13	10	9	8
	0.10	61	44	36	28		0.10	11	9	8	7
0.60	0.01	71	55	47	38						
	0.02	64	49	42	34						
	0.05	55	41	34	27						
	0.10	47	35	29	22						

Table A.7e. Binomial Sample Size for Each of Two Independent Proportions, Two-Tailed Test ($P_1 = 0.25$)

P_2	Alpha	Beta 0.01	0.05	0.10	0.20	P_2	Alpha	Beta 0.01	0.05	0.10	0.20
0.30	0.01	3867	2878	2411	1902	0.65	0.01	73	56	48	39
	0.02	3486	2552	2114	1639		0.02	66	50	43	34
	0.05	2965	2110	1714	1291		0.05	57	42	35	28
	0.10	2550	1764	1404	1025		0.10	49	36	29	23
0.35	0.01	1023	765	643	509	0.70	0.01	58	45	38	32
	0.02	923	679	564	440		0.02	52	40	34	28
	0.05	786	563	459	348		0.05	44	33	28	22
	0.10	678	472	378	278		0.10	38	28	23	18
0.40	0.01	476	357	301	240	0.75	0.01	46	36	31	26
	0.02	430	317	265	207		0.02	42	32	27	22
	0.05	366	264	216	165		0.05	35	27	23	18
	0.10	316	221	178	133		0.10	31	23	19	15
0.45	0.01	278	209	177	141	0.80	0.01	37	29	25	21
	0.02	251	186	156	123		0.02	34	26	23	19
	0.05	214	155	127	98		0.05	29	22	19	15
	0.10	185	130	105	79		0.10	25	18	16	12
0.50	0.01	182	138	117	94	0.85	0.01	30	24	21	18
	0.02	165	123	103	82		0.02	27	21	19	16
	0.05	141	102	85	65		0.05	23	18	15	13
	0.10	121	86	70	53		0.10	20	15	13	10
0.55	0.01	129	98	83	67	0.90	0.01	25	20	17	15
	0.02	117	87	74	59		0.02	22	18	15	13
	0.05	99	73	60	47		0.05	19	15	13	11
	0.10	86	61	50	38		0.10	16	13	11	9
0.60	0.01	96	73	62	51	0.95	0.01	20	16	15	13
	0.02	86	65	55	44		0.02	18	15	13	11
	0.05	74	54	45	36		0.05	15	12	11	9
	0.10	64	46	38	29		0.10	13	10	9	7

Table A.7f. Binomial Sample Size for Each of Two Independent Proportions, Two-Tailed Test ($P_1 = 0.30$)

P_2	Alpha	Beta 0.01	0.05	0.10	0.20	P_2	Alpha	Beta 0.01	0.05	0.10	0.20
0.35	0.01	4251	3163	2650	2089	0.70	0.01	74	57	49	40
	0.02	3832	2804	2322	1800		0.02	67	51	43	35
	0.05	3259	2318	1882	1416		0.05	57	42	36	28
	0.10	2803	1937	1541	1124		0.10	49	36	30	23
0.40	0.01	1108	827	695	550	0.75	0.01	58	45	38	32
	0.02	999	734	610	475		0.02	52	40	34	28
	0.05	851	608	496	376		0.05	44	33	28	22
	0.10	733	510	408	300		0.10	38	28	23	18
0.45	0.01	508	381	321	255	0.80	0.01	46	36	31	25
	0.02	459	338	282	221		0.02	41	32	27	22
	0.05	391	281	230	175		0.05	35	26	22	18
	0.10	337	236	190	141		0.10	30	22	19	15
0.50	0.01	293	220	186	149	0.85	0.01	36	29	25	21
	0.02	264	196	164	129		0.02	33	26	22	18
	0.05	225	163	134	103		0.05	28	21	18	15
	0.10	194	137	111	83		0.10	24	18	15	12
0.55	0.01	190	144	122	98	0.90	0.01	29	23	20	17
	0.02	172	128	107	85		0.02	26	21	18	15
	0.05	147	106	88	68		0.05	22	17	15	12
	0.10	127	90	73	55		0.10	19	15	13	10
0.60	0.01	133	101	86	69	0.95	0.01	23	19	17	14
	0.02	120	90	76	60		0.02	21	17	15	13
	0.05	103	75	62	48		0.05	18	14	12	10
	0.10	89	63	52	39		0.10	16	12	10	9
0.65	0.01	98	75	64	52						
	0.02	88	66	56	45						
	0.05	75	55	46	36						
	0.10	65	47	38	30						

Table A.7g. Binomial Sample Size for Each of Two Independent Proportions, Two-Tailed Test ($P_1 = 0.35$)

P_2	Alpha	Beta				P_2	Alpha	Beta			
		0.01	0.05	0.10	0.20			0.01	0.05	0.10	0.20
0.40	0.01	4540	3377	2828	2229	0.70	0.01	98	75	64	52
	0.02	4092	2993	2478	1920		0.02	88	66	56	45
	0.05	3479	2474	2008	1511		0.05	75	55	46	36
	0.10	2992	2067	1644	1198		0.10	65	47	38	30
0.45	0.01	1168	872	732	579	0.75	0.01	73	56	48	39
	0.02	1053	774	642	500		0.02	66	50	43	34
	0.05	897	641	522	395		0.05	57	42	35	28
	0.10	772	537	429	316		0.10	49	36	29	23
0.50	0.01	530	397	334	265	0.80	0.01	56	44	38	31
	0.02	478	352	294	230		0.02	51	39	33	27
	0.05	407	293	239	182		0.05	44	33	27	22
	0.10	351	246	197	146		0.10	38	28	23	18
0.55	0.01	302	227	192	153	0.85	0.01	44	34	30	25
	0.02	272	202	169	133		0.02	40	31	26	22
	0.05	232	168	138	106		0.05	34	26	22	18
	0.10	200	141	114	85		0.10	29	22	18	15
0.60	0.01	194	147	124	100	0.90	0.01	35	27	24	20
	0.02	175	130	109	87		0.02	31	24	21	18
	0.05	149	109	90	69		0.05	27	20	18	14
	0.10	129	91	74	56		0.10	23	17	15	12
0.65	0.01	134	102	87	70	0.95	0.01	28	22	19	16
	0.02	121	91	76	61		0.02	25	20	17	14
	0.05	104	76	63	49		0.05	21	16	14	12
	0.10	89	64	52	40		0.10	18	14	12	10

Table A.7h. Binomial Sample Size for Each of Two Independent Proportions, Two-Tailed Test ($P_1 = 0.40$)

P_2	Alpha	Beta 0.01	0.05	0.10	0.20	P_2	Alpha	Beta 0.01	0.05	0.10	0.20
0.45	0.01	4732	3520	2947	2322	0.75	0.01	96	73	62	51
	0.02	4265	3119	2582	2001		0.02	86	65	55	44
	0.05	3626	2578	2093	1573		0.05	74	54	45	36
	0.10	3118	2153	1713	1248		0.10	64	46	38	29
0.50	0.01	1204	898	754	597	0.80	0.01	71	55	47	38
	0.02	1086	797	662	515		0.02	64	49	42	34
	0.05	924	660	538	407		0.05	55	41	34	27
	0.10	796	553	442	325		0.10	47	35	29	22
0.55	0.01	540	405	341	271	0.85	0.01	54	42	36	30
	0.02	488	359	299	234		0.02	49	37	32	26
	0.05	415	298	244	186		0.05	42	31	26	21
	0.10	358	250	201	149		0.10	36	27	22	17
0.60	0.01	305	229	193	154	0.90	0.01	42	33	28	24
	0.02	275	204	170	134		0.02	38	29	25	21
	0.05	235	169	139	107		0.05	32	24	21	17
	0.10	202	142	115	86		0.10	28	21	17	14
0.65	0.01	194	147	124	100	0.95	0.01	32	26	22	19
	0.02	175	130	109	87		0.02	29	23	20	17
	0.05	149	109	90	69		0.05	25	19	16	14
	0.10	129	91	74	56		0.10	22	16	14	11
0.70	0.01	133	101	86	69						
	0.02	120	90	76	60						
	0.05	103	75	62	48						
	0.10	89	63	52	39						

Table A.7i. Binomial Sample Size for Each of Two Independent Proportions, Two-Tailed Test ($P_1 = 0.45$)

P_2	Alpha	Beta				P_2	Alpha	Beta			
		0.01	0.05	0.10	0.20			0.01	0.05	0.10	0.20
0.50	0.01	4828	3591	3007	2369	0.75	0.01	129	98	83	67
	0.02	4352	3182	2635	2041		0.02	117	87	74	59
	0.05	3700	2630	2135	1605		0.05	99	73	60	47
	0.10	3181	2197	1747	1273		0.10	86	61	50	38
0.55	0.01	1216	907	762	603	0.80	0.01	92	70	60	49
	0.02	1097	805	668	520		0.02	83	63	53	43
	0.05	933	667	543	411		0.05	71	52	44	34
	0.10	804	558	446	328		0.10	61	44	36	28
0.60	0.01	540	405	341	271	0.85	0.01	67	52	45	37
	0.02	488	359	299	234		0.02	61	46	39	32
	0.05	415	298	244	186		0.05	52	39	33	26
	0.10	358	250	201	149		0.10	45	33	27	21
0.65	0.01	302	227	192	153	0.90	0.01	51	39	34	28
	0.02	272	202	169	133		0.02	46	35	30	25
	0.05	232	168	138	106		0.05	39	29	25	20
	0.10	200	141	114	85		0.10	34	25	21	16
0.70	0.01	190	144	122	98	0.95	0.01	38	30	26	22
	0.02	172	128	107	85		0.02	35	27	23	19
	0.05	147	106	88	68		0.05	30	23	19	16
	0.10	127	90	73	55		0.10	26	19	16	13

Table A.7j. Binomial Sample Size for Each of Two Independent Proportions, Two-Tailed Test ($P_1 = 0.50$)

P_2	Alpha	Beta				P_2	Alpha	Beta			
		0.01	0.05	0.10	0.20			0.01	0.05	0.10	0.20
0.55	0.01	4828	3591	3007	2369	0.80	0.01	122	93	79	64
	0.02	4352	3182	2635	2041		0.02	110	83	70	56
	0.05	3700	2630	2135	1605		0.05	94	69	57	45
	0.10	3181	2197	1747	1273		0.10	82	58	48	37
0.60	0.01	1204	898	754	597	0.85	0.01	86	66	56	46
	0.02	1086	797	662	515		0.02	78	59	50	40
	0.05	924	660	538	407		0.05	66	49	41	32
	0.10	796	553	442	325		0.10	57	42	34	26
0.65	0.01	530	397	334	265	0.90	0.01	62	48	41	34
	0.02	478	352	294	230		0.02	56	43	37	30
	0.05	407	293	239	182		0.05	48	36	30	24
	0.10	351	246	197	146		0.10	42	30	25	20
0.70	0.01	293	220	186	149	0.95	0.01	46	36	31	26
	0.02	264	196	164	129		0.02	41	32	27	23
	0.05	225	163	134	103		0.05	35	27	23	18
	0.10	194	137	111	83		0.10	31	23	19	15
0.75	0.01	182	138	117	94						
	0.02	165	123	103	82						
	0.05	141	102	85	65						
	0.10	121	86	70	53						

**Table A.7k. Binomial Sample Size
for Each of Two Independent Proportions,
Two-Tailed Test ($P_1 = 0.55$)**

P_2	Alpha	Beta			
		0.01	0.05	0.10	0.20
0.60	0.01	4732	3520	2047	2322
	0.02	4265	3119	2582	2001
	0.05	3626	2578	2093	1573
	0.10	3118	2153	1713	1248
0.65	0.01	1168	872	732	579
	0.02	1053	774	642	500
	0.05	897	641	522	395
	0.10	772	537	429	316
0.70	0.01	508	381	321	255
	0.02	459	338	282	221
	0.05	391	281	230	175
	0.10	337	236	190	141
0.75	0.01	278	209	177	141
	0.02	251	186	156	123
	0.05	214	155	127	98
	0.10	185	130	105	79
0.80	0.01	171	129	110	88
	0.02	154	115	97	77
	0.05	132	96	79	62
	0.10	114	81	66	50
0.85	0.01	113	86	73	60
	0.02	102	77	65	52
	0.05	87	64	53	42
	0.10	75	54	44	34
0.90	0.01	78	60	51	42
	0.02	71	54	46	37
	0.05	60	45	38	30
	0.10	52	38	31	24
0.95	0.01	55	43	37	31
	0.02	50	38	33	27
	0.05	43	32	27	22
	0.10	37	27	23	18

**Table A.7l. Binomial Sample Size
for Each of Two Independent Proportions,
Two-Tailed Test ($P_1 = 0.60$)**

P₂	Alpha	Beta			
		0.01	0.05	0.10	0.20
0.65	0.01	4540	3377	2828	2229
	0.02	4092	2993	2478	1920
	0.05	3479	2474	2008	1511
	0.10	2992	2067	1644	1198
0.70	0.01	1108	827	695	550
	0.02	999	734	610	475
	0.05	851	608	496	376
	0.10	733	510	408	300
0.75	0.01	476	357	301	240
	0.02	430	317	265	207
	0.05	366	264	216	165
	0.10	316	221	178	133
0.80	0.01	256	193	164	131
	0.02	232	172	144	114
	0.05	198	143	118	91
	0.10	171	121	98	74
0.85	0.01	155	118	100	81
	0.02	140	105	89	70
	0.05	120	88	73	57
	0.10	104	74	60	46
0.90	0.01	101	77	66	54
	0.02	91	69	58	47
	0.05	78	58	48	38
	0.10	68	49	40	31
0.95	0.01	68	53	45	37
	0.02	62	47	40	33
	0.05	53	39	33	27
	0.10	46	34	28	22

Table A.7m. Binomial Sample Size for Each of Two Independent Proportions, Two-Tailed Test ($P_1 = 0.65$)

P_2	Alpha	Beta 0.01	0.05	0.10	0.20
0.70	0.01	4251	3163	2650	2089
	0.02	3833	2804	2322	1800
	0.05	3259	2318	1882	1416
	0.10	2803	1937	1541	1124
0.75	0.01	1023	765	643	509
	0.02	923	679	564	440
	0.05	786	563	459	348
	0.10	678	472	378	278
0.80	0.01	433	325	274	219
	0.02	391	289	242	190
	0.05	334	240	197	151
	0.10	288	202	163	122
0.85	0.01	229	173	147	118
	0.02	207	154	130	102
	0.05	177	129	106	82
	0.10	153	109	88	67
0.90	0.01	136	104	88	72
	0.02	123	93	78	62
	0.05	105	77	64	50
	0.10	91	65	54	41
0.95	0.01	86	66	57	46
	0.02	78	59	50	41
	0.05	67	50	42	33
	0.10	58	42	35	27

**Table A.7n. Binomial Sample Size
for Each of Two Independent Proportions,
Two-Tailed Test ($P_1 = 0.70$)**

P2	Alpha	Beta			
		0.01	0.05	0.10	0.20
0.75	0.01	3867	2878	2411	1902
	0.02	3486	2552	2114	1639
	0.05	2965	2110	1714	1291
	0.10	2550	1764	1404	1025
0.80	0.01	915	685	576	456
	0.02	826	608	506	395
	0.05	704	504	412	313
	0.10	607	423	339	250
0.85	0.01	380	286	241	193
	0.02	343	254	213	167
	0.05	293	212	174	134
	0.10	253	178	144	108
0.90	0.01	196	149	126	102
	0.02	178	133	112	89
	0.05	152	111	92	71
	0.10	131	94	76	58
0.95	0.01	113	87	74	60
	0.02	102	77	66	53
	0.05	88	65	54	43
	0.10	76	55	45	35

**Table A.7o. Binomial Sample Size
for Each of Two Independent Proportions,
Two-Tailed Test ($P_1 = 0.75$)**

P2	Alpha	Beta			
		0.01	0.05	0.10	0.20
0.80	0.01	3386	2522	2114	1668
	0.02	3053	2236	1853	1438
	0.05	2597	1850	1504	1134
	0.10	2235	1547	1233	901
0.85	0.01	783	586	494	392
	0.02	707	521	434	340
	0.05	603	433	354	270
	0.10	520	363	292	216
0.90	0.01	316	238	202	162
	0.02	285	212	178	140
	0.05	244	177	146	113
	0.10	211	149	121	91
0.95	0.01	157	120	102	83
	0.02	142	107	90	72
	0.05	122	90	75	58
	0.10	106	76	62	48

Table A.7p. Binomial Sample Size for Each of Two Independent Proportions, Two-Tailed Test ($P_1 = 0.80$)

P_2	Alpha	Beta			
		0.01	0.05	0.10	0.20
0.85	0.01	2810	2094	1756	1388
	0.02	2534	1858	1541	1198
	0.05	2157	1538	1252	945
	0.10	1856	1287	1027	753
0.90	0.01	627	471	397	316
	0.02	566	419	349	274
	0.05	483	348	286	219
	0.10	417	293	236	176
0.95	0.01	241	183	155	125
	0.02	218	163	137	109
	0.05	187	136	113	88
	0.10	162	115	94	72

Table A.7q. Binomial Sample Size for Each of Two Independent Proportions, Two-Tailed Test ($P_1 = 0.85$)

P_2	Alpha	Beta			
		0.01	0.05	0.10	0.20
0.90	0.01	2137	1595	1340	1060
	0.02	1928	1416	1176	916
	0.05	1642	1174	957	725
	0.10	1415	984	787	579
0.95	0.01	447	337	285	228
	0.02	404	300	252	199
	0.05	345	251	207	160
	0.10	299	212	172	130

Table A.7r. Binomial Sample Size for Each of Two Independent Proportions, Two-Tailed Test ($P_1 = 0.90$)

P_2	Alpha	Beta			
		0.01	0.05	0.10	0.20
0.95	0.01	1368	1025	863	686
	0.02	1235	911	760	595
	0.05	1054	758	621	474
	0.10	910	637	513	381

Program AP.1. BASIC Program for Michael's Normality Test

```
100 REM                    CALCULATION OF VALUES FOR
110 REM                  MICHAEL'S STABILIZED NORMAL
120 REM                     PROBABILITY  PLOT
130 REM
140 REM         Adapted  from  Nelson,  Lloyd S.,    "A
150 REM         Stabilized Normal Probability Plotting
160 REM         Technique", Journal  of  Quality Tech-
170 REM         nology, 21, July 1989 (213-215). Copy-
180 REM         right 1989 by the American Society for
190 REM         Quality  Control; reproduced  with per-
200 REM         mission.
210 :
220 DIM Y(100)
230 DEF FNA(X)=ATN(X/SQR(1-X^2))
240 LPRINT CHR$(27)"&a"8"L"
250 DEF FNB(X)=A1+B1*X^C1
260 DEF FNC(X)=A2+B2*X^C2
270 DEF FND(X)=A3+B3*LOG(X)^C3
280 LET PI=3.14159265#
290 :
300 DATA 1.5,0.0,4.5,-1.5,4.0,0.5,-8.0,2.5,-2.0,-1.5,
310 DATA 2.57,3.57,-4.43,-1.43,4.07,-1.43,-2.93
320 LET N=17
330 FOR J=1 TO N
340     READ Y(J)
350     LET T1=T1+Y(J)
360     LET T2=T2+Y(J)^2
370 NEXT J
380 LET MEAN=T1/N
390 LET SD=SQR((T2-T1^2/N)/N)
400 LET SD1=SD*SQR(N/(N-1))
410 LPRINT "MEAN=" ;MEAN;" STD. DEV.=";SD1
420 LPRINT
430 FOR J=1 TO N-1
440     FOR K=J TO N
450         IF Y(J)=<Y(K) THEN 500
460         LET A=Y(J)
470         LET Y(J)=Y(K)
480         LET Y(K)=A
490     NEXT K
```

Program AP.1. (*Continued*)

```
500 NEXT J
510 LPRINT"    OBS.";"    X'";"    Y'";
520 LPRINT"    ABS. DIFF."
530 LPRINT"--------------------------------"
540 FOR J=1 TO N
550     LET X=(2/PI)*FNA(SQR((J-.5)/N))
560     LET X1=INT(1000*X+.5)/1000
570     LET Z=(Y(J)-MEAN)/SD
580     LET S=0
590         FOR K=1 TO 12
600             LET F1=SIN(K*Z*SQR(2)/3)
610             LET F2=EXP(-(K^2/9))/K
620             LET S=S+F1*F2
630         NEXT K
640     LET P=.5+(Z/(3*SQR(2))+S)/PI
650     LET Y1=(2/PI)*FNA(SQR(P))
660     LET Y2=INT(1000*Y1+.5)/1000
670     LET D=ABS(X1-Y2)
680     LET U$="###.###    .###    .###    .###"
690 LPRINT USING U$;Y(J),X1,Y2,D
700 NEXT J
710 LPRINT
720 LET A1=1.44846
730 LET B1=.660325
740 LET C1=.294099
750 LET A2=1.35578
760 LET B2=.64518
770 LET C2=.293011
780 LET A3=1.93521
790 LET B3=.110589
800 LET C3=1.74233
810 LET Z$="MAX. ABS. DIFF."
820 LET D1=1/(FNB(N)^2)
830 LET D2=1/(FNC(N)^2)
840 LET D3=1/(FND(N)^2)
850 LPRINT"  GOODNESS OF FIT CRITICAL VALUES"
860 LPRINT"           ALPHA    .10    .05    .01"
870 LET W$="    .###    .###    .###"
880 LPRINT Z$;
890 LPRINT USING W$;D1,D2,D3
900 LPRINT CHR$(12)
910 END
```

Program AP.2. BASIC Program for the Wilcoxon Rank Sum Test

```
100 REM                    WILCOXON'S RANK SUM TEST
110 REM                       William M. Wooding
120 REM                    Final Revision, March, 1992
130 :
140 PRINT "Enter title of job (one line or less):"
150 LINE INPUT TITLE$
160 PRINT "Identification of treatments:"
170 LINE INPUT "Treatment A (smaller group): ";TREATA$
180 LINE INPUT "Treatment B (larger or equal group): ";TREATB$
190 LPRINT "WILCOXON RANK SUM TEST: ";DATE$
200 LPRINT TITLE$
210 LPRINT
220 LPRINT
230 '
240 '    INPUT DATA:
250 DIM Y(100), R(100)
260 '
270 INPUT "Enter number of data in smaller array (m): ";M
280 '
290 INPUT "Enter number of data in larger array (n): ";N
300 '
310 PRINT
320 PRINT "Enter data, smaller array first (one #/line):"
330 PRINT
340 FOR I=1 TO (M+N)
350      INPUT Y(I)
360 NEXT I
370 '
380 '    RANK ALL DATA
390 '
400 NL = 0
410 NS = 0
420 '
430 FOR I = 1 TO (M+N)
440      FOR J = 1 TO (M+N)
450           IF Y(J) < Y(I) THEN LET NL = NL + 1
460           IF Y(J) = Y(I) THEN LET NS = NS + 1
470 NEXT J
480           R(I) = (2*NL + NS + 1)/2
490           NL = 0
500           NS = 0
510 NEXT I
520 '
530 '    PRINT THE ARRAYS OF DATA AND THEIR RANKS
540 '
550 LPRINT "          TREATMENT A",,"          TREATMENT B"
560 LPRINT "     DATA", "    RANKS",,"     DATA", " RANKS"
570 LPRINT
580 LET AA$ = "####.#"
590 LET BB$ = "####.####"
600 LET CC$ = "#.####"
610 '
```

Program AP.2. (*Continued*)

```
620 FOR I = 1 TO M
630     LPRINT USING BB$; Y(I);
640     LPRINT SPACE$(5);
650     LPRINT USING AA$; R(I);
660     LPRINT SPACE$(20);
670     LPRINT USING BB$; Y(I+M);
680     LPRINT SPACE$(5);
690     LPRINT USING AA$; R(I+M)
700 NEXT I
710 '
720 IF M = N THEN GOTO 810
730 IF M < N THEN GOTO 750
740 '
750 FOR I = (2*M+1) TO (M+N)
760     LPRINT SPACE$(41);
770     LPRINT USING BB$; Y(I);
780     LPRINT SPACE$(5);
790     LPRINT USING AA$; R(I)
800 NEXT I
810 '
820 '    CALCULATE STATISTICS
830 '             SUMS AND MEANS
840 '
850 SUMA = 0
860 SUMB = 0
870 SUMRA = 0
880 SUMRB = 0
890 '
900 FOR I = 1 TO M
910     LET SUMA = SUMA + Y(I)
920     LET SUMRA = SUMRA + R(I)
930 NEXT I
940 '
950 FOR I = (M+1) TO (M+N)
960     LET SUMB = SUMB + Y(I)
970     LET SUMRB = SUMRB + R(I)
980 NEXT I
990 '
1000     ABAR = SUMA/M
1010     BBAR = SUMB/N
1020     RABAR = SUMRA/M
1030     RBBAR = SUMRB/N
1040     '
1050     '           PROBABILITIES
1060     '
```

Program AP.2. (*Continued*)

```
1070     WM = SUMRA
1080     NN = M + N
1090     EWM = (M/2)*(NN + 1)
1100     VWM = ((M*N)/12)*(NN+1)
1110     Z = (WM - EWM)/SQR(VWM)
1120     '
1130     R# = 0.2316419
1140     B1# = 0.31938153#
1150     B2# = -0.356563782#
1160     B3# = 1.781477937#
1170     B4# = -1.821255978#
1180     B5# = 1.330274429#
1190     '
1200     FZ = EXP(-Z^2/2)SQR(2*3.141592654#)
1210     T = 1/(1 + R#*ABS(Z))
1220     '
1230     P = FZ*(B1#*T + B2#*T^2 + B3#*T^3 + B4#*T^4 + B5#*T^5)
1240     PP = 2*P
1250     '
1260     LPRINT
1270     LPRINT
1280     LPRINT
1290     LPRINT "GROUP A ("TREATA$"):"
1300     LPRINT ,, "SUM = ";SUMA
1310     LPRINT ,, "MEAN = ";ABAR
1320     LPRINT ,, "RANK SUM = ";SUMRA
1330     LPRINT ,, "RANK MEAN = ";RABAR
1340     LPRINT ,, "NUMBER OF DATA = ";M
1350     '
1360     LPRINT
1370     LPRINT "GROUP B ("TREATB$"):"
1380     LPRINT ,, "SUM = ";SUMB
1390     LPRINT ,, "MEAN = ";BBAR
1400     LPRINT ,, "RANK SUM = ";SUMRB
1410     LPRINT ,, "RANK MEAN = ";RBBAR
1420     LPRINT ,, "NUMBER OF DATA = ";N
1430     '
1440     LPRINT
1450     LPRINT "ABAR - BBAR = ";ABAR - BBAR
1460     '
1470     LPRINT "PROBABILITY (1-TAIL) = ";
1480     LPRINT USING CC$; P
1490     LPRINT "PROBABILITY (2-TAIL) = ";
1500     LPRINT USING CC$; PP
1510     LPRINT "(Normal approximations)"
1520     LPRINT CHR$(12)
1530     END
```

Program AP.3. BASIC Program for Normal Approximation Using Logistic Distributions

```
100 '     PROGRAM AP.3
110 '         Using a logistic approximation to the
120 '         standardized normal distribution, this
130 '         program approximates Z, given P(x), or
140 '         P(x), given Z.  Z is a point on the ab-
150 '         scissa of the standardized normal dis-
160 '         tribution curve which marks the start
170 '         of an upper tail area of the curve (to
180 '         its right), in standard deviation units.
190 '         P(x) is the probability density value,
200 '         equal to that tail area.  The accuracy
210 '         declines at very low and high probabil-
220 '         ity values.  In the most widely used
230 '         range, between 0.050 and 0.200, proba-
240 '         bilities are given accurately to three
250 '         or more decimal places, but Z values
260 '         are limited to about two.
270 '
280 '         To use, with GW BASIC loaded, load the
290 '         program, type RUN, and follow the in-
300 '         structions on the screen.
310 '
320 '         REFERENCE: Tiemstra, Peter J., "Meas-
330 '         uring the Performance of Inspection
340 '         and Sorting Systems", Journal of Qual-
350 '             ity Technology, 13, No. 3, 1981.

360 '         Program by W.M.Wooding, 1983.
370 '
380 '
390 CLS
400 PRINT   "This program calculates one-tailed Z,"
410 PRINT   "a value on the standardized normal ab-"
420 PRINT   "scissa, given the normal probability"
430 PRINT   "density, P(x).  If Z is given, P(x) is"
440 PRINT   "obtained.  As many solutions as desired"
450 PRINT   "may be gotten without restarting the"
460 PRINT   "program."
470 PRINT
480 PRINT      "To calculate Z, ENTER a capital Z,"
490 PRINT   "then the value of P(x)."
500 PRINT
```

Program AP.3. (*Continued*)

```
510 PRINT          "To calculate P(x), ENTER a capital"
520 PRINT    P, then the value of Z."
530 PRINT
540 INPUT ANS$
550 INPUT X
560 IF ANS$ = "Z" THEN P = X ELSE Z = X
570 IF ANS$ = "Z" THEN GOTO 710
580 '
590 '                **CALCULATION OF P**
600 U = Z*(3*Z^2 + 67)/42
610 P = EXP(U)/(EXP(U) + 1)
620 PRINT
630 PRINT "The value of Z was given as "; Z
640 LPRINT "The value of Z was given as "; Z
650 PRINT "The corresponding probability is approx. "; P
660 LPRINT "The corresponding probability is approx. "; P
670 PRINT: LPRINT
680 GOTO 820
690 '
700 '                **CALCULATION OF Z**
710 U = LOG(P/(1-P))
720 V = -7*U
730 W = 67/9
740 S = SQR(V^2 + W^3)
750 Z = (S - V)^(1/3) - (S + V)^(1/3)
760 PRINT: LPRINT
770 PRINT "The value of P(x) was given as "; P
780 LPRINT "The value of P(x) was given as "; P
790 PRINT "The corresponding Z value is approx. "; Z
800 LPRINT "The corresponding Z value is approx. "; Z
810 PRINT: LPRINT
820 INPUT "Do another? (ENTER capital Y or N)"; ANS$
830 IF ANS$ = "N" THEN 860
840 PRINT "Choose again:"
850 GOTO 480
860 END
```

Program AC.1. HP-42S Calculator Program Probability Points– Normal Distribution

```
01  LBL "NORMPR"          Program name
02  MVAR "LLIM"           Menu variable
03  MVAR "ULIM"              "
04  MVAR "ACC"            "
05  MVAR "X"                 "
06  PGMINT "AREA"         Calls AREA program
07  INTEG "X"             Integrates results from AREA
08  END
```

Program AC.2. HP-42S Calculator Program: AREA Subprogram

```
01  LBL "AREA"            Program name
02  MVAR "X"              Menu variable (integrand)
03  PI                    Function pi
04  2                     Enters number (2)
05  x                     Multiply pi by 2
06  SQRT                  Take square root
07  1/x                   Inverse
08  RCL "X"               Recall X
09  X↑2                   Square the result
10  +/-                   Change sign
11  2                     Number 2
12  ÷                     Divide by 2
13  E↑X                   Antilog of natural log
14  x                     Multiply
15  END                   End of program
```

Bibliography:
Selected Books for Reference

PURPOSES AND ARRANGEMENT

The books listed here have been chosen for your reference and further study. Many of them, as well as all the items in the reference lists appearing at the ends of most of the chapters, serve also as references in the text.

Most of the books listed in this bibliography have been selected for their clarity and their emphasis upon applied rather than theoretical experimental design and statistics. Comments are included with each entry to assist you in making selections. Those that are particularly recommended are marked with asterisks. The listings were compiled while keeping in mind that you may not have had preparation in statistics. Therefore, most of the books listed are those judged to be understandable and useful with little or no preparation except a reading of this book and a willingness to study. One or two more advanced books are listed, however, because they are unique.

In addition to the various clinical trial, experimental design, and statistics listings, there are five categories that are included because I personally find them useful and feel that you may, also. These consist of the "Graphical Data Display" section, which includes three unique volumes, and the books listed in "Guides to Good Writing," which I have found invaluable in my technical writing. In addition, there is a section entitled "Medical References." You are probably familiar with most or all of these, and they are listed more as recommended sources for a statistician working in medical statistics than for medical or paramedical workers. None of them are medical texts. A fourth section "Computer Software," does not comprise books, but lists three software packages suitable for desktop computers. One of these, SYSTAT, includes versions that will run on a variety of other machines as well. If your firm has a statistics department, that organization will undoubtedly already possess one or more favorite packages, but you may wish to have one or more of those listed for your own desktop machine. Finally, five volumes are listed in a "Miscellaneous" group. Three were included as general interest material, and may be read for pleasure as well as information.

The emphasis in this book is on study planning and experimental design, although there are two chapters on statistical analysis. You might therefore wonder at the substantial number of volumes on statistics that are listed. These were included (a) to supply those who are interested with a good choice of references on analysis to compensate for the lack in this book, and (b) because many of the cited volumes also contain useful material on design.

In the following sections, the listings are in the form of (a) major categories comprising arrangements by subject, and (b) within each section, alphabetical listings arranged according to the senior or sole author's names. The reference numbers are enclosed in square brackets, and these are used throughout the text when an item in this bibliography is cited, to distinguish them from citations of the periodical literature listed at the ends of most chapters, which use parentheses. Not every book in this bibliography is necessarily referenced in the text.

LISTINGS

Clinical Trials

[1] Cox, Kenneth R., *Planning Clinical Experiments*, Charles C. Thomas, Springfield, Ill., 1968.
Old but still useful. Elementary level; one chapter on simple analysis.

[2] Friedman, Lawrence M., Curt D. Furberg, and David L. DeMets, *Fundamentals of Clinical Trials*, John Wright, PSG, Boston, 1983.
Elementary treatment. Some simple analysis. The authors are at NIH (not in industry).

[3] Meinert, Curtis, L., *Clinical Trials, Design, Conduct and Analysis*, Oxford University Press, New York, 1986.
Very thorough descriptions of the nontechnical and organizational aspects of large trials. All but one of 14 trials discussed, however, appear not to be industrial. The designs illustrated are very simple, and are limited to parallel studies only. There is a small amount of elementary statistics. Excellent reference lists.

[4]* Pocock, Stuart, *Clinical Trials, A Practical Approach*, John Wiley, New York, 1983.
An outstanding elementary and practical book. Covers most important aspects of clinical studies with varying degrees of thoroughness. Much less emphasis upon experimental designs than this book. A little very easy statistics in 3 of its 15 chapters. Highly recommended.

[5] Shapiro, Stanley H., and Thomas A. Louis, Eds., *Clinical Trials, Issues and Approaches*, Marcel Dekker, New York, 1983.
A fine book, informative, and well-written. None of the authors is employed in industry, although all are very well-known and several of them do industrial consulting.

Clinical Trial Design and Statistics

[6]* Bailar, John C., III. and Frederick Mosteller, Eds., *Medical Uses of Statistics*, NEJM Books (New England Journal of Medicine), Waltham, Mass., 1986.
Chapters by many of the best-known people in the field. Easy reading. Highly recommended.

[7] Bolton, Sanford, *Pharmaceutical Statistics, Practical and Clinical Applications*, 2nd ed., Marcel Dekker, New York, 1990.
Bolton's textbook was received when the preparation of the present volume was in its later stages, and I have not read it yet. Although the author's statement in his preface, to the effect that it appears to be "the only textbook on statistical applications in the pharmaceutical sciences," is arguable in view of Fleiss' and Pocock's books, which follow, it is certainly one of the few, and appears to be a thorough and competent exposition of elementary statistics oriented toward the drug industry. There are two chapters on design. The text should be easily understandable to a reader of this book.

[8]* Fleiss, Joseph L., *The Design and Analysis of Clinical Experiments*, John Wiley, New York, 1986.
This is unquestionably the best modern work on design and analysis for clinical trials, but the reader must have some undergraduate preparation in statistics. If you have such a background or the equivalent, it is very highly recommended.

[9] McMahon, F. Gilbert, Ed., *Importance of Experimental Design and Biostatistics*, Futura, Mount Kisco, N.Y., 1974.
A well-integrated collection of brief chapters by well-known authors in the field of clinical trials, including both industrial and government representatives. Easy reading.

[10] Woolson, Robert F., *Statistical Methods for the Analysis of Biomedical Data*, John Wiley, New York, 1987.
This book is a very well-written text, done from the point of view of elementary medical statistics. Exercises are included. It is intended for the same audience as this volume (medical researchers) as well as students.

Experimental Designs

[11]* Cochran, William G., and Gertrude M. Cox, *Experimental Designs*, 2nd ed., John Wiley, New York, 1957.
This is the bible of applied experimental design, and, despite its age, it should be on your desk if you get no other book on design. Not restricted to clinical trials. Very highly recommended. It is now available in paperback.

[12]* Cox, D. R., *Planning of Experiments*, John Wiley, New York, 1958.
A deservedly famous book by a statistician known all over the world. Easily readable by any professional research person. The mathematics is very elementary, and the book is entirely devoted to design (no analysis). Not specific to clinical trials. High recommended. It is now available in paperback.

[13]* Daniel, Cuthbert, *Applications of Statistics to Industrial Experimentation*, John Wiley, New York, 1976.

Very precise and complete. The best modern volume on experimental design. The author has worked in and with industry for most of his life. Not biologically oriented.

[14]* Davies, Owen L., Ed., *Design and Analysis of Industrial Experiments*, 2nd ed., Hafner, New York, 1960.
As thorough as Cochran and Cox [11], and second only to that book in usefulness. Contains the best practical treatment of factorial designs in print. Not especially biologically oriented. Easy to understand. Highly recommended, if you can find one (may be out of print).

[15] Diamond, William J., *Practical Experiment Designs for Engineers and Scientists*, Lifetime Learning, Belmont, Cal., 1981.
A unique book. Substantial amount of math, but all algebra. If you do not mind the necessary math, it is strongly recommended.

[16] Fisher, Sir Ronald A., *The Design of Experiments*, 7th ed., Hafner, New York, 1960.
Most statisticians consider Fisher, together with Gosset (Student) to be the founders of modern small sample statistics and experimental design. Among many other contributions, Fisher was the man who originated the concept of randomized assignments in experimental designs, the analysis of variance, and many other fundamental ideas and procedures of modern applied statistics. The book is not very mathematical, but it must be read slowly and carefully to fully absorb Fisher's ideas.

[17] Whitehead, John, *The Design and Analysis of Sequential Clinical Trials*, John Wiley, New York, 1983.
Very thorough and quite advanced. In spite of this, it is listed here because it is the only volume on this subject in print, at this writing. There is some treatment of this topic in Armitage (cf. item [18], which follows) and Armitage wrote a book on the subject some years ago. Sequential trials are very rare in industrial drug testing today.

Clinical Trial and Medical Statistics

[18] Armitage, P., *Statistical Methods in Medical Research*, John Wiley, New York, 1971.
A famous and comprehensive text. Easy to understand if read carefully.

[19]* Buncher, C. Ralph, and Jia-Yeong Tsay, Eds., *Statistics in the Pharmaceutical Industry*, Marcel Dekker, New York, 1981.
An outstanding collection by many well-known authors. The level of the material varies with subject and author. Very practical and highly recommended.

[20]* Colton, Theodore, *Statistics in Medicine*, Little Brown, Boston, 1974.
One of the best. A bit limited in breadth, but understandable to the layman in statistics if read seriously. Very readable style. Does not include treatment of analysis of variance. Highly recommended.

[21] Feinstein, Alvan R., *Clinical Biostatistics*, C. V. Mosby, Saint Louis, 1977.
Useful, elementary, entertaining reading.

[22] Hill, Sir Austin Bradford, *Principles of Medical Statistics*, 8th ed., Oxford University Press, New York, 1967.
Probably the first, and certainly one of the most famous texts in medical statistics. Very elementary, but very comprehensive.

[23]* Inglefinger, Joseph A., Frederick Mosteller, Lawrence A. Thibodeau, and James H. Ware, *Biostatistics in Clinical Medicine*, Macmillan, New York, 1983.
A very thorough elementary book by well-known authorities. Covers some topics not common among other listings in this bibliography.

[24] Lee, Elisa T., *Statistical Methods for Survival Data Analysis*, Lifetime Learning, Belmont, Cal., 1980.
This is a comprehensive, clear, and well-written textbook on a subject that is important for some types of clinical trials.

[25] Mainland, Donald, *Elementary Medical Statistics*, 2nd ed., W. B. Saunders, Philadelphia, 1963.
Nearly as famous as Hill [22]. The arrangement of the material (questions and answers) is unusual, but the material is very elementary and very common-sense.

[26] Miller, Rupert G., Jr., *Beyond ANOVA, Basics of Applied Statistics*, John Wiley, New York, 1986.
A fine book, and very practical, written by a wise and broadly read statistician who was well-known in the field.

Sample Size Estimation

[27]* Cohen, Jacob, *Statistical Power Analysis for the Behavioral Sciences*, 2nd ed., Lawrence Erlbaum, Hillsdale, N.J., 1988.
The most comprehensive of the surprisingly few books devoted to this important subject (I am aware of only two others, one of which is out of print). Relatively easy to read, once you have read the present volume. There is one unusual concept, the effect size, to get used to. See the comments in Chapter 15 about Cohen's book and the corresponding computer program. The program is listed as item [67]. A necessity for your library. Very highly recommended.

[28] Kraemer, Helena Chmura, and Sue Thiemann, *How Many Subjects? Statistical Power Analysis in Research*, Sage, Beverly Hills, 1987.
This is the only modern book besides Cohen of which I am aware. It comprises a short monograph, covering a number of topics related to the title. See Bratcher et al., cited in Chapter 15, reference (5).

Biostatistics

[29]* Bliss, C. I., *Statistics in Biology*, Vol. 1, McGraw-Hill, New York, 1967.
See comments under the next item [30]. Highly recommended.

[30]* Bliss, C. I., *Statistics in Biology*, Vol. 2, McGraw-Hill, New York, 1970.
This and Vol. 1 [29] are the most comprehensive textbooks available that are specifically oriented to biostatistics. They stress applications, and can be read without earlier preparation in statistics. Of course, like all statistics texts, they cannot be read like a novel; they must be studied. High recommended.

[31] Lewis, Alvin, *Biostatistics*, 2nd ed., Van Nostrand Reinhold, New York, 1984.
A well-written, very elementary textbook.

General Statistics

[32] Box, George E. P., William G. Hunter, and J. Stuart Hunter, *Statistics for Experimenters*, John Wiley, New York, 1978.
A fine professional book. Includes chapters on design as well as statistical analysis. All three authors are prominent in the applications of statistics in the physical sciences. William Hunter died a few years ago.

[33]* Dixon, Wilfred J., and Frank J. Massey, Jr., *Introduction to Statistical Analysis*, 4th ed., McGraw-Hill, New York, 1983.
This book is one of the hardy perennials, as famous and widely used as Snedecor and Cochran [38], and as comprehensive as that book and Neter, Wasserman, and Kutner [37]. It is well worth a place on your desk. Highly recommended.

[34]* Draper, Norman, and Harry Smith, *Applied Regression Analysis*, 2nd ed., John Wiley, New York, 1981.
This elementary text is the definitive work in its field. You need a prior acquaintance with elementary statistics. Requires matrix algebra, but the authors present a course in that topic in Chapter Two. Highly recommended.

[35] Fisher, Sir Ronald A., *Statistical Methods for Research Workers*, 14th ed., Hafner, 1973.
The first edition of this book was, I believe, the first book on applied statistics in science published in the twentieth century. Fisher was the pioneer who discovered the analysis of variance and many other techniques. This book first appeared in 1924 and for many years was probably the most popular applied statistics book of all time. It was published not only in English, but in French, German, Spanish, Italian, and Japanese. It is still a useful reference for the applied scientist.

[36]* Mandel, John, *The Statistical Analysis of Experimental Data*, Dover, New York, 1984 (Originally published in 1964 by Wiley-Interscience.)
An unusual approach to statistical analysis, written for the practitioner in the physical and biological sciences. Stresses models, measurement, and curve fitting. Highly recommended.

[37]* Neter, John, William Wasserman, and Michael H. Kutner, *Applied Linear Statistical Models*, 3rd ed., Richard D. Irwin, Homewood, Ill., 1990.
Although most of the examples in this book are business rather than science-related, this is the most comprehensive and clearly presented modern text on applied statistics of which I know. It covers regression, analysis of variance, and some experimental design in one volume of 1127 pages. Some background in statistics is desirable before tackling it. It has been criticized as being repetitive, but I find that technique to be helpful in fixing important points in the mind. Very highly recommended.

[38]* Snedecor, George W., and William G. Cochran, *Statistical Methods*, 7th ed., Iowa State University Press, Ames, 1980.
This book is widely regarded as the best elementary and intermediate textbook of applied statistics in print for the physical and biological sciences. Snedecor has been dead for a number of years, and Cochran wrote most of this edition and was

coauthor of the previous one. He died before completing the present volume, and it was completed by David F. Cox. It ranges from the elementary to intermediate level. This is the best, in my opinion. If you get no other statistics book, get this.

An eighth edition appeared in 1989 from the same publisher. The preface states that it was written by several members of the Iowa State Department of Statistics. It contains some material that does not appear in the earlier ones. However, I have read this as well as several of the earlier editions, and I am of the opinion that the seventh edition is the best.

Nonparametric and Discrete Data Analysis

[39]* Conover, W. J., *Practical Nonparametric Statistics*, 2nd ed., John Wiley, New York, 1980.
This is the latest and most up-to-date, as well as the most popular book on this subject as of this writing. Highly recommended.

[40] Fienberg, Stephen E., *The Analysis of Cross-Classified Categorical Data*, The MIT Press, Cambridge, Mass., 1977.
This is a simplification of and introduction to material presented more exhaustively elsewhere, especially in Bishop, Fienberg, and Holland (MIT Press, 1975), which is the definitive work in the field of log-linear models. This technique is a method of analyzing contingency tables (especially multifactor) by an ANOVA-like procedure.

[41]* Fleiss, Joseph, L., *Statistical Methods for Rates and Proportions*, 2nd ed., John Wiley, New York, 1981.
This is the definitive modern work on this subject. It is especially appropriate for workers in medical statistics who must use nonnormal responses such as the binomial. There is also useful elementary information about sensitivity and specificity of diagnostic procedures, and on probability. Highly recommended.

[42]* Freeman, Daniel H., Jr., *Applied Categorical Analysis*, Marcel Dekker, New York, 1987.
A valuable and comprehensive textbook on a subject highly relevant to the analysis of clinical trial data: responses in terms of dichotomous (binomial or yes/no) scales and multinomial (multiple-integer) scales, such as scores. The examples principally use nonexperimental data, with which we have not been concerned here, but this book is nevertheless highly recommended.

[43] Hollander, Myles, and Douglas A. Wolfe, *Nonparametric Statistical Methods*, John Wiley, New York, 1973.
This is another fine general reference (written as a textbook, for classroom use) among the small group of extant texts on this topic.

[44] Maxwell, A. E., *Analysing Quantitative Data*, John Wiley, New York (and Methuen, London), 1961.
Old but good. All about contingency tables, explained very simply, in a few pages. No material on log-linear models, because it predates them.

[45] Siegel, Sidney, *Nonparametric Statistics for the Behavioral Sciences*, McGraw-Hill, New York, 1956.
I believe this is the earliest volume completely devoted to "nonparametric" tests. It was a fine book, but has now been more or less replaced by Conover [39]. Included here because there are very few applied books on this topic.

[46] Wilcoxon, Frank, and Wilcox, Roberta, *Some Rapid Approximate Statistical Procedures*, Lederle Laboratories Division, American Cyanamid Company, Pearl River, N.Y., 1964.
This is the fourth or fifth edition of a pamphlet first published by Wilcoxon at Lederle in the 1940s. Wilcoxon's original paper was published in 1945, and is referenced at the end of Chapter 14 of this book. Frank Wilcoxon was the inventor of the Rank Sum and Signed Ranks tests, and was a famous authority on "nonparametric" testing in general.

Statistical Tables

[47]* Beyer, William H., Ed., *Handbook of Tables for Probability and Statistics*, 2nd ed., Chemical Rubber, Cleveland, 1968.
Probably the most comprehensive set of tables available for practical work. This edition is still the current one as of this writing (1992). Included is much material on experimental design, as well as analysis, tables of random flat and random normal numbers, and many other statistical tables. An essential reference. Highly recommended.

[48] Fisher, Sir Ronald A., and Frank Yates, *Statistical Tables for Biological, Agricultural and Medical Research*, 6th ed., Hafner, New York, 1963.
One of the two oldest and most famous modern compilations of statistical tables. The other is Pearson and Hartley [51]. Very readable and useful. This was the first set of tables available for its purposes of which I am aware, and until Pearson and Hartley appeared, the only one for some years.

[49]* Moses, Lincoln E., and Robert V. Oakford, *Tables for Random Permutations*, Stanford University Press, Stanford, Cal., 1963.
This is the only book I know of which is entirely devoted to presenting sets of random permutations. It is a great time-saver, and nearly essential if you are designing many randomized blocks or similar trials. Its use is described in some of the examples in this book. Highly recommended.

[50] Owen, D. B., *Handbook of Statistical Tables*, Addison-Wesley, Reading, Mass., 1962.
A useful and compact set of tables. A number of them are unique in that they are more complete than the usual tables, and so require less interpolation. For example, the t table is tabulated by sequential degrees of freedom up to 100, before a sparser tabulation is begun. The book also contains tables difficult to find elsewhere.

[51] Pearson, E. S., and H. O. Hartley, Eds., *Biometrika Tables for Statisticians*, Vol. I, Biometrika Trust, University College, London (3rd ed. reprinted with corrections), 1976.
This and Vol. II [52] are the most complete of all the compilations of tables that I know of that are available in English. They are the standard in the statistics profession. The nonstatistician may find them a bit difficult to use, however. Some of the other volumes listed in this section (with the exception of Fisher and Yates [48]) use these as their source, and you may find some of those easier to use.

[52] Pearson, E. S., and H. O. Hartley, Eds., *Biometrika Tables for Statisticians*, Vol. II, Biometrika Trust, University College, London (reprinted with corrections), 1976.
See notes under Vol. I [51].

[53]* Rohlf, F. James, and Robert R. Sokal, *Statistical Tables*, 2nd ed., W. H. Freeman, San Francisco, 1981.
This is a small and most usefully arranged set of general tables. The common tables, like the normal, F, t, and chi squared, are particularly easy to use. The volume was originally issued as a companion to Biometry, The Principles and Practice of Statistics in Biological Research, *a fine statistics text by the same authors, now in its second edition* (1981), *but this book can be purchased separately.*

Statistical and Mathematical Reference Books

[54] Abramowitz, Milton, and Irene A. Stegun, Eds., *Handbook of Mathematical Functions*, John Wiley, New York, 1984. Originally issued by the U.S. National Bureau of Standards Applied Mathematics Series #55, 10th ed., 1972. Now available from Dover Publications, Mineola, N.Y.
A giant volume of 1046 *pages. Almost every function or table conceivable.*

[55] Gellert, W., S. Gottwald, M. Hellwich, H. Kastner, and H. Kustner, Eds., *The VNR Concise Encyclopedia of Mathematics*, 2nd ed., Van Nostrand Reinhold, New York, 1989.
Another giant of a book, beautifully illustrated, well worth a place on your shelf.

[56] James, Glenn, and Robert C. James, *Mathematics Dictionary*, 4th ed., Van Nostrand Reinhold, New York, 1976
A useful book for your office shelf.

[57]* Kotz, Samuel, and Norman L. Johnson, Eds.-in-Chief, and Campbell B. Read, Assoc. Ed., *Encyclopedia of Statistical Sciences*, John Wiley, New York, nine vols., 1982–1988 (with a supplement volume issued in 1989).
I believe this is the only modern set of its kind in English. It is a tremendous resource, and should be available to anyone concerned with statistics. Highly recommended.

Medical Reference Books

[58]* Barnhart, Edward R., Publisher, *Physician's Desk Reference*, current edition, Medical Economics, Oradell, N.J. (issued annually; the 1993 edition is the 47th).
The unique guide to ethical drugs in America. You probably have it already, but, if not, and you work with prescription drugs, you probably need it. Highly recommended.

[59]* Barnhart, Edward R., Publisher, *Physician's Desk Reference for Nonprescription Drugs*, current edition, Medical Economics, Oradell, N.J. (issued annually; the 1993 edition is the 14th).
This, like [58], *is equally useful if your trials are concerned with OTCs and proprietaries. Highly recommended.*

[60] Berkow, Robert, Ed.-in-Chief, *The Merck Manual of Diagnosis and Therapy*, 15th ed., Merck Sharp and Dohme Research Laboratories Division, Merck & Co., Rahway, N.J., 1987.
The well-known guide, organized by type of disorder. Includes clinical laboratory test information.

[61]* Cutler, Anne G., Managing Ed., *Stedman's Medical Dictionary*, 24th ed., Williams & Wilkins, Baltimore, 1981.
A good dictionary, one of the two best-known medical dictionaries available (the other is Dorland's). Highly recommended.

[62] Windholz, Martha, Ed., *The Merck Index*, 11th ed., Merck & Co., Rahway, N.J., 1989.
A dictionary or handbook of substances used as drugs. Chemically oriented. The compounds are listed by their generic as well as their Geneva names, where applicable. Most organics, inorganics, and even mixtures of materials are listed if they have been used now or in the past as medicinal materials. Descriptions of the chemical, physical, and pharmacological properties are given, as well as structures. Very useful if you need such information in your work.

Graphical Data Display

[63]* Cleveland, William S., *The Elements of Graphing Data*, Wadsworth Advanced Books and Software, Monterey, Cal., 1985.
This volume is the first and only one of its kind. Anyone who uses plots or graphs of any type in reports, or in papers or books for publication, should have it. For the first time, it reduces the art of the display of graphical information to an empirical discipline. Very highly recommended.

[64]* Tufte, Edward, R., *The Visual Display of Quantitative Information*, Graphics Press, Cheshire, Conn., 1983.
This book is another very unusual volume on the subject of graphics. More than Cleveland [63], Tufte relies on illustrations of the use and misuse of graphics that respectively inform and mislead. Not quite as overtly scientifically oriented as Cleveland's book, but just as valuable. And not only is it very instructive, but it is a true enjoyment to read and/or peruse. Also very highly recommended.

[65]* Tufte, Edward R., *Envisioning Information*, Graphics Press, Cheshire, Conn., 1990.
Categorizes methods of presenting information by means other than language. Beautifully illustrated. As instructive and useful as Tufte's earlier book [64].

Computer Software

[66]* Wilkinson, Leland, *SYSTAT: The System for Statistics*, and *SYGRAPH: The System for Graphics*, SYSTAT, Evanston, Ill., 1990. In addition, the following supplements, which are of interest in some clinical studies, are available, among others, and can use SYSTAT files: *Design* (a program for estimating sample sizes, calculating tables of expected mean squares, setting up randomization plans, and obtaining orthogonal polynomials by Gerald Dallal); and *Survival* (a survival analysis program by Dan Steinberg and Phillip Colla).
In my opinion, SYSTAT is one of the best, perhaps the best available statistical analysis system. It surpasses in completeness, clarity, accuracy, and precision some of the widely known mainframe systems. It is now available for DOS systems (IBM-type desktops), Apple equipment, VAX/VMS, and Data General machines. Wilkinson is a well-known and very competent practitioner. Highly recommended.

[67]* Borenstein, Michael, and Jacob Cohen, *Statistical Power Analysis: A Computer Program*, Lawrence Erlbaum, Hillsdale, N.J., 1988.
This program embodies the methods and procedures in Cohen's book [27]. *Highly recommended.*

[68]* Galen Research, *Electronic Tables*, S. E. Warner Software, Salt Lake City, 1990.
Many tables that you would otherwise find only in the volumes listed in the earlier "Statistical Tables" section can be accessed rapidly with this inexpensive software. Parameters of 19 *probability distributions, as well as some special functions, are available, most to many more decimal places than you (or I) will ever need. Highly recommended.*

Guides to Good Writing

[69]* Fowler, H. W., 2nd ed., revised by Sir Ernest Gowers, *A Dictionary of Modern English Usage*, Oxford University Press, New York, 1987.
This is an extraordinary directory of style, syntax, and grammar—far more than a dictionary despite its name. It is arranged alphabetically as a series of short (and some not so short) essays. You can read it as you would a novel or an encyclopedia, but with greater profit. Very highly recommended.

[70] Laird, Charlton, updated by William D. Lutz, *Webster's New World Thesaurus*, Simon & Schuster, New York, 1985.
In my opinion, this is the best of the new "dictionary" type of thesauri. However, all of these are about on a par with the better thesauri offered by the popular word processors. None is as complete or effective as the standard Roget (see [72]). *If you are in a hurry, you may find a word you can use. I list it here because using it is better than using no thesaurus, and less work than using Roget.*

[71]* Mish, Frederick C., Ed.-in-Chief, *Webster's Ninth New Collegiate Dictionary*, 9th ed., Merriam-Webster, Springfield, Mass., 1989.
This is the standard "small" dictionary (only 1568 *pages), and the next best thing to the Merriam-Webster "big one.") Highly recommended.*

[72]* Roget, P. M., *Roget's International Thesaurus*, 4th ed., Peter M. Chapman, Ed., Thomas Y. Crowell Company, New York, 1977.
Like "Webster's" dictionaries, there are many "Roget" thesauri in the bookstores, but this is the standard and the best. Most people who write anything other than personal letters need it even if they have a thesaurus of sorts on their word processor. This book is more useful and much more complete than the "dictionary" types. Very highly recommended.

[73]* Strunk, William, Jr., and E. B. White, *The Elements of Style*, 3rd ed., Macmillan, New York, 1979.
This is the best-known style manual. Only 85 *pages. Unless you are sure you don't need it, you do! Highly recommended.*

[74]* Tichy, H. J., *Effective Writing for Engineers, Managers, Scientists*, 2nd ed., John Wiley, New York, 1988.
Tichy is Professor Emeritus of the Herbert H. Lehman College of the City University of New York, and has been well-known for years as a consultant to industry. There are several volumes on technical writing on my shelves. This is the best work on the subject I have ever read. Very highly recommended.

Miscellaneous

[75]* Box, Joan Fisher, *R. A. Fisher, The Life of a Scientist*, Wiley, New York, 1978.
The jacket of this book states that "R. A. Fisher's pivotal role in developing theories and methods of science affects everyone doing research today ..." Box is one of Fisher's daughters, and presents a fine and technically oriented story of her father's life, with emphasis on his work in statistics. You should find it enjoyable and interesting. Highly recommended.

[76] Ritschel, W. A., *Handbook of Basic Pharmacokinetics*, 2nd ed., Drug Intelligence Publications, Hamilton, Ill., 1980.
A convenient and clearly presented monograph on the principles and theory of drug action in the human body. Important if you do or plan to do bioavailability or "bioequivalence" tests.

[77] Stigler, Stephen M., *The History of Statistics: The Measurement of Uncertainty before 1900*, Harvard University Press, Cambridge, Mass., 1986.
Well-done and interesting history. The author is a statistician at the University of Chicago, and the book discusses developments with technical detail. Any reader of the present book should have no trouble following it, however. The title hints that a second volume covering events, theory and techniques after 1900 may be forthcoming.

[78] Tallarida, Ronald J., and Rodney B. Murray, *Manual of Pharmacologic Calculations With Computer Programs*, Springer-Verlag, New York, 1981.
A useful handbook of methods, equations and algorithms, including some statistics. The level varies according to subject.

[79] Tanur, Judith M., *Statistics: A Guide to the Unknown*, 3rd ed., Brooks/Cole, Pacific Grove, Cal., 1989.
A delightful and readable compilation; each chapter by a well-known statistician. Each tells the story of an unusual or remarkable statistical investigation or similar subject. Primarily intended for students, to show the breadth and variety of statistical accomplishments, but so interestingly done that almost anyone will find it enjoyable reading.

Index

*Now available in a lower priced paperback edition in the Wiley Classics Library.